Marie D. Jones

Natural Health

Your Complete Guide to Natural Remedies and Mindful Well-Being

ABOUT THE AUTHOR

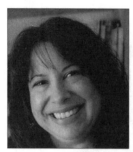 **Marie D. Jones** is the author of over twenty nonfiction books, including Visible Ink Press' *Earth Magic: Your Complete Guide to Natural Spells, Potions, Plants, Herbs, Witchcraft, and More; The New Witch: Your Guide to Modern Witchcraft, Wicca, Spells, Potions, Magic, and More; Disinformation and You: Identify Propaganda and Manipulation;* and *The Disaster Survival Guide: How to Prepare for and Survive Floods, Fires, Earthquakes and More.* A former radio show host, she has been interviewed on more than two thousand radio programs worldwide, including *Coast-to-Coast AM, The Shirley MacLaine Show,* and *Midnight in the Desert,* and she has also contributed to dozens of print and online publications. Jones makes her home in San Marcos, California, and is the mom to one very brilliant son, Max.

Please visit us at www.visibleinkpress.com.

Natural Health

Visible Ink ®
43311 Joy Rd., #414
Canton, MI 48187-2075

Visible Ink Press is a registered trademark of Visible Ink Press LLC.

Most Visible Ink Press books are available at special quantity discounts when purchased in bulk by corporations, organizations, or groups. Customized printings, special imprints, messages, and excerpts can be produced to meet your needs. For more information, contact Special Markets Director, Visible Ink Press, www.visibleinkpress.com, or 734-667-3211.

Managing Editor: Kevin S. Hile
Cover Design: Graphikitchen, LLC
Page Design: Cinelli Design
Typesetting: Marco Divita
Proofreaders: Larry Baker, Shoshana Hurwitz
Indexer: Larry Baker
Cover images: Shutterstock.

Paperback ISBN: 978-1-57859-555-6
Hardcover ISBN: 978-1-57859-773-4
eBook ISBN: 978-1-57859-781-9

Cataloging-in-Publication data is on file at the Library of Congress.

Printed in the United States of America.

10 9 8 7 6 5 4 3 2 1

TABLE OF CONTENTS

PHOTO SOURCES

Botanicus.org: p. 394,
Daderot (Wikicommons): p. 299.
DPic (Wikicommons): p. 253.
Frank and Frances Carpenter Collection, Library of Congress: p. 36.
Institute of Advanced Studies in Culture: p. 6.
Phil Konstantin: p. 308.
Sean Markwei: p. 26.
Shutterstock: pp. 3, 9, 12, 15, 17, 21, 23, 29, 30, 32, 40, 43, 51, 53, 56, 58, 61, 64, 66, 68, 72, 74, 76, 79, 82, 84, 88, 91, 99, 103, 104, 107, 109, 112, 114, 119, 121, 124, 127, 129, 132, 135, 137, 139, 142, 146, 148, 150, 155, 158, 161, 164, 168, 169, 173, 179, 183, 185, 189, 196, 198, 202, 205, 209, 212, 217, 218, 224, 227, 233, 237, 240, 245, 247, 248, 255, 259, 265, 267, 270, 275, 278, 281, 285, 289, 291, 295, 297, 301, 304, 310, 313, 321, 327, 330, 331, 334, 337, 339, 342, 345, 347, 354, 355, 357, 359, 361, 364, 366, 369, 372, 375, 384, 387, 389, 391, 395, 397, 400, 403, 406, 408, 416.
Visible Ink Press: p. 325.
Marcus Wieman: p. 23.
Public Domain: p. 96.

DISCLAIMER

Information in this book is not meant as a replacement for medical treatment, nor is it intended to substitute for the advice of your physician. It is meant for educational and information purposes only. If you have any questions about your health, please always seek help from a health care professional.

INTRODUCTION

Our ancestors lived off the land. They hunted prey for food and cloth-ing, using skins for shelter from the elements. They picked berries and plants for sustenance, and, most likely through trial and error, knew which were not to be consumed. They knew where the good, clean water sources were (the ones not being used by hungry lions and tigers), and how to use plants and leaves and parts of trees to heal wounds. Everything they needed was provided by nature.

They worked with the cycles of nature, the sun and moon phases and the seasons. There was a time to hunt and a time to grow, a time to move and a time to stay put. Their connection to the planet and its forces, laws, and cycles was strong and uninterrupted by the distrac-tions of our modern times.

Today, unless we hunt, have our own land to farm, and collect our own rainwater, most of us won't go to such trouble as to acquire our own food, water, and the fabrics we wear. We buy them at stores, or we order them online to be delivered to our doorstep. When we don't feel well or need to dress a wound, we go to the store and buy pills and bandages and ointments. For more serious ailments, we go to the doctor and do what they tell us, often without questioning it or asking for a second opinion.

It's premade, prefabricated, processed, put together, produced, and promoted to us.

With such ease at our fingertips, we must wonder why humanity is so sick and tired? We must ask, if everything has been made so easy for us to get, why is our health suffering? If all the stress and strain has been taken out of daily existence, why are we so burdened with disease, stress, and lack of well–being?

Maybe it's time we get back to basics and take another long look at what our planet has to offer.

Nature doesn't need us. It can survive just fine—in fact, thrive—without human interference. But maybe we need nature more than we thought we did. Modern life is all about comfort and ease, quick fixes, and instant gratification. When we feel sick, we are told to take pills. When we can't sleep, we are told to take pills. When we have no joy in our lives, we are told to take pills. There seems to be a pill for everything these days, and in many cases, ten pills. Big Pharma has stepped forward as our savior, health advisor, doctor, and therapist, all rolled into one big industry that doesn't care about us beyond the extent that we can continue using their products.

Health care has become sick care, with little in the way of advice on how to truly get and stay healthy. Lifestyle takes a back seat to a readily written-out prescription, and diet and exercise are after-thoughts after we've been saddled with ten different pills to make our boo boos better. Our bodies and minds are objects to be altered with chemicals; our spirits are the targets of stressful distractions meant to keep us from realizing we have the power.

We *do* have the power to take back our health and our lives.

Have you ever wondered why, despite the proliferation of drugs on the market and advertisements suggesting you "ask your doctor if _____ is right for you," people are sicker than ever? Why, with so many choices in pharmaceuticals, are the rates of heart disease, cancer, diabetes, and auto-immune diseases rising, along with allergies, respiratory diseases, COPD, obesity…? Shouldn't we be getting healthier with so many magic pills to choose from? With such an abundance of food choices at the grocery stores and access to water through our faucets and plastic bottles and jugs, shouldn't we be healthy and lean and strong? With a gym on every corner, along with a personal trainer, shouldn't we all be lean? There are so many books, videos, programs, products, pills, methods, and treatments that it's exhausting to list them all; they are pushed on us via the media and sold to us via our allopathic, Westernized medical system. You'd think we would all be living long, satisfying lives well into our 100s.

Instead, we are still dying young, or living to an old age but barely able to function physically or mentally. The older we get, the more that ails us, and the more doctors pile on the meds and the surgeries and the treatments. Even our children are popping pills for attention, focus, and for just being wild, free, unruly children. We are overmedicated but constantly under the weather.

Yes, there are times when a pill or prescription is a lifesaver, such as during a heart attack or to lower dangerously high blood pressure; this book does not deny that fact. Yes, there are times when a doctor or surgeon can save a life. But all too often we are pushed toward the halls and rooms of allopathic medicine and told to take handfuls of pills with deadly side effects or lack of safety studies, even though there are solutions to our problems that offer far fewer, if any, side effects. Naturopathic medicine will never replace allopathic medicine entirely, but at least it will walk alongside it as a powerful alternative. In many cases, it might even pull ahead and win the race when it comes to the holistic health of the body, mind, and spirit.

Shouldn't we at least give it a chance? If you care about your health, perhaps it's time to go back to the garden and revel in and relish the gifts that Earth has to offer. Because those gifts are numerous and include greater well-being for the physical vessel we call our bodies and for the brains that power them, as well as our much-neglected spirits, a more natural health equation could brings us back into balance.

Don't throw out all your meds or tell your general doctor to take a hike. This book asks only that you open your mind to another side of healthy living that does not come from a chemical warehouse or a pharmaceutical rep's briefcase. There is plenty of room for both, but shouldn't you at least have the choice, the knowledge, and the power to decide which route you wish to take toward a life of greater health and well-being? No prescription is needed, other than your time, focus, and willingness to learn.

Throughout this book, I will cite scientific studies to back up the claims made by natural health modalities and techniques. Always talk to your doctor about trying anything new with herbs, exercise, or diet, and, if possible, find a doctor who is a naturopath or at least willing to embrace natural remedies. Be your own advocate, and if something doesn't resonate don't try it. At the very least, this book will offer plenty of methods and ways to improve health on many levels and bring back a harmonious balance to your life.

Whether you have too much stress, cannot sleep at night, are looking for forms of exercise that are not brutal and injurious, or want to start a practice of gratitude, it's all here. Allow this book to be your "feel good" manual to help you on your journey and share it with others you love and care about.

Before you reach for a pill to stop a headache or some junk food to comfort you during a stressful time, stop and look here for a better choice, a better alternative, one that will both deal with the problem at hand and nourish you in general. Too often, we turn to the fast fixes in life, only to find out later they came with baggage that ruins our well-being down the road. That's not healthy living. That's putting a bandage on a wound that, once it festers, could lead to a dangerous infection or inflammation later.

Your health choices should not be aimed at merely covering up symptoms. Healing happens on a much deeper level. It is worth your time and effort to seek out something better that will change the way you live for long-lasting health.

You deserve to be healthy. You deserve to be well. You deserve a longer life with a sharper mind, a stronger body, and a resilient spirit. You deserve each gift the natural world has to offer.

Let's go see what those gifts are.

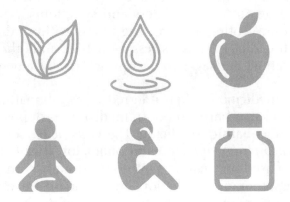

What Is Natural Health?

The word "natural" means "existing or caused by nature, not made or caused by humankind" when used as an adjective. It can also mean something that agrees with the character or makeup of something, an inherent characteristic. Either way, it refers to the realm of nature rather than the world of the manufactured and engineered. Natural health, therefore, is the health inherent to us when we are born before our bodies, minds, and spirits are assaulted by chemistry. Our bodies have built-in systems for keeping us well, for fighting diseases, and for healing us.

However, the proliferation of toxins in our world often disrupts those natural forces within, leaving us filled with toxic chemicals and suffering the effects of exposure to chemicals in our food, water, air, soil, and products we consume, including, ironically, the medications that are supposed to make us well. Nature may have cures for all that ails us, but we sabotage nature with the products of our human quest for faster, simpler, easier, and cheaper.

Naturopathic (alternative) medicine, or naturopathy, suggests nonchemical and nonmedical methods of dealing with diseases and illness, but naturopathic doctors are trained in both conventional and alternative medicine. They see both sides of the same fence, the fence that should be about healing, but in conventional medicine of today, it often only leads to more sickness and symptoms. Naturopathy is the system of preventing and treating illness without drugs, usually by incorporating diet, exercise, stress reduction, and other modalities such as meditation, massage, and acupuncture, to name just a few.

Western medicine is often referred to as "allopathic" medicine, which means science-based, modern medicine, as opposed to "osteopathic" or "homeopathic" medicine. The word itself comes from the Greek words *allos*, for "opposite," and *pathos*, for "to suffer." Allopathic medicine is focused on treating symptoms, usually with pharmaceuticals, surgeries, therapies, radiation, and standard treatments, sometimes focused on suppressing the symptoms rather than allowing the body's own natural immune defenses to spring into action. Other words for allopathic medicine include conventional medicine, orthodox medicine, mainstream medicine, and biomedicine. The healers in allopathic medicine are doctors, nurses, surgeons, pharmacists, and other healthcare professionals. Again, allopathic medicine has its place in the quest for health and is the world of cutting-edge science, technologies, and treatments that can prolong and save lives. To remove a cancerous tumor, you want a surgeon, not a meditation coach. To stop a stroke, you want a hospital setting with medications meant to prevent further damage or even death.

Osteopathic and homeopathic medicine ... embrace the body's innate abilities and immune system and look to cure the actual root cause of disease instead of just treating and easing symptoms.

Allopathic medicine has its place, it's just not the only place. Osteopathic and homeopathic medicine, on the other hand, embrace the body's innate abilities and immune system and look to cure the actual root cause of disease instead of just treating and easing symptoms. Osteopathy is a medical practice that emphasizes the treatment of medical disorders through the manipulation and massage of the bones, joints, and muscles. Homeopathy refers to a 200-year-old system created in Germany by a physician named Samuel Hahnemann that posits the body can cure itself often by using small amounts of natural substances like plants or minerals to stimulate the body's own healing processes. Homeopathy believes that something that causes symptoms in a healthy person can be treated with a small dose of something that triggers those same symptoms. In the end, it triggers the body's natural defense system to kick into gear and take care of the original problem. An example of homeopathy might be using red onion, which causes the eyes to water, to treat allergies, which have the same symptom.

The Empire Fights Back: A Brief History of Suppression

Nature has provided cures for thousands of years. Plants, roots, and herbs have been used as far back as 5000 B.C.E. by the Sumerians, who made them the basis of their healing methods. Ancient texts and cuneiforms show images of herbs and make mention of their use for salves, balms, and their use in food to heal. The first herbal concoction goes back as far as 162 C.E. by the great physician

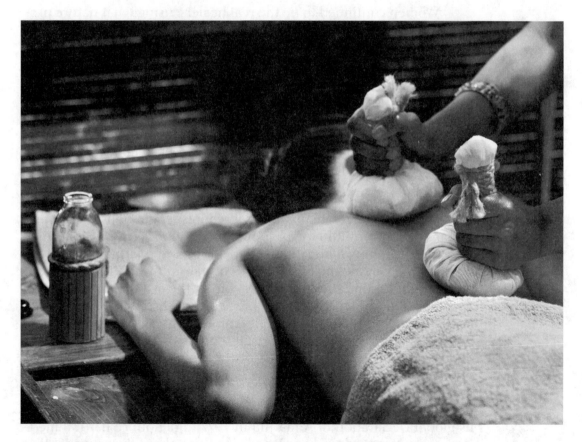

A woman receives an herbal massage from an Ayurvedic practitioner. These traditions date back many centuries and are still used as part of Chinese and Indian cultures.

Galen, and both ancient Chinese and Indian Ayurvedic traditions have used herbs and plants for healing for thousands of years as well as indigenous cultures the world over. This was later adopted in Western medicinal traditions in ancient Rome, Greece, and throughout Europe.

Both women and men used these natural healing methods, but eventually, natural methods such as kitchen witchery became more the work of women until men took over "medicine," especially around the twelfth century when pressure from the Church and the transition from matriarchal to patriarchal societies and spiritual traditions occurred. By the thirteenth century, the Church had become more accepting of medicinal practices in general, but female healers had been relegated to the "underground" and called "witches," while men alone could practice openly.

Women continued to be the real healers, using what nature provided, but it wasn't until modern times that they were able to openly practice both traditional and natural medicine. Colleges and universities that offered medical schools were male dominated, but today, it is leaning more toward women graduates. Natural medicine and holistic healing have also, since the nineteenth century, become far more acceptable, preferable to many, and open to both genders. However, the American Medical Association (AMA) mentioned in its 1847 founding documents code of ethics that members who consulted with or practiced any kind of homeopathy would be booted from the association.

Until about 1910, many medical schools taught holistic therapies and modalities until the AMA joined forces with John D. Rockefeller, who was becoming a huge force in the booming pharmacological industries, to evaluate the effectiveness of natural health therapies that were taught around the country. Of course, the evaluation was a total rejection of natural medicine and pushed drug–based medicine, which Rockefeller would greatly benefit from. Congress then allowed the AMA the power to decertify medical schools that taught such classes and did not meet the standards of their new and approved, drug–oriented medicine.

This was followed by the World Health Organization releasing its global Declaration of Alma Ata in 1977 to denounce natural medicine and promote drug–based medicine throughout the countries that were a part of the United Nations.

It wasn't until the 1950s and into the 1960s that modalities such as chiropractic, midwifing, and other natural approaches began to gain a foothold on people who did not want to turn their lives over to the growing Big Pharma stronghold. This progress was fought the whole time by pharmaceutical companies, doctors, the complicit Food and Drug Administration (FDA), and researchers who all did not want to lose business or profit by allowing chiropractors to help alleviate pain or allow midwives to help women have safer births. The battle continued as natural cures for diseases like cancer were silenced, censored, and blocked at every angle to keep the public beholden to the power of conventional medicine.

As cancer rates and types increased, the AMA worked with the FDA and various cancer organizations to make sure natural cure claims were shut down....

As cancer rates and types increased, the AMA worked with the FDA and various cancer organizations to make sure natural cure claims were shut down, even going so far as to harass doctors and practitioners who made such claims, even get their licenses to practice revoked or worse. In one case, described in "Suppression of Highly Effective Natural Medicine & Alternative Medicine" from *The Natural Guide*, a man named Harry Hoxsey, who operated 17 alternative health clinics in the 1950s, was the victim of a vicious attack by the AMA because of an herbal formula he had used on thousands of cancer patients, many of whom had claimed they were cured.

Hoxsey was arrested over 100 times, and each time he was jailed, hundreds of his patients would rally around the prison and pray for his release. In court, not one of his patients ever testified against him, yet the harassment continued until he sued the AMA for slander and libel.

In 1953, Benedict Fitzgerald Jr., special counsel to the U.S. Senate Commerce Committee, conducted an in–depth investigation and concluded that the FDA, AMA, and National Cancer Institute conspired to suppress a fair investigation of Hoxsey's treatments. His clinics flourished after that, and he successfully treated over 12,000 patients.

Sadly, the FDA shut down all his clinics by 1960, stating that cancer had no cure and that Hoxsey's practice was illegal. His head nurse ended up moving to Mexico and opening a thriving clinic in Tijuana. From that point on, natural cures for cancer were deemed illegal in the United

The Rockefeller Connection

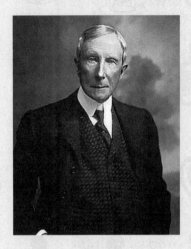

John D. Rockefeller Sr.

John D. Rockefeller Sr. (1839–1937) was the first billionaire in the United States, and his family is one of the wealthiest and most powerful families on the planet. Rockefeller might be said to have been responsible for the decline of alternative and holistic medicine. Before he became a huge force in the petrochemical industry, which began around 1900, people were still able to access natural health doctors and therapies. However, Rockefeller saw the potential of monopolizing the oil, chemical, and medical industries all at the same time, using petrochemical-based medicines and treatments that could be patented and, therefore, sold for huge profits. Natural remedies came from nature and couldn't be patented; therefore, it wasn't possible to exploit them for huge financial gain. Big Pharma was born.

Rockefeller's desire to monopolize medicine relied on him having no real competition with natural health doctors, though, so he got together with his friend, steel industry magnate Andrew Carnegie, and the two of them plotted. From the Carnegie Foundation, they sent a man named Abraham Flexner around the country to visit medical schools and hospitals and report back. Flexner had no medical background at all, but he was trained in psychology and had a reputation for his evaluation skills, critical thinking, and dislike for traditional education. This report became known as the Flexner Report and was the first big step in Big Pharma's stranglehold on the medical industry. Of course, the report was filled with all the ways medical institutions must be reorganized, centralized, and vastly improved, and soon, over half of all medical schools had shut down due to the negative report. The Flexner Report successfully eliminated most natural medical schools and established the new biomedical model of pharmaceuticals and drugs as the gold standard of medical training.

As a result of the report, many doctors were jailed for practicing natural medicine. To look like the hero after all these schools and practices closed, Rockefeller then came to the rescue, donating over $100 million to selected hospitals and medical schools and forming a front group called the General Education Board, which was instrumental in making sure all students at medical universities received the same homogenized education, one that was approved by Rockefeller and his new Big Pharma machine. The students all learned about patented medicines. Natural health had no place in Rockefeller's plans. In 1913, Rockefeller founded the American Cancer Society, which has been accused of focusing more on diseases than cures, and pushes chemotherapy, surgeries, and radiation over natural, holistic lifestyle therapies.

If one man could be pinpointed as heralding the birth and ascension of Big Pharma, it was John D. Rockefeller. His power and wealth made it all but impossible to stop him.

States, and any amount of force was used to stop those who claimed they could cure the disease. Granted, quacks and hoaxers in the natural health world make claims they cannot back up to take people's money, but how different is this from the Big Pharma companies that do the exact same thing, often with much deadlier side effects?

It does come down to money. Alternative and natural health methods do not make money for Big Pharma, and with such a powerful lobbying stronghold on our political system, it's no surprise that natural cures and healings are shunned and called "pseudoscience" and worse. By simply dismissing all-natural health as a big hoax, the conventional medicine "mafia" has been able to keep a strong grip on what doctors learn in college, what they are allowed to offer to patients, the proliferation of drugs and pharmaceuticals, and the focus on cut/slash/burn treatments for cancer, even today when people have the power of the internet and access to more information than ever in our history.

Yet, throughout the 1970s to today, more and more people have been seeking out other ways of being healthy that don't involve a handful of pills and surgical procedures. With the advent of the internet, things really changed, as people could now find more and more information about holistic and natural health with a few clicks of the keyboard, including real scientific studies being done on herbal remedies, alternative treatments, and healing that defied what the AMA and Big Pharma were pushing: dependency on conventional medicine alone.

Today, a great awakening is happening as people realize that the conventional way hasn't been working very well. The top three causes of death are heart disease, cancers, and medical error. Today, people can look up their own information, do their own research, investigate, and advocate for themselves, even as the world of Big Pharma and Big Medicine fights back by lobbying Congress with more money and perks, buying more media advertising, and now, in the year 2021, working with Big Tech such as Twitter, Facebook, Instagram, and other social media sites to censor, block, warn, and take down for good any person or site that they can find that promotes natural health, asking questions about vaccine ingredients and drug side effects, questioning the narrative of mainstream media, demanding transparency and answers about COVID-19 inconsistencies and who makes money off of which vaccines and treatments, and everything else that falls outside the acceptable boundaries of conventional medicine.

This censorship has become so tyrannical in 2021 alone when hundreds of voices were silenced and deplatformed, including some top researchers and studies conducted at major universities and institutions, simply because they did not go along with what was being parroted on mainstream media and the halls of politics. It has caused untold thousands of deaths by preventing people from accessing information about cures and treatments for diseases and ailments because to do so would mean less profit for the pharmaceutical companies, health insurance companies, and doctors and surgeons who have no interest in curing patients, only keeping them.

Somehow, natural medicine has found a way to rise above the censorship and political and media manipulations and not be silenced. This is because for so many people, it works. We as a nation get sicker and sicker by the year, but more resources exist for those who choose a more holistic approach to taking care of themselves and their loved ones. This does not mean they disregard conventional medicine in its entirety but that they understand that the body has its own healing forces and an immune system that should be cultivated, nourished, strengthened, and empowered and that healing doesn't end where the body ends but also includes attention to the mind, the emotions, the spirit, and the soul.

When it comes to many diseases of the past, things like better sanitation, improved nutrition, cleaner air and water, and refrigeration to prevent food spoilage all go a long way toward keeping the human body in a better position to fend off viruses and germs. Treating nu-

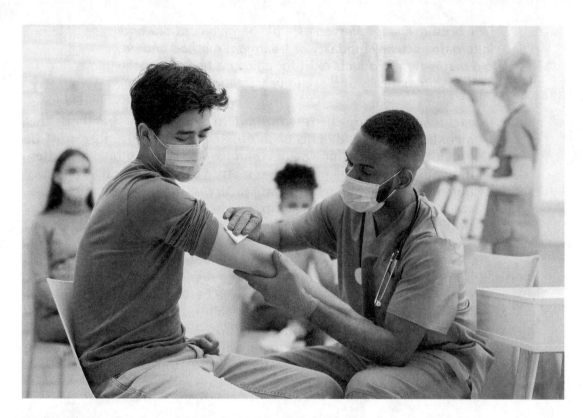

Modern medicine has devised a COVID-19 vaccine using the mRNA technique, but could other, more natural vaccines and treatments be safer than what the medical community is promoting?

trition deficiencies and removing toxins helps decrease the risk of developing illnesses or lessening the impact of those already being experienced, and it is not always necessary to rush out for the latest pill, vaccine, or surgery. In developing nations, lack of the above is what often leads to major outbreaks of disease, but the people in poorer countries tend to die of all causes in greater numbers without good food, clean air and water, and basic sanitation and waste removal as the foundations of public health. Even the act of hand-washing has gone a long way toward improving health standards. Doctors in the past didn't wash their hands after performing autopsies, then they would go deliver babies. This led to a high infant mortality rate that could have been prevented with one simple act.

The bottom line is, everyone should be given options and alternatives to any modality or treatment method and be told that natural products exist for pain or a bad cold rather than automatically and

The bottom line is, everyone should be given options and alternatives to any modality or treatment method and be told that natural products exist for pain or a bad cold rather than automatically and exclusively treating them with

exclusively treating them with modern, conventional methods that include a host of side effects and toxic chemicals. Choices must be provided. Naturopathic doctors train in both conventional and alternative medicine and must have many years of clinical experience under their belts before they can practice so they can approach a disease or illness from two angles instead of just one, expanding the possibilities of finding a great path to treatment and a cure.

In the end, those choices must work. In the nineteenth century, homeopathy began to flourish, and the death rates from diseases like cholera, scarlet fever, and typhoid were between one–eighth to one–half those in conventional hospitals. By the year 2008, more than 38 percent of adults in the United States had used some form of alternative medicine, and today, those rates are much higher, thanks in part to the power of social media to share and spread information and personal experiences.

The Whole Being

Natural healing and medicine can be one of these or all of these, but they are always nature based. Holistic medicine refers to treating the whole being rather than just the parts that are diseased or infected and looks at body, mind, and spirit as one unit that if any part is not healthy, it causes the entire being to be unhealthy. Allopathic medicine tends to treat just the "parts," and holistic medicine treats the whole of the parts. Holistic health involves five different aspects:

- Physical
- Mental
- Emotional
- Spiritual
- Social

When any of the above is out of balance or "dis–eased," it can affect the entire being, thus the idea of treating the whole of the person and not just the physical pain, or the emotional trauma, caused by an accident or illness. This is not to say you need holistic treatment for a broken ankle. In some situations, it is all about a part of the body, but for diseases like cancer, heart disease, diabetes, and others that have many aspects in play, in general, it always helps to look at how it affects the entire person. Treating a cancer victim only by cutting out the tumor and not recognizing the need for therapy, counseling, breath work, meditation, and dealing with stress and anxiety does not make the victim that much stronger or more resilient and does nothing toward an overall sense of well-being.

Some natural modalities involve manipulating and working with energies, frequencies, sound, light, color, heat, touch, and massage. Ancient Chinese herbal medicine, acupressure, acupuncture, Reiki, hands-on healing, reflexology, Ayurveda, and even the use of chiropractic manipulations are all included under the natural health umbrella.

Complementary medicine is another term that includes natural tools and modalities to complement the body's own defenses and immune abilities rather than compete with them. The name also refers to healing that can complement allopathic treatments such as meditation and stress relief after a heart attack operation or using acupuncture with cognitive behavioral therapy for anxiety or depression. It is possible for the two to find middle ground for the betterment of the patient.

These types of medicine approaches were once never taught in universities and medical schools, although that is changing as more clinics open and more hospitals include these natural approaches in their comprehensive patient care programs.

Never Mess with Your Health

This is a book that emphasizes natural health and healing, but a place always exists for traditional medicine, and you must never ignore signs and symptoms that require a visit to a doctor, urgent care, a call to 911, or a ride to the hospital emergency room. Natural healing works wonders for so many things, as this book will prove, but if you have the following symptoms, don't rely on herbal remedies to do what modern medicine may be better at:

- Any broken bone or sprain that might require surgery
- Deep lacerations that will need stitches
- Bleeding that does not stop or worsens

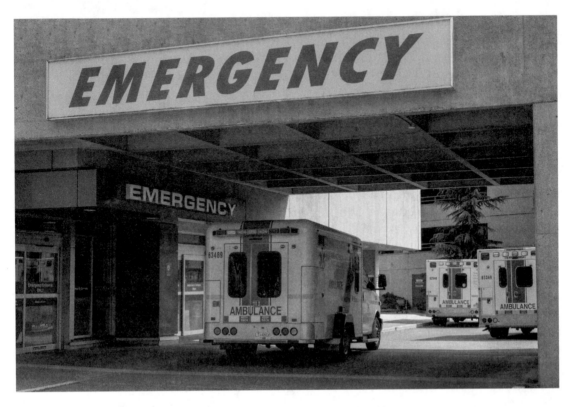

Natural health solutions can be wonderful alternatives to modern medicine, but in many cases, such as life-or-death emergencies, go to an emergency room and seek immediate help.

- Blood in the stool, urine, ears, or vomit
- Loss of consciousness
- Delirium
- Fever above 103 degrees, especially in children, that is not alleviated with other methods
- A tumor or lump in breast or lymph nodes
- Discoloration of skin or extremely pale skin
- Bluish lips
- Confusion and slurring of words
- Heart pain and chest pressure, especially if it radiates to the arms, jaw, or neck
- Dizziness that lasts more than an hour or so and has no discernable cause
- Suspected food poisoning or chemical poisoning of a household cleaner or toxic product

- Suicide ideation and talk or attempts at suicide
- Drug overdose, street and prescription
- Alcohol sickness
- Possible internal injuries from an accident or fall

Of course, if you have a horrible flu that isn't going away, you may want to check in with your doctor. If you have been diagnosed with a disease or illness such as diabetes, cancer, heart disease, Parkinson's, or any other chronic issue, it must involve your doctor and a team of specialists so you can make the best plan of action for your treatment. If you suspect you or someone you love is having a heart attack or stroke, call an ambulance immediately. This is not a time to mix up an herbal tea or syrup; it's a life-or-death situation that requires medical intervention in a hospital setting.

 Just because you prefer natural healing modalities does not mean you should shun these traditional modalities completely.

Surgery is a must for removing tumors and cancer, for putting in a stent or pacemaker, or for fixing a hernia. Just because you prefer natural healing modalities does not mean you should shun these traditional modalities completely. Sometimes, you will need a surgeon to do what needs to be done; no natural poultice or salve exists that can correct a leg length discrepancy, remove a painful bunion, or fix a broken collarbone.

Don't be stupid with your health. When in doubt, call the doctor or go the ER. If it's serious, don't go it alone. Ways exist to combine natural health and traditional health, as you will see. But remember that a time and a place exist for everything, even prescription medications when you are seriously ill and need them for initial treatment.

An Integrative Approach

All-natural healing methods take an integrative approach to the human body. Integrative medicine offers doctors and practitioners trained to treat the whole, much like holistic health care. The therapies they use integrate physical, emotional, and sometimes spiritual tools for healing and advocate some allopathic treatments, too. Integrative medicine combines the best of both worlds and involves:

- Alternative medical systems and methods that originated outside of Western medicine such as Ayurveda and Chinese herbalism and medicine
- Body–mind methods and interventions that focus on mental, spiritual, and emotional approaches such as support groups, classes, journaling, and prayer work
- Energy-based therapies that work with sound vibrations, light, heat, electromagnetic fields, and healing touch, including hands-on healing and Reiki
- Biological-based therapies that focus on diet, the use of herbs and plants, and aromatherapy
- Manipulative/body-based therapies such as massage therapy, deep-tissue therapy, and chiropractic medicine

The mindset behind these therapies is that disease must be treated holistically rather than part by part. Health is like the foundation of a house. If it is not sturdy and secure, the walls and ceiling won't stand. You must first and foremost heal the causes of disease and recognize that all the parts and systems work together, so fixing just one doesn't fix the whole. An individual organ is not the whole being. Yes, treat the individual organ, but don't leave it at that. Look

A healthy flow of life energy means less stress and less inflammation in the body because of stress. Acupressure has been shown to release endorphins for a feeling of well-being and less pain.

to see where in the entirety of the body, and the mind and spirit, the root cause still lingers, then treat that.

Some of the more popular and widely used therapies are presented here, and many will be further expanded upon later in the book.

Acupressure

Acupressure is a form of traditional Chinese medicine that uses pressure on the body's energy points, or meridians, that carry and hold life energy, known as chi or qi. We become ill when the energy is blocked or misdirected and out of balance. Applying pressure via the practitioner's fingers or thumbs directly on meridian points frees up the trapped or blocked chi and allows it to flow unimpeded to restore the body to health. Acupressure can be used on everything from muscle pain to insomnia to allergies and can also alleviate anxiety and depression. A healthy flow of life energy means less stress and less inflammation in the body because of stress. Acupressure has been shown to release endorphins for a feeling of well-being and less pain.

Several recent scientific studies back up the use of acupressure to overcome insomnia, stop pain, and provide immediate relief for

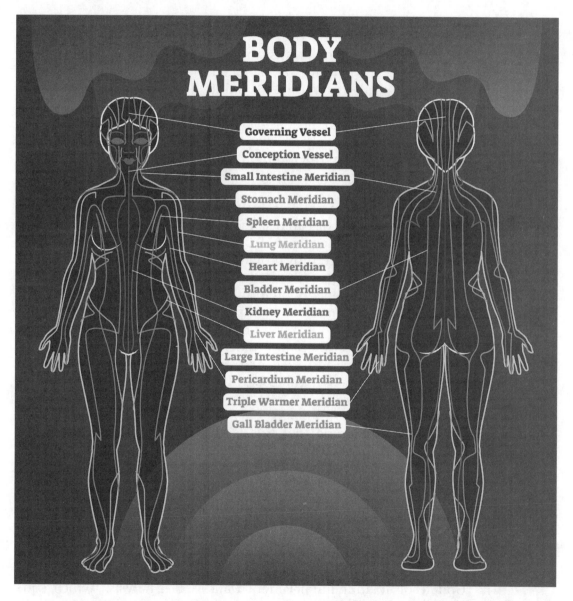

BODY MERIDIANS

Governing Vessel
Conception Vessel
Small Intestine Meridian
Stomach Meridian
Spleen Meridian
Lung Meridian
Heart Meridian
Bladder Meridian
Kidney Meridian
Liver Meridian
Large Intestine Meridian
Pericardium Meridian
Triple Warmer Meridian
Gall Bladder Meridian

The body has 14 "meridians," according to those who practice acupuncture, and each one, when stimulated, affects a specific part of the body.

anxiety. A 2013 study by M. Carotenuto et al. titled "Acupressure Therapy for Insomnia in Adolescents: A Physomnographic Study" resulted in deeper sleep for the study subjects, and a 2015 study featured in the journal *Pain Management Nursing* titled "Effects of Acupressure on Anxiety: A Systematic Review and Meta–Analysis" found that acupressure relieved anxiety and improved mental health.

Acupuncture

Like acupressure, this is an ancient Chinese healing method that involves the placement of small, thin needles on specified areas of the body called acupuncture points. This stimulates the nerves and muscles and allows for the release of healing chemicals that can alleviate chronic pain, headaches, inflammation, and even arthritis. Acupuncture is so widely practiced that many health insurance companies cover sessions, including for things like general anxiety and depression.

The foundation of acupuncture, like acupressure, is that the body's energy, called qi, can become blocked, and the positioning and turning of the tiny needles helps to unblock the channel so the qi energy flows naturally, thus providing healing. The needles direct the qi energy to different bodily organs or functions and can also be used to drain out excess energy buildup in the body. The pins are located along the body's 14 meridian points, which affect different organ functions, including the kidneys, liver, heart, spleen, and lungs. The needles are placed just below the skin's epidermis layer, so no bleeding occurs. Some practitioners add heat or electrical charges along with the needles or accompanying massage. In China, acupuncture is used as a form of anesthesia.

Some may argue that this is all just the placebo effect, but science backs up acupuncture's ability to battle many types of pain. The October 12, 2012, issue of *JAMA Internal Medicine* featured a study called "Acupuncture for Chronic Pain: An Individual Patient Data Meta–Analysis" that found acupuncture had positive results alleviating PMS, neck pain, chronic pain, and osteoarthritis, and another 2016 study with 2,349 participants found it worked on chronic and tension headaches. The May 1, 2018, issue of *Journal of Pain* features another study by Andrew Vickers et al. called "Acupuncture for Chronic Pain: Update of an Individual Patient Data Meta–Analysis," which concluded that no placebo effect was involved and that acupuncture worked on pain, even long-term pain.

Acupressure and acupuncture are probably the most widely studied alternative treatments in the scientific community and prove to be effective modalities for healing of the body and the mind. Even over a decade ago, the World Health Organization recognized these modalities as beneficial for treating over 100 conditions from migraines to asthma to neuralgia to back pain to sore throats to anemia to myopia to ulcers … the list goes on. They have even been successful for helping people stop smoking and for treating alcoholism and have been used to help AIDS patients strengthen their immune systems and alleviate many uncomfortable symptoms.

Aromatherapy

Smell is powerful. Aromatherapy uses essential oil extracts from plants to help people relax, sleep better, relieve pain, and improve mood and well-being. Oils can be diffused in burners, massaged into the skin as creams or balms, or put into bathwater. This practice goes back over 5,000 years. We will get more into this subject later in the book, but is any science behind the use of plant parts and extracts made of roots, leaves, seeds, and blossoms to achieve better health?

A 2017 study titled "Effects of Aromatherapy on Sleep Quality and Anxiety of Patients" in the BACCN *Nursing in Critical Care* journal found that in a clinical setting, patients with heart disease who used lavender aromatherapy were better able to sleep and experienced less anxiety. Another 2017 study called "Evidence-Based Complementary and Alternative Medicine" found that nurses who worked the night shift were better able to sleep after a massage with sweet marjoram essential oil.

Our sense of smell is powerful and, when we smell the right things, can calm us or give us energy. Some smells that formulate an essential oil blend excite the body and awaken the brain, others sedate or calm it, and knowing which ones do what is, pun intended, essential.

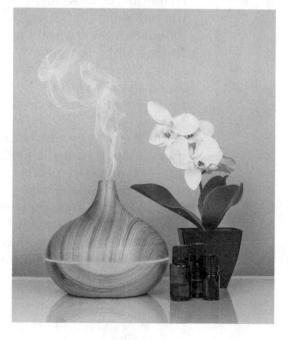

Pleasant aromas have been shown to reduce stress and soothe emotions.

More on which essential extracts work for what in a later chapter.

Ayurvedic Medicine

Ayurveda originated over 3,000 years ago and is still widely practiced today all over the world. Many of the methods that belong to Ayurveda predate written records and were passed down from generation to generation via word of mouth. This healing method is more than just one thing. It involves specialized diets, use of herbs, massage, and other ways of balancing the body, mind, and spirit for holistic well-being. Yoga is part of the Ayurveda program and is mentioned in many texts to address physical and mental health issues such as high blood pressure, insomnia, stress, and depression.

Ayurveda consists of three main types of treatment: elimination therapies, pacification therapies, and nourishing therapies. An Ayurvedic physician or practitioner will prescribe a patient a treatment that is individualized and directed toward the ailment and could include the use of herbs for healing inflammation; some compound of herbs and metals for constipation; a lifestyle program of diet and exercise; body manipulation; therapies using oils to detox the body of chemicals; or movement to rebalance and bring greater harmony to the individual and increase their well-being. The foundation of this modality is the restoration of balance in the body. Often, this involves using holistic treatments, meditation, diet, massage, breathing, and herbal therapies to remove toxic buildup that brings about imbalance and disharmony to the body, mind, and spirit. Herbal therapy is used to restore those balances and increase energy and vitality.

One of the most widely studied herbs is turmeric, which is a mainstay of Ayurvedic medicine's plant-based dietary system for its anti-inflammatory powers, as is the practice of oil pulling, in which the patient swishes 1 tablespoon of coconut oil through their teeth and around the mouth to pull out bacteria and lessen the impact of plaque. Like ancient Chinese medicine, the old is new again as the internet and YouTube how-to videos have made oil pulling all the rage again for those wishing to find natural alternatives to expensive dental bills.

Biofeedback

We can control our bodily processes with our minds and breathing, and biofeedback proves it. Bodily processes that are involuntary include our heart rate, blood pressure, breathing, and skin temperature, but biofeedback allows us to take control and improve health conditions by learning how to relax and perform mental and breathing exercises to control the body. Done with a specific machine, which can now be purchased for the home, the patient is hooked up to the machine via electrodes on the skin, and they follow along to instructions via a therapist or a video or audio guide.

The process puts you in touch with your body and teaches you how you can control even involuntary processes by being aware of your mood, thoughts, and breathing. Doing so provides you with a sense of power over your own health and well-being, and many studies have shown that those who use biofeedback can rid themselves of stress, anxiety, depression, overwhelm, and tension headaches and also improve mental and physical performance.

A 2016 study titled "Biofeedback Training and Tension-Type Headaches," published in the National Library of Medicine database, found that this is an effective treatment for all types of headaches. The good news is that you no longer need to buy an expensive biofeedback machine as prices have become more user-friendly, and you might even be able to get a device from your health insurance company (they often send free blood pressure monitors and such if your doctor has deemed it necessary).

The good news is that you no longer need to buy an expensive biofeedback machine as prices have become more user-friendly, and you might even be able to get a device from your health insurance company....

Bodywork

This umbrella term refers to a number of therapies and treatments that involve working with the human body. This can be in the form of breath work, massage, energy medicine, exercise therapy, manipulative therapies, and somatic therapies. Bodywork is hugely popular in the United States as an alternative way to achieve balance and health. Bodywork looks at the body as a whole unit, combined with the mind and spirit, to seek holistic harmony and healing. Some modalities involve the use of manipulating the electromagnetic fields of the body around the heart and the brain.

Bodywork can involve hands-on touch or nontouch therapies. Some of the most widely known types of nontouch bodywork include breath work, Reiki, qigong, tai chi, energy healing, therapeutic touch, and yoga. Those involving touch and manipulation include chiropractic medicine, reflexology, shiatsu, massage, posture integration, deep tissue massage, somatic experiencing, craniosacral therapy, and the methods that go by the names Bowen Technique, Alexander Technique, Rolfing, Feldenkrais Method, and Hakomi Method.

- Alexander Technique: Restores balance, flexibility, and ease of movement via activities that release tension and increase energy levels. This includes movements to improve posture and coordination and relieve pain. It was created by Frederick Matthias Alexander, who believed his poor posture led to the loss of his voice during public speaking events. It can be applied to everyday activities, too, such as rising from a sitting position properly, and teaches overall movement efficiency for well-being of the body and mind.

- Feldenkrais Method: Created by nuclear physicist Moshe Feldenkrais after he suffered a sports injury, this technique uses movement training, gentle touch, and verbal instruction to restore range of motion and functional integration. The first form of the Feldenkrais Method focuses on the practitioner's touch to improve breathing and body alignment. The second form focuses on slow, nonaerobic motions that help the subject relearn proper body movement.

- Hakomi Method: This is a type of psychotherapy that is body based and uses body–mind awareness and touch to explore buried beliefs and influence them for lasting, positive changes. It involves altered states of consciousness to allow the patient to access core beliefs; they are then instructed on how to shift so they are empowering, not destructive.

- Esalen Massage: Swedish massage that is influenced by the teachings of Esalen leaders Charlotte Selver and Bernie Gunther, who taught sensory awakening. It's massage with a philosophy behind it, a type of meditation combined with touch to quiet the mind and bring about present–moment awareness.

- Craniosacral Therapy: Sort of a light chiropractic touch therapy focused on the brain and spinal cord to break up trapped stress and negative energy and improve health and immune functioning.

- Stone Therapy: Heated and cooled stones are applied to the body, sometimes during a massage, to relieve stiffness and sore muscles.

- Lymphatic Massage: This massage is focused on using gentle and precise massage movements to assist the flow of the body's lymphatic fluids.

- Rolfing: Created by biochemist Dr. Ida Rolf, this therapy aligns the body segments through deep massage and manipulation of the connective tissue called fascia. Each session might focus on a different part of the body that has become tight or rigid from injury or trauma. Practitioners must be certified by the Rolf Institute in Boulder, Colorado.

- Shiatsu: A massage therapy that works with the body's energy meridians. It is done fully clothed. The practitioner presses on the meridian points and stretches and opens them to release blocked energy and bring back natural flow, similar to acupressure.

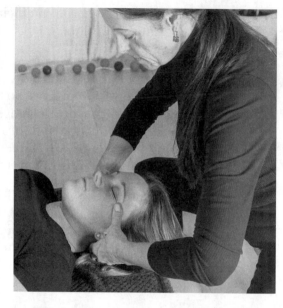

In shiatsu massage, the practitioner presses on certain points in the body to release blocked energies.

- Watsu: Shiatsu massage done in a warm pool of water.

- Kinesiology: A diagnostic system that looks at individual muscle function to determine what the patient needs for healing and well-being. Practitioners test strength and mobility of muscles and muscle groups and analyze posture and walking gait. Treatment involves diet, exercise, muscle and joint manipulation; this is one alternative therapy that is widely accepted and used in allopathic medicine and dentistry.

Botanical/Herbal Medicine

Long before any society had allopathic, drug-focused treatments for diseases, people used what nature had to offer in the form of herbs and plant parts to create remedies and medicinals for whatever ailment presented itself. This practice has continued to evolve and today is used by more and more people eager to shun pharmaceuticals with their pages of side effects in favor of Earth's own prescription medications.

Herbalists were the apothecaries of old and the first pharmacists, who knew which plant part did what and how to blend them for the best effect. Whether in the form of dried powder, tincture, herbal teas, infusions, concoctions and decoctions, salves and balms, or any other form possible, the vast and extensive world of plant life created a vast and extensive herbal medicine foundation that practitioners use and continue to add to.

Many women accused of witchcraft throughout history were herbalists, who understood how to heal fellow villagers with plants grown in the woods or in pots on the hearth and were known as "kitchen witches" or "practical witches." Kitchen witches of today use herbs in cooking, spell work, and for healing and look to the foundational wisdom of their ancestors while adding their own modern spin on things, even sharing remedies and recipes on the internet and social media.

Those who seek to "live off the land" become adept at herbal medicine, too, as do those who have been sickened or injured by modern drugs and treatment methods or experienced failure with treatments only to become sicker than ever. They believe nature knows best and that if the earth made it, it will and does work.

Chiropractic

Chiropractic medicine has become widely accepted as both a singular and a complementary form of treatment. It still carries a little of the "natural medicine" stigma, but chiropractors are required to attend medical school and then some to become qualified to practice. Chiropractors learn to adjust and manipulate the body by applying controlled force with their hands, the most common treatment involving spinal adjustments to reduce stress and head, neck, and shoulder pain. Joint movement from this type of therapy also loosens and relaxes tight muscles and joints and can restore more mobility and range of motion and improve back pain and posture issues.

Chiropractors learn to adjust and manipulate the body by applying controlled force with their hands, the most common treatment involving spinal adjustments to reduce stress and head, neck, and shoulder pain.

When joint movement is restricted by a variety of factors, the surrounding tissue becomes inflamed. This can happen either in a singular event like a car accident, over time from heavy gym weight use or repetitive stress, or poor posture for long periods such as sitting at a cubicle all day and then at home.

A November 2013 study for the *Journal of Manipulative and Physiological Therapies* found that chiropractic adjustments are efficient at reducing neck and lower back pain. Other studies concluded the same; this is why this type of treatment is hugely popular today: because it works. Word of caution: because these manipulations can result in terrible injury if done by someone untrained, always check the practitioner's background and education and seek out references and reviews from people who have had adjustments.

EFT

Emotional freedom technique (EFT) is an alternative treatment that is often referred to as "tapping." It is very popular today as a method for reducing physical pain, emotional stress, and PTSD. It has been used successfully for years to help alleviate anxiety and PTSD, with plenty of research to back it up. Developed by a man named Gary Craig, the method involves disrupting both the energy behind an issue and the negative emotions and thoughts associated with it. On his website, Craig writes, "EFT breathes fresh air into the healing process by borrowing from the Chinese meridian system. While acupuncture, acupressure and the like have been primarily focused on physical ailments, EFT stands back from this ancient process and points it also at emotional issues. These, in turn, often provide benefits for performance and physical issues. EFT combines the physical benefits of acupuncture with the cognitive benefits of conventional therapy for a much faster, more complete treatment of emotional issues, and the physical and performance issues that often result."

Tapping along the body's meridian energy points is key, and you can't wing it. A process must be followed for beneficial results. You use your fingertips to tap, like a form of acupressure. First, you identify the issue you want to "tap on." Is it an illness, a fear or phobia, or a bad habit? You do one issue at a time, and you can repeat the process as many times as needed to disrupt the brain's responses to the issue and find healing.

Using an instructional video or working with someone who is an expert at tapping, you then come up with a phrase or sentence that will explain the

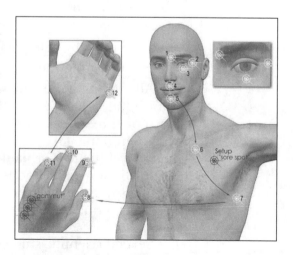

Many of the body points manipulated in EFT are around the face, especially around the eyes.

issue you are working on. You acknowledge the issue, and you accept yourself as is. So, your phrase might be something like "Even though I fear spiders, I deeply and completely accept myself" or "Even though I have issues with my adult son, I deeply and completely accept myself." Then, you begin tapping as follows.

The sequence is:

- karate chop (KC): small intestine meridian
- top of the head (TH): governing vessel
- eyebrow (EB): bladder meridian
- side of the eye (SE): gallbladder meridian
- under the eye (UE): stomach meridian
- under the nose (UN): governing vessel
- chin (CH): central vessel
- beginning of the collarbone (CB): kidney meridian
- under the arm (UA): spleen meridian

Begin tapping the karate chop point while saying your setup phrase three times. Then, tap each following point seven times, moving down the body in this order:

- eyebrow
- side of the eye
- under the eye
- under the nose
- chin
- beginning of the collarbone
- under the arm

After tapping the underarm point, go back to the top of the head to finish the sequence, remembering to repeat the phrase each time, or two or three times, at each tapping point; the frequency is up to you. When done, take a deep breath and check in with yourself. Do you still feel the fear or pain you were tapping on with the same intensity? Did some relief occur? Some people tap once and find full relief. Others must do it several times. No wrong way exists if you follow the correct sequence.

Several scientific studies back up EFT's claims to reduce anxiety and PTSD, including a 2013 randomized controlled trial published on PubMed titled "Psychological Trauma Symptom Improvement in Veterans Using Emotional Freedom Techniques: A Randomized Controlled Trial" that showed veterans suffering from PTSD had a significant reduction in psychological stress after just one month of tapping. Half of the study participants were relieved enough that they were diagnosed as no longer having PTSD. Another 2016 study showed that EFT decreased general anxiety significantly compared to other types of treatment.

The great thing about EFT is that you can learn to do it on your own and it's free. It has no side effects, and plenty of instructional videos are available as well as online EFT trainings and courses.

Energy Medicine

Energy healing or medicine is an umbrella term that includes a variety of therapies and techniques that manipulate and influence the body's energy fields. Considered pseudoscience by many in the allopathic medicine field, those who have used energy healings tell a different story of success, health, and a return to balance and harmony of body and mind.

Several scientific studies back up EFT's claims to reduce anxiety and PTSD.... The great thing about EFT is that you can learn to do it on your own and it's free.

Some of the healing types that fall under this umbrella are resonance therapy, sound therapy, light therapy, hands-on healing, Reiki, touch therapy, vibrational healing, distance healing, magnet therapy, color therapy, breath work, chakra balancing, qigong and tai chi, psychic healing, therapeutic touch, aura balancing and cleansing, crystal healing, meditation, acupuncture, acupressure, Puranic energy work, intuitive medicine, EFT (tapping), and any therapy that involves energy points or meridians on the body.

A lot of debate has occurred over whether or not the placebo effect is at work with energy healing or if the body truly can be healed and empowered by the manipulation of its energy fields. The brain and the heart both have their own electromagnetic fields and we are surrounded by EMF, so it seems natural that our health would be directly tied to the presence and flow of energy in and around us.

Science might have a lot to learn about how the body interacts with its own energy fields and those it comes in contact with, and it behooves modern researchers to pursue studies and clinical trials. Energy healing can involve devices and machines that are often inexpensive or some that are pretty pricey, and the methods can be done alone with training or under the guidance of a knowledgeable practitioner. Energy healing might include a strong spiritual or religious element to work both the body and the spirit in tandem or not, and it might require one session or 20. Few insurance companies would cover energy healing except for sound and light therapy, Reiki (which is used in hundreds of hospitals), and many forms of massage, so check with your general doctor and insurance company if you need the healing for physical pain and injury.

As always, do your research.

Hands-on Healing

Hands-on healing (aka "laying-on of hands") is a religious healing method involving laying the hands on the body to remove or extract illness and the demons that cause it. Hands-on healing doesn't have to be a religious act and was once practiced widely in the past, mainly in rural areas, where the vestiges of religious healing were still a part of everyday life. The concept behind it was that a trained healer

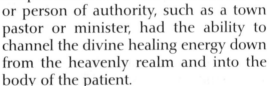

or person of authority, such as a town pastor or minister, had the ability to channel the divine healing energy down from the heavenly realm and into the body of the patient.

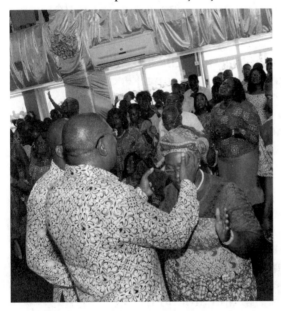

Dr. Ebenezer Markwei of Living Streams International in Accra, Ghana, practices the laying-on of hands on one of his followers.

Some religious sects used snakes and more extreme forms of hands-on "healing," and the result was not always positive. Today, hands-on healing still occurs in many churches, big and small, across the country, and plenty of people who feel they have the gift of channeling such energy via their hands offer their services to those who believe. It's no different from Reiki, really, when the religious extremism is left out of the equation. To those who experience a hands-on healing by someone they trust and believe in, it works, suggesting a strong "power of suggestion" influence.

Belief is powerful, and if someone believes they are being healed of cancer or a skin ailment, they very well may convince their bodies to do the work of healing.

Hydrotherapy

Hydrotherapy is an umbrella term for a host of methods and treatments that use water for healing, both internally and externally. This includes things like saunas, hot springs, steam baths, foot baths, sitz baths, colonics, and contrast therapy. Some of these forms are used in allopathic medicine, but others have taken on the label of pseudoscience.

Water is life giving. We are conceived in water and stay there, being nourished and nurtured, until we come down the birth canal. The human body is up to 60 percent water, with the brain and heart composed of 73 percent water, the skin 64 percent, the muscles and kidneys about 79 percent, and the bones about 31 percent. No wonder water continues to help us heal. We can go days, weeks, even months without food but only three days without water.

Hot water helps superficial blood vessels dilate, activates the sweat glands, removes toxins from tissues, and eases and loosens tight joints. Cold water constricts blood vessels and assists blood flow away from an inflamed area.

A nineteenth-century Bavarian monk named Father Sebastian Kneipp is considered the father of hydrotherapy. He used "contrast hydrotherapy," which alternates hot and cold water, a treatment method still used today. Hydrotherapy became popular in the United States when John Henry Kellogg of the Kellogg cereal family later attempted to prove its scientific merits at Michigan's Battle Creek Sanitarium. This method would remove toxins from the body and help drain the lymphatic system. Today, hot mineral baths are one of the most popular forms of hydrotherapy throughout Europe and the United States as well as treatments using flotation tanks, specified tubs, whirlpool baths, and wrapping compresses made of hot or cold water around a body part to increase circulation or lessen inflammation.

The principle behind water healing therapies is the use of temperature to induce a reaction in the body. Hot water helps superficial blood vessels dilate, activates the sweat glands, removes toxins from tissues, and eases and loosens tight joints. Cold water constricts blood vessels and assists blood flow away from an inflamed area. Just immersing the body into a bath of water helps relax muscles, relieve joint pain, and bring calm and serenity to the mind and spirit. Adding a bit of aromatherapy to the water treatment increases relaxation levels and relieves stress.

Balneotherapy, which dates to 1700 B.C.E., involves soaking in mineral waters or natural mineral hot springs to treat everything from back pain to arthritis. Mineral baths are known to have many healing properties and can also strengthen the immune system. The skin benefits greatly from water, prompting practitioners to use balneotherapy for treating rashes, acne, and swelling. The use of mud packs, soaks, wraps, and douches are often called spa therapy today.

Other types of hydrotherapy include colonic cleanses and irrigations to rid the digestive system of toxins, aquatic therapy and exercise (a 2018 study in *Clinical Rehabilitation* found that aquatic exercise done twice weekly reduces pain and improves joint function in patients with osteoarthritis), foot baths to reduce swelling and pain and balance circulation, therapeutic baths to treat skin conditions and stress, steam baths to relieve the skin of toxins, saunas and ice baths, sitz baths to treat issues of the sexual organs and rectum, whirlpool therapy to increase circulation and improve tissue repair, and Watsu, a massage that is done while you float in a pool of warm water.

People with rheumatoid arthritis can benefit from hydrotherapy, as shown in a 2016 review published in the Cochrane Database of Systematic Reviews stating aquatic exercise can improve pain and increase the quality of life for people with knee and hip osteoarthritis. A 2017 review in the *Journal of Strength and Conditioning Research* found that cold-water immersion improved the recovery time for sports-related issues and extreme physical activity.

However, some groups of people should not use this modality or should check with their doctors first, including pregnant women, those with high blood pressure and existing heart disease, those with kidney disease, cancer patients, and those who have experienced thrombosis.

Hypnotherapy

Imagine the power of the human voice healing illnesses and overcoming phobias and addictions. Hypnotherapy uses hypnosis to bring about a state of deep relaxation to access the subconscious, where entrenched programming and beliefs can be exposed and dealt with, especially those that cause imbalance, disease, and trauma.

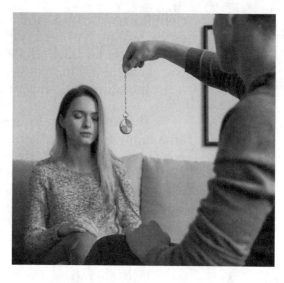

A professional hypnotherapist can help change unwanted thoughts, habits, and behaviors and increase your self-awareness by using the power of suggestion when you are in the hypnotic state. At this time, the brain is hugely accepting and lacks the normal censoring quality of the awakened state, yet you are always in control, so don't be afraid when under hypnosis.

Hypnotherapy is not about mind control but, rather, it relaxes the patient and makes their subconscious more accessible to a therapist's treatment.

Hypnotherapy has been tremendously successful in healing depression, anxiety, PTSD, panic attacks, insomnia, overcoming smoking, overeating, addictions, and facing phobias to lessen their impact. The biggest problem with this natural healing therapy is the patient's willingness to overcome any anxieties about being "put under." No, you won't turn into a clucking chicken unless that is okay with you! It is much less obtrusive than people expect and nothing like the crazy Vegas-style comedy shows.

Hypnotherapy is a direct line to the part of the mind that programs our lives but that we cannot reach or change much by sheer willpower or intellectual understanding.

Light Therapy

The use of natural light and artificial light as therapies for a host of diseases makes sense, as no life on our planet would survive without adequate sunlight. We are more closed in and locked inside than ever, and the rise of cancers, heart disease, and other illnesses are often linked to the lack of vitamin D in our bodies. Light is, like water, life, and we get too little of it or too much of the damaging "tech gadget" blue light that is damaging to our DNA.

Our ancestors knew the power of light and practiced what was once called "heliotherapy" in ancient Greece, ancient Egypt, and an–

cient Rome. The Incas and Mayas who worshipped the sun gods knew of the healing power of light. India spoke of healing with light in texts that date as far back as 1500 B.C.E. and mentioned combining herbs with light for a skin treatment. Other such mentions are found in Buddhist literature and ancient Chinese medicinal writings.

The first person to develop a modern method of light therapy, also known as phototherapy, was Niels Finsen, a Faroese physician who used short-wavelength light to treat lupus vulgaris and red light to treat smallpox lesions. He became known as the father of light therapy and received the Nobel Prize for Physiology or Medicine in 1903 for his discoveries. However, later research proved light therapy obsolete for treating smallpox and other diseases, proving the science is never settled.

Light therapies involve using a range of light frequencies along the spectrum to cure and heal skin ailments, seasonal depression, anxiety, neonatal jaundice, and cancers. Light can also heal wounds and reset our circadian rhythm to help us get better sleep and ward off insomnia. Blood irradiation light therapy kills viruses and cancerous cells in the blood.

Many treatments involve the use of ultraviolet light, which is great for healing skin conditions such as eczema, acne, psoriasis, and vitiligo. Narrowband UVB light is specifically effective and assists the body in the production of vitamin D. Full-body light therapy can be performed in a medical facility or at home but is not to be mistaken with tanning beds, which use high-powered UVA light and can cause cancer.

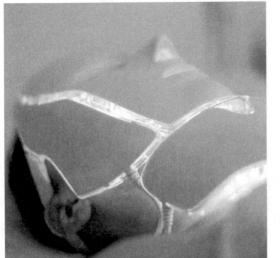

A woman is shown here undergoing light therapy to treat a facial skin condition.

Blue- and red-light therapies have been used to treat acne vulgaris to some effectiveness, but not enough long-term research has been done to show they work better than any other acne treatments. Laser therapy has been researched as a treatment for chronic wounds, and high-powered lasers have successfully been used to close wounds in a clinical setting instead of using stitches.

Light therapy seems to most benefit mental health, especially seasonal affective disorder (SAD), which strikes so many in the darker winter months. Light therapies also help reset the body's internal clock, especially the use of morning light to regulate the circadian rhythms needed for adequate sleep. For some people, just going outside and standing in the morning sun for 10 minutes does wonders to keep the body's clock running.

Blue- and red-light therapies have been used to treat acne vulgaris to some effectiveness, but not enough long-term research has been done to show they work better than any other acne treatments.

Babies born with jaundice from excess bilirubin, a yellow pigment found in the liver, are treated with white-light phototherapy, which transforms the bilirubin into a compound the infant can easily excrete through the urine and stools.

Research suggests that light delivered at a frequency of 40 flashes per second can restart the natural 40-hertz gamma rhythm of the brain and diminish toxic levels of amyloid plaques, proteins that harm brain function and memory. A reduction of these proteins can lead to improvements of symptoms of Alzheimer's disease.

The many methods of light therapy include the use of light boxes, photodynamic therapy, natural exposure, and artificial sun lamps. Too much sunlight can be risky, and too much ultraviolet light does cause damage to the skin and erythema, even at lower exposure times, so it is better to turn to the experts, who will also be able to better protect you from possible eye damage from intense light exposure.

The best thing about light therapy is that you don't have to pay huge fees to doctors or buy expensive machines if you don't want to. Just open the door and go outside in the sun for a while, and your mood and energy level are both sure to lift.

Massage Therapy

Massage therapy is used to treat a variety of issues from anxiety to pain control, muscle injury and stiffness, and emotional and mental illnesses like PTSD. It is a technique that reduces tension and brings about a sense of calm via the manipulation of muscles by rubbing, pressing, patting, and kneading and by the use of hot stones and essential oils. Often, massage is coupled with aromatherapy for a powerful healing therapy. The benefits of touch and smell include helping the body relax, which decreases anxious and fearful thoughts and manages the rise of adrenaline and the fight–or–flight response in those with anxiety disorders. Often, music is played to help calm the mind during massage.

It is important to try a few different massage therapy locations and professionals to find the right fit that works best for you. Never give your time or business to someone who is rude, rushes you along to accommodate other customers, or has no licenses to show their training. Always look for a licensed or certified massage therapist who has proof of standards and requirements for their state licensure. Licensed massage therapists can be found through the National Certification Board for Therapeutic Massage & Bodywork and the American Massage Therapy Association.

You may feel some soreness in the days following massage therapy, but you should never feel pain or discomfort during or after a massage. Talk to your doctor before getting a massage, especially if you have an existing muscular condition or are pregnant. By lowering stress hormones, regular massages can improve general health and well-being as well as relieve muscle pain and tension, improve circulation, and increase flexibility. It also helps lower blood pressure and heart rate, decrease muscle tension and pain, decrease aches including headaches, increase positive mood, and improve sleep. Massage is best done by trained therapists who use several methods or styles depending on what the goal is. Many insurance companies cover massage therapy, thanks to a large body of research that shows how effective it is.

Some of the more popular massage styles are:

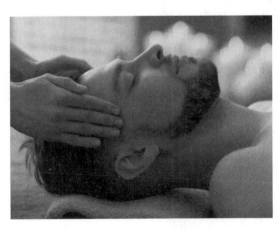

Massage therapy can obviously help with muscle aches and pains, but it also can work to destress you, treating everything from anxiety to depression and PTSD.

*   Swedish massage: This is the most popular type of massage to relax the body and mind. A total body massage is when a person lies on the massage table as a trained massage therapist slowly works through different muscle groups. It improves circulation and blood flow, relieves mental stress, and reduces muscle pain and tension.

- Deep tissue: This style has the massage therapist using more pressure and intensity when working through the deep muscles to release muscle knots associated with physical discomfort, stress, and headaches.

- Sports massage: Used by athletes, sports massage focuses on preparing muscles for intense training as well as helps muscles recover and heal after intense performance or injury.

- Hot stone massage: Hot stones are placed at various pressure points on the body to relieve tension and revitalize circulation.

- Chair massage: Used mainly for neck, upper back, and shoulder massages that don't require you to lie on a table. This is not a full-body massage.

- Thai massage: Invigorates your entire body by manipulating muscles via massage and yoga poses. Your therapist uses your whole body to loosen your joints and muscles. This form of massage is relaxing and energizing.

Those who get regular massages swear by their ability to bring a state of calm and peace back to the mind, body, and spirit, especially after a hectic or challenging time.

In a study titled "Effectiveness of Therapeutic Massage for Generalized Anxiety Disorder: A Randomized Controlled Trial" published in the *International Journal of Depression and Anxiety* on May 27, 2010, 68 people with generalized anxiety disorder showed that massage worked on par with other relaxation therapies but was far less expensive and more cost effective. Another study, "Effect of Massage Therapy on Pain, Anxiety, Relaxation, and Tension after Colorectal Surgery: A Randomized Study," showed that massage may be beneficial during postoperative recovery for patients undergoing abdominal colorectal surgery.

Massage has been studied frequently in many different clinical settings for heart patients, cancer patients, and mental illness patients and has shown consistently to be a boost to healing and well-being. Those who get regular massages swear by their ability to bring a state of calm and peace back to the mind, body, and spirit, especially after a hectic or challenging time. Massage is one of the most popular and widely used therapies for healing and well-being with ancient roots and is readily found in most communities with a little research (look for reviews on sites like Yelp, too). After a rough day at the office or dealing with the chaos of raising kids at home, having a massage can keep burnout at bay. Some workplaces even bring in a masseuse weekly for employees to use on their breaks, so why not ask your supervisor about this? A 15–minute chair massage can lead to greater productivity and better attitudes around the office and is well worth the cost.

While you can watch a few instructional videos on how to give someone a decent shoulder massage, it isn't advisable to go beyond that because of the possibility of injury or muscle bruising. Massage therapy in general has relatively few negative side effects, mainly feeling too much pain and discomfort after having a session (indicating an inexperienced therapist) or any contraindications that might occur with prescription medications or medical conditions, so ask your doctor about those issues before starting this type of therapy.

Massage satisfies our need for touch.

Meditation

Like mindfulness, meditation is widely practiced by those who are religious, spiritual, or simply focused on relaxation and centering for mental and physical health. The word "meditation" comes from the Latin verb *meditari*, which means "to think, contemplate, and ponder." Many different types of meditation exist according to region and religion, and meditation is also a part of traditional yoga practices. The word has become an umbrella term for a variety of methods of getting into a relaxed and peaceful state of being in the present moment.

Mindfulness meditation is meant to bring an increased awareness to the present and an expansion of consciousness to embrace your surroundings, all while using the power of your breath. In this state, thoughts and emotions are only observed, not judged or stressed over. Each thought is like a cloud that gently passes across the mind and exits, keeping the mind focused on the breath.

Many people use a mantra or a sacred word or phrase to assist them in meditation. You can silently say the mantra to yourself as you go deeper or say it out loud, but always stay focused on the breath. Mantra meditation is a favorite in yoga classes and Western meditation centers along with guided or visual meditations where you listen to a voice assisting you on a visual journey to a sacred place you can visit again and again when you need to find a calm center. These types of meditation engage all your senses, and often in the deep calm, you will experience intuitions or inspirations. Not everyone experiences this every time they meditate, but the purpose is to create a quiet and calm center within which can be returned to at any time.

The most popular type of meditation is Transcendental Meditation, which uses a repeated mantra that is given to you by a master meditator. You repeat this assigned and sacred mantra silently as you work with the breath to achieve a state of profound inner peace and calm.

Meditation can be about focusing the mind and attention on something such as a candle flame or the movement of water on the surface of a pond, or it can be about working with the breath to achieve an altered state of consciousness and deep relaxation. Witches use a form of focused meditation when they scry with a crystal ball or mirror or read tea leaves to achieve a heightened state of awareness in which they can access information and insight from a higher source, the universe, or the gods and goddesses.

Movement meditations consist of things like walking and run-ning, paying attention to the present moment and what you are ex-periencing with the five senses, and practices like tai chi and qigong, two Eastern movement practices. Tai chi is a gentle, flowing series of postures and movements that are a martial art, done in a graceful and slow manner. Deep breathing during tai chi creates a powerful sense of calmness and inner strength. Qigong works with the energy of qi or chi that permeates all things. It is also a movement practice that combines meditation with physical exercises and breathing for bal-ance and harmony of the body, mind, and spirit and is a part of tra-ditional Chinese medicine.

Native American Traditional Healing

Native American and indigenous traditional healing methods strongly focus on the body, mind, and spirit as a cohesive unit and include a spiritual aspect of the connection between the person and the Great Spirit as a higher force and guide. They put great emphasis on herbs and plants as remedies, smudging and burning of sage and incense, dancing and chanting to achieve a higher state of conscious-ness and honor the Great Spirit, storytelling and ceremonial practices, a reverence for nature and her gifts, and a sense of community and connection to others.

Each tribe may have its own regional practices and traditions, but the fundamentals are the same. A local medicine healer, male or female,

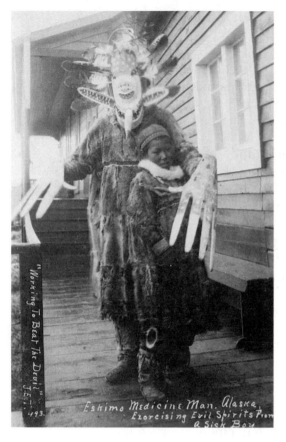

"Working To Beat The Devil" J.E.T. 493.

Eskimo Medicine Man, Alaska, Exorcising Evil Spirits From a Sick Boy

A Yup'ik medicine man is shown here trying to expel evil spirits from a boy in 1890s Nushagak, Alaska.

takes care of the people of the village or town much like a local general doctor, but a strong emphasis is also placed on the individual taking responsibility for his or her health and well-being.

In shamanic cultures, a medicine man or woman will alter their conscious state with rhythmic drumming, rattling, or chanting to "journey" into an internal reality made of three levels—the upper world, the middle world, and the lower world—where they meet with animal, human, and spirit guides to assist in healing a patient. They may also engage in a deeper, more intense "soul retrieval" for those who are very sick. They seek the wisdom and gifts of nature and other entities and come back to waking consciousness with a plan for treatment, usually involving herbal concoctions and remedies.

Other indigenous cultures may perform rituals or ceremonies to a deity or deities to ask for help to heal a village member or impart wisdom to share with the patient. This is another way of accessing a higher force or power to glean knowledge and ask for assistance and is usually performed by the tribal elders or the older and wiser members of the community.

Nutritional Therapy

Food is medicine, and we will explore this in detail in the next chapter. The use of food and nutrition to heal is common sense and as old as time. We are what we eat, and luckily, if we make the right choices, nature has provided us with foods that can heal us and make us live longer.

Osteopathy

This type of medical treatment focuses on the manipulation and massage of bones, joints, and muscles. Osteopathic doctors are required to have the same level of medical school studies as a traditional M.D. and is one of the two types of physicians who are licensed to practice medicine and surgery in the Western Hemisphere. Osteopaths focus on the whole body and how the structure of the body, skeletal and muscular, is interdependent with the other parts of the body. Where chiropractors focus on the spine and adjustments of the neck and joints, osteopathy focuses on the muscle tissue and bones.

The techniques used were founded by Andrew Taylor Still, who believed that a tissue layer called myofascial continuity linked every part of the body to the other. It was the role of the osteopath to look for an osteopathic lesion, now called somatic dysfunction, so that it could be manipulated and corrected. Osteopathic manipulative treatment (OMT) is known for treating back pain and musculoskeletal issues.

Today, osteopathic medicine is still practiced, but many doctors combine it with more traditional treatments such as pharmaceuticals, surgeries, diet, exercise, and rehabilitation and therapy. A systematic review and meta-analysis of 15 randomized controlled trials did find in 2014 that OMT reduced pain and improved functional status in acute and chronic nonspecific lower back pain as well as moderate-quality evidence that it also reduced lower back pain in postpartum and pregnant women.

Ozone Therapy

Ozone is a colorless gas made up of three oxygen atoms. Administering ozone gas into the body is a therapy that has been used to treat illnesses and wounds. Despite a warning in 2019 from the FDA that ozone is toxic and has no known medical applications, other studies have shown that it can treat several medical conditions by stimulating the body's own immune system, such as a 2017 study for *Medical Gas Research* titled "Ozone Therapy: An Overview of Pharmacodynamics, Current Research, and Clinical Utility." Ozone can also be used for purposes of disinfection of wounds.

In a hospital setting, the gas used is made from medical-grade sources of oxygen. Medical ozone has been used for over 100 years, so a history exists of benefits to the therapy. When the ozone gas meets the body's fluids, more proteins and red blood cells are created, and this increases the levels of oxygen in the body. A 2017 study titled "Dental Applications of Ozone Therapy: A Review of Literature" for the *Saudi Journal of Dental Research* showed that it can render inactive bacteria, viruses, fungi, protozoa, and yeast growth. Ozone therapy has been examined and used to fight the recent COVID-19 virus to some success.

Ozone therapy helps those with breathing disorders because it increases oxygen levels in the blood and reduces stress load on the lungs. Intravenous ozone therapy, which involves injections of ozone and blood, can treat COPD. However, ozone should not be inhaled and can damage the lungs, and the EPA advises against using ozone air purifiers in the home for this reason.

Ozone therapy has showed some success in reducing the risk of diabetes complications as indicated in a 2018 study in the *Journal of Cellular Physiology* titled "Therapeutic Relevance of Ozone Therapy in Degenerative Diseases: Focus on Diabetes and Spinal Pain." Ozone gas can correct oxidative stress and trigger the immune system and the body's natural antioxidants to reduce the presence of inflammation. Ozone therapy also helps heal foot ulcer wounds and reduce infection rates, and because it does stimulate the immune system, it has shown success with those with immune disorders like HIV.

Intravenous ozone therapy, which involves injections of ozone and blood, can treat COPD. However, ozone should not be inhaled and can damage the lungs....

Although this therapy has been researched quite a bit, it is still necessary to be cautious when seeking out a practitioner, and it is important to check their background and history. Also, check with your general doctor and insurance company because it is not considered a widely used form of therapy, as it is risky, and the FDA has stated that it can irritate the lungs and cause fluid buildup, so be careful and practice due diligence when considering this route.

The Power of Touch

Whether you're getting a relaxing massage or a hug from a friend, something healing about caring touch affects the body and the brain. A good hug calms anxiety, boosts mood, balances the immune system, and lowers blood pressure by reducing the stress hormone cortisol and releasing oxytocin, the "feel-good" hormone that increases feelings of well-being and positivity. Oxytocin is responsible for the bonding feelings between lovers and between mothers and their infants while breastfeeding and hugging their babies closely.

During touch, changes occur to the brain pattern activity as well as increased levels of dopamine and serotonin, neurotransmitters that regulate mood and relieve stress and anxiety. The thalamus, the emotional hub of the brain, sends impulses of calm and happiness during touch and fosters a sense of being cared for and loved.

People need touch to alleviate loneliness and negative feelings. Touch, especially good hugs, provide connection and human interaction. A prolonged deep hug can do wonders for the worst mood or to lift sadness as a way of showing support and concern. Just as we are told to pet our dogs and cats to lower our blood pressure and heart rate, a hug can do the same, especially when it is "safe" and nonsexual and lasts more than a few seconds. Therapeutic touch and hugs work well to relieve pain and fibromyalgia and to decrease fear.

According to an article titled "Why You Should Get (and Give) More Hugs" by Erica Cirino for the April 11, 2018, issue of *Healthline*, we need many hugs or other forms of nurturing touch and nonsexual soothing each day to survive and thrive, and in the United States, people tend to be touch deprived. We need to learn to give and ask for hugs during the day from those nearest to us, as science proves that regular hugs from the people closest to us can have positive effects on the brain and body. This is especially important when we are upset, and a good hug allows us to release pent-up fear and anger. Even hand-holding and head-stroking count as therapeutic touch, and some children love to have their arms tickled or backs scratched as a soothing mechanism that many parents can attest works.

Reflexology

Reflexologists apply pressure with their hands to different points on the body, such as the hands, feet, and ears, that are linked to the nervous system or various organs. An example is applying pressure to the arch of the foot to assist in bladder function and requires the reflexologist have a solid understanding of which points on the body correspond to which organs. A typical session is like both massage and acupressure and can relieve stress; get rid of asthma; treat diabetes, anxiety, depression, and tension; improve mood; and assist in better sleep. Yes, you can do reflexology on yourself, but it works so much better when you are able to fully relax and allow someone else to apply the

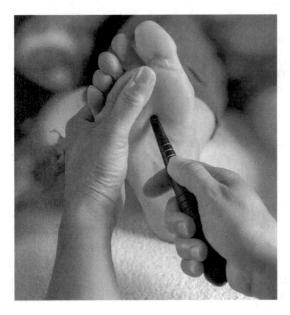

Reflexology is similar to accupressure in that the reflexologist applies pressure to specific points of the body. Reflexology differs from accupressure in that it focuses on the feet while accupressure covers the entire body.

pressure. You might also do it wrong and create more pain and bruising.

Several scientific studies support the use of reflexology for reducing stress and reducing the effect of chemotherapy, including a 2017 study published in the *Asia Pacific Journal of Oncology Nursing* called "The Effect of Reflexology on Chemotherapy-induced Nausea, Vomiting, and Fatigue in Breast Cancer Patients."

Reiki

This Japanese energy–healing technique involves the laying of hands over different areas of the body to manipulate and balance the "life force" and restore harmony and good energy to the body. This brings about healing of the body, mind, and spirit and can increase vitality, too. The philosophy behind Reiki is that the body's depletion of energy invites disease and illness, so the energy must be restored. Interestingly, Reiki can be done without the person's hands ever touching your body, as they are not manipulating the body itself but the life force, and can even be done long distance, such as via Zoom video or over the phone.

A 2015 analysis published in the *Journal of Evidence-Based Integrative Medicine* by David E. Manus, Ph.D., found that Reiki does provide relief from pain and anxiety in post–op and cancer patients. A September 2017 review of 13 studies for the same publication found that Reiki was more effective than placebos for pain, anxiety, depression, and well-being and had "broad potential" as a complementary health therapy.

Resonance

The body responds to resonance, vibration, and frequency. Whether as light, sound, or energy, this concept is at the heart of many ancient healing traditions. If we can align the body's own vibratory frequencies with those associated with healing, perhaps we can achieve health and well-being without drugs or harsh treatments, restoring the self to its own natural and harmonious balance.

Nicole La Voie, a French–Canadian mother, is considered one of the founders of resonance healing. She was employed as an X–ray technician, and when her son was born with glandular system failure, she wondered if her excessive exposure to radiation was to blame. She studied homeopathy, became a Reiki master, and created a sound therapy system based upon a specific system of vibrational frequencies, called sound wave energy, using it to help her own son. She likened the human body to a symphony, with each cell having its role in the overall orchestration. "When a musician (organ or system) produces a sour note, we bring them back into harmony by helping them to retune their instrument or refocus their attention." The sound wave energy system uses frequencies between 15 and 33 hertz to achieve balance and peace of mind.

If we can align the body's own vibratory frequencies with those associated with healing, perhaps we can achieve health and well-being without drugs or harsh treatments....

Dr. Peter Guy Manners, a 1950s British naturopath, used entrainment, where weaker pulsations fall under the influence of stronger ones, believing that specific resonant frequencies were associated with healthy tissues and organs. Finding the right frequencies became known as sympathetic resonance. This research was expanded upon by Robert Monroe in the 1960s at the Monroe Institute in Virginia. The end goal was to figure out how to apply specific frequencies to sync with the body's own, rid it of disease and toxins, and restore health.

Sound, even light, are not the only modalities for syncing vibrations and bodily resonance for ultimate well–being. Bioresonance uses electric, magnetic, or electromagnetic fields to cure disease and can reactivate the natural resonance of human cells by utilizing a machine with magnetic mats to pulse electromagnetic energy into the affected area.

This brings us to the work of royal Raymond Rife in the early twentieth century. He was born in 1888 and studied at Johns Hopkins. During his lifetime, he invented several medical devices, including the incredibly complex universal microscope in 1933, which had nearly 6,000 different parts and was capable of magnifying objects 60,000 times their normal size. Until recently, this was the only microscope that could view a virus, and Rife used it to study viruses and how they influenced the body. He also heavily influenced research in optics, electronics, radiochemistry, biochemistry, ballistics, and aviation.

His focus was on how to destroy killer viruses. He used resonance to intensify the virus's natural frequency so that it could be observed. He then increased the oscillation rate until the virus was destroyed from structural breakdown. He called this oscillation rate the mortal oscillatory rate (MOR). Surprisingly, he discovered that no damage was done to the surrounding tissue during the process.

Rife generators sold today use the frequencies that he discovered worked best on viruses, even cancer. Though he had many adherents who insisted that his machines cured them, his work was considered highly controversial, and the FDA cracked down on the sale of his devices. People today can find a Rife generator but should make sure it is not a cheap knockoff. Do your due diligence.

The entire body resonates at different frequencies. Light, sound, energy, magnetics, electricity, music, and harmonics are all ways of finding the restoration and synchronization of the natural and inherent vibrations of well-being once disease has been introduced. The system seeks harmony, and with the use of vibrational therapies and healing methods, it can find it and be healed.

Sound Therapy

Just as light can heal, so can sound. Sound therapy can include everything from chanting to music therapy to sound baths, where the body is surrounded by specific frequencies that have healing powers. Sound not only emits a reaction but creates a response. Sound waves that are designed to focus on specific ailments and issues are directed at the patient and permeate the body and mind, which is why so many spas and healing centers feature sound healing rooms and experiences and YouTube is filled with sound therapy frequency videos with millions of views each.

Whether Tibetan bowls or beautiful wind chimes, classical music or the natural sounds of a forest canopy, what we hear directly influences our health and well-being. Ask anyone who lives near a construction site or a busy airport, and they will tell you how an overwhelm of sound can hurt, not heal, when it is not aligned to the frequencies that bring pleasure and calm. Phone apps that provide white noise, rain sounds, storm sounds, and waves crashing on the beach are hugely popular as sleep and relaxation aids. Sound matters.

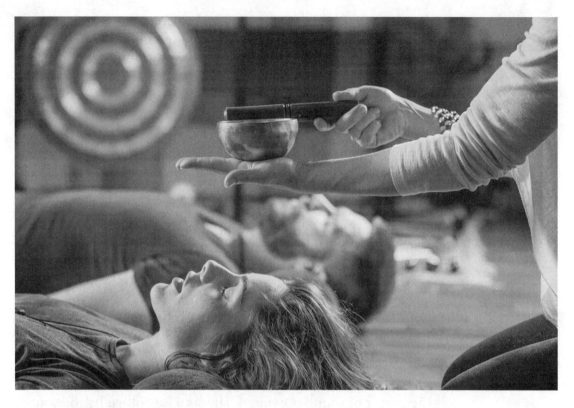

A Tibetan singing bowl is one tool that can be used in the practice of sound therapy, which uses the healing powers of sound frequencies.

Sound therapy is a sensory therapy, like massage, and affects the brain in a positive way to increase the capacity for relaxation, help memory recall, and assist the right brain and left brain to achieve a more harmonious balance. Binaural beats are a popular method, using two separate tones played in each ear that present as a single tone to synchronize brainwaves and bring about a euphoric or deeply relaxed state. Repetitive sound such as chanting, rattles, and drumming can put you in an altered state of consciousness and assist in other healing methods like hypnosis or visualization and meditation. Ambient background music and white noise are often used by people experiencing insomnia.

Even the sound of your breath moving through your body during yoga or meditation is a type of sound therapy. The point is to use sounds of any kind that resonate with the person to achieve an immersive state where the body, mind, and spirit are affected positively and the sound vibrations work on every level of the body, down to the cellular level, to soothe, massage, and restore. You can try sound therapies on your own; many websites provide samples or free downloads, and the American Music Therapy Association provides resources for finding sound therapy practitioners in your state should you wish to go that route.

You can try sound therapies on your own; many websites provide samples or free downloads, and the American Music Therapy Association provides resources for finding sound therapy practitioners in your state....

Scientific studies involving sound therapy for the relief of physical and psychological pain have been numerous, including one from the University of California that found that meditating accompanied by Tibetan bowls decreased anger and stress noticeably. Another study at Germany's University of Bonn looked at 30 separate studies that found evidence that binaural beats reduced anxiety, and an analysis of 400 studies by McGill University found that listening to music and playing it yourself improved overall mental and physical health.

The power of sound is evident. The soul is soothed by the sound of birds chirping in the treetops and stressed by the sound of traffic and honking horns all day. Sometimes, no sound at all is truly golden.

Traditional Chinese Medicine

Traditional Chinese medicine is an ancient practice that has evolved over the last several thousand years and is still practiced widely today all over the world. It involves the use of diet, herbs, mind/body work, movement such as tai chi, acupuncture, acupressure, and traditional Chinese medical remedies, many of which are passed down via writings and books or taught to subsequent generations. Just as with Western allopathic doctors, Chinese medical practitioners know how to diagnose and treat diseases and ailments via a long history of tried-and-true methods and modalities.

The overall goal is to achieve balance and harmony of the body's energy systems and to treat the patient holistically as a whole person desiring the full spectrum of well-being. Herbal remedies are a main fixture of Chinese medicine as a frontline treatment or today as a complementary treatment with allopathic medicine.

Yoga

Yoga is a philosophy, an art, and also a way to connect to one's body and be healthy physically and mentally. For a discussion on yoga, please see "The Power of Movement" chapter.

Choosing a Practitioner

When choosing a naturopathic or holistic doctor or therapy, the same rules apply as with choosing a general doctor. Do a lot of research, get reviews and recommendations, and check into their backgrounds and training. *Consumer Reports* magazine offers "4 Tips for the Smart and Safe Use of Alternative Medicine" suggesting you do your own research, be choosy, consider any costs to you or insurance issues, and look at the bigger picture when it comes to your overall treatment.

- Do your own research: Try to find out what's known about the safety and efficacy of any treatment you're considering as well as any supplements or herbal remedies you are given. Look for reputable sources, such as the National Center for Complementary and Integrative Health, and talk to your primary care provider, too. Learn about the treatment method being suggested on your own, and don't always leave it all up to someone else to be your best advocate.

- Be choosy about who you choose: Make sure he or she is credentialed, with a state license where appropriate. Check with your primary care doctor to ask for a referral. Be skeptical of someone who tries to sell you additional products (although this should not be a deal breaker, as many conventional doctors now sell skin care lines and diet products) or sign you up for a long-term treatment plan (beyond four to eight sessions) or recommends that you forgo all conventional treatments, including life-saving surgery. Check reviews on Yelp and other sites, too. These can be valuable for finding out problems before you go for a first visit.

- Consider the cost: Ask about the price up front for an office visit and ongoing treatment and check beforehand with your insurance company to see if it is covered. Also, talk to your provider about nonpharmaceutical options that are more likely to be covered by insurance, including cognitive behavioral and physical therapy.

- Don't shun convention completely: Both conventional and alternative medicine have a time and place. For more serious health problems, of course, check with your general doctor, too, espe-

cially if they might require surgery. Always check with a pharmacist for interactions with your current meds and herbs and dietary
supplements.

According to *The Alternative Health and Medicine Encyclopedia* by
James E. Marti, the American Holistic Medical Association (AHMA) has
a series of questions you should ask before deciding to choose a holistic physician (including a few of this author's, too):

- Do you feel comfortable and cared for when you visit the office?

- Is your appointment time honored, or do you have to wait?

- How do you feel when you are in the environment?

- Is the practitioner accessible?

- Is the practitioner sensitive enough to place his/herself in your
  position regarding your fears and anxieties about an illness or
  proposed treatment?

- Is the practitioner healthy, or is he/she overweight, smokes, drinks,
  shows signs of overwork or stressed out?

- Is the office clean and the staff friendly?

- Do they openly inform you of their background, training, and
  clinical experience?

- How long have they been in business?

- What successes have they had with your specific condition?

- Did the physician fully diagnose your condition?

- Did the physician order expensive tests?

- Did the practitioner prescribe pharmaceuticals with known side
  effects?

- Do you trust both the physician's tone and the therapy outlined
  for you?

- Were you given a reasonable amount of time to evaluate the
  course of treatment and recommendations before you began, or
  did you feel rushed into it?

Ideally, these are questions to ask any doctor or practitioner,
conventional or natural. It all comes down to being your own best
advocate and using discernment. If it doesn't feel right, don't do it. If
the person makes you uncomfortable or suggests things that don't
resonate, find someone else. Never be fooled by a white coat making
bad suggestions, no matter who they are or what the plaques on their
wall say.

The Power of Social Media

One of the best ways to find someone who is a great fit is to check with friends on social media. You can also find review sites, and often, the practitioners have a Facebook page or Twitter account where you can interact and ask questions. Some holistic doctors host YouTube channels filled with free content. Don't be afraid; this author has found some amazing and helpful holistic and natural doctors, chiropractors, dieticians, herbalists, scientists, and researchers offering free and empowering content, often with scientific sources included. Others shun social media, but you can always find reviews on Facebook, Yelp, and other sites, and ask around for local recommendations on a neighborhood app called Nextdoor, a great place to find out who is in your immediate area.

If you find a doctor or practitioner you love or a treatment method that works well, spread the word so others can benefit.

Don't just share bad news or leave bad reviews. If you find a doctor or practitioner you love or a treatment method that works well, spread the word so others can benefit. The same goes for reading books or watching videos. Leave a review, even if just a few lines, for the next person who is on the quest for an alternative to the conventional, traditional medical arena.

You can even check your local Chamber of Commerce and Better Business Bureau on Facebook and Twitter to see if anyone has lodged formal complaints against a business or practice. You would never pick a conventional doctor by closing your eyes and pointing to a random name on a list, so don't do the same when looking for a naturopathic doctor. This is your body and your health we are talking about, and no one will care as much about it as you.

What Is Well-Being?

The *Merriam-Webster* dictionary defines well-being as "the state of being happy, healthy, or prosperous." Perhaps it is a combination of all three. Happiness alone sounds perfect, but if you are not healthy, you will have struggles and suffering. Having your health but living in poverty and having no food to feed your children limits your ability to find true inner peace and outer security. Being rich but miserable, well, we have many examples of that with celebrities, corporate executives, athletes, and others who have amassed great wealth but are alcoholics, drug addicts, abusers, criminals, and mentally ill. Finding a coherence of all these factors, or at least an acceptance of them, goes a long way toward making the best out of even the worst of situations.

Total well-being can encompass many different levels, including emotional, physical, spiritual, social, career/purpose, and societal satisfaction with life. Let's start with these:

- Emotional: Focuses on coping with stress and stress-management skills, relaxation, boosting self-love and self-esteem, and learning to control emotions to feel better.

- Physical: Focuses on the function of the body via diet, exercise, stress management, sleep, building good habits, and being healthy.

- Spiritual: Focuses on finding a deeper connection to life and others, a sense of inner knowing, a connection to a higher source, and gleaning wisdom from that source.
- Social: Focuses on our connections to family and friends and groups of people, going to school and taking classes, traveling and visiting places, and having fun experiencing life with others in social settings.
- Career/Purpose: Focuses on what we do for work or a vocation and finding purpose and meaning in using our gifts, skills, and talents for our own benefit and the benefit of others.
- Societal: Focuses on being a productive and positive member of a community, contributing to society at large, and experiencing other cultures and environments to enrich and expand our awareness.

If one is out of whack, the whole tower of cards can come tumbling down if we are not careful. At the same time, well-being can begin in one or more of those areas and spread to the greater whole. The choice is up to us and rests strongly on our outlook, perspective, and attitudes about ourselves and our lives.

Well-being is a state of mind, a state of being that takes "all of the above" into consideration and finds ways to bring balance and, in the absence of balance, to find that still center within to operate from.

Don't be intimidated into thinking your life has to be perfect in all these areas to experience well-being. It helps, but it's probably a goal that few can reach. So many times throughout our lives, we may have a few imbalances, and those may shift as we experience different circumstances. We may be healthy and rich one year, then struggling and sick the next. Well-being is also the ability to adapt to our circumstances and find the gifts they offer.

Some poor people are able to experience a deep state of well-being, and some people fighting cancer can find incredible peace. Well-being is a state of mind, a state of being that takes "all of the above" into consideration and finds ways to bring balance and, in the absence of balance, to find that still center within to operate from.

When we experience more well-being as individuals, it adds to our overall public health. We put into the system healthier behaviors, longer lives, more happiness and energy, stronger productivity, and deeper social connections, which empower the collective. A sick society is made up of sick individuals, and when they become healthier and stronger, society does, too. Then, we have stronger families and better policies, and we put more care into how we are building the future for our children. We take better care of the planet when we take better care of ourselves. It's positive spillover that contributes benefits to local communities, states, the country, and the world.

Well-being, according to the Centers for Disease Control and Prevention, is defined as:

- Physical well-being
- Economical well-being
- Social well-being
- Development and activity
- Emotional well-being
- Psychological well-being
- Life satisfaction
- Domain-specific satisfaction
- Engaging activities and work

The above constitute the elements of a life well lived, but if that appears to be a tall order, again, it is possible to improve some levels and, therefore, the whole will be all the better for it. This applies to individuals and to society at large, and you can see from this list that when even one of these is ignored, suppressed, or diminished, the population suffers. Though the CDC's list is more about public health policy, it is a good indicator of the areas we can focus on in our quest for greater life satisfaction, happiness, and well-being. Considering things like genetics and personality, income and work, age and gender, and quality of relationships, we can see that one group of people may deal with some specific challenges more than others.

You can increase your own level of well-being and that of those around you

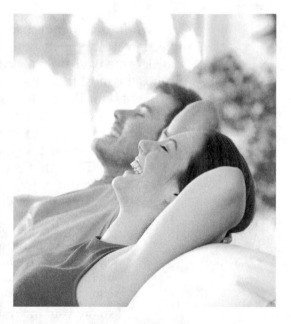

To achieve a full sense of well-being, all aspects of your life—physical, social, career, emotional, psychological, and so on—need to be in balance.

and your community. It does take work, a skill set, and a little time to override patterns of behaviors and actions that have led to your lack of well-being. Learning, consistency, and patience are definitely possible, and this book is filled with ideas and methods you can try for increasing your own happiness, health, and sense of purpose. It takes effort to adopt new habits and skills, so don't be hard on yourself if a year has gone by and you still feel you aren't living at an optimal level. It no doubt took years to bring you to where you are now, so don't be afraid to make the time commitment required in order to level up.

As they say, the time will pass anyway.

Tools for Finding Your Purpose

A 2010 study published in *Applied Psychology* found that individuals with high levels of eudemonic well-being, which involves a sense of purpose along with a sense of control and meaning, tend to live longer and have a greater sense of overall well-being. A 2016 study published in the *Journal of Research and Personality* found that individuals who feel a sense of purpose make more money than individuals who feel as though their work lacks meaning.

Finding your purpose and passion in life requires a lot of self-reflection and some work to uncover the real you beneath the you that you became over time based on the ideas and perceptions of others, but it is the most fulfilling work you can ever do. Finding your purpose isn't just about doing things that make you happy or having fun or even about giving and being charitable to make a difference in the world. Purpose is like your sigil, or the mark you seek to make and leave upon the world. It's your song, your motto, your logo, your story, and the great "why" that drives your desires, actions, and behaviors.

Here are some tips to help you find your purpose and cultivate it:

- Meet new people and engage in new activities: While you may believe your purpose is linked to childhood delights, and it well may be, often when we engage in something new that expands our horizons, we find the elusive nature of our purpose. New people may spark new interests.
- Explore your interests: Don't just read about things or look them up on the internet. Get out there and explore new and old interests in a more hands-on manner. Get your feet wet and your hands dirty and dig into life.

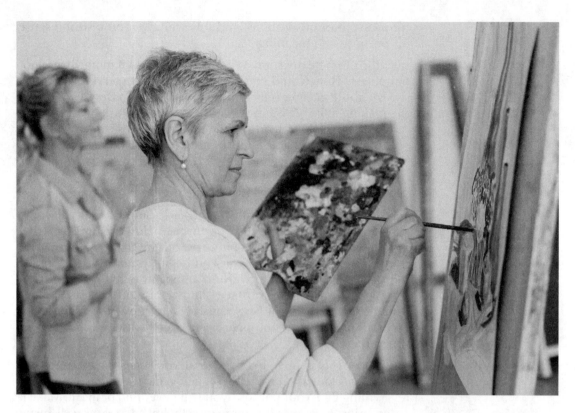

One excellent way to achieve well-being is to explore and pursue personal interests that have nothing to do with a career or doing necessary, day-to-day tasks.

- Ask people what you are good at: The people closest to you can often see skills, gifts, and talents that you are oblivious to or take for granted. Ask people you trust what they think you excel at and what you do that makes them and others feel good. Look for the gold in the perceptions of others while not adopting or attaching to what they think you are. The goal here is not to let others define you but to see how you shine through the eyes of others.

- Look at what bothers you: Yes, the things you rail against, complain about, and bring out the social justice warrior within are often keys to pet causes and passions that you may want to explore further. If animal abuse enrages you, can you find purpose in working to stop abuse or work with abused animals? If you are all about finding a cure for cancer, how can you put that passion into actions you can take to help the cause? If you are always complaining about the litter in your local park, can you make it your purpose to clean up your environment in small and large ways? What injustices make you angry? Find ways to become a proactive part of solutions, and this will give you a strong sense of purpose and meaning.

- Ask the ultimate question: What would you do if money were not an object? How would you spend your time if you didn't have to worry about paying bills and making a living? How would you be making a life? This is a powerful question to ask because it removes a huge obstacle to seeking greater purpose: having to earn your keep. Money and finances are one of the biggest blocks to aligning our lives to a greater purpose. You can always do things without money to move toward a sense of meaning in your life, but you have to ask, and answer, the question first.

- Make a list or journal about what obstacles and excuses you come up with that keep you from your purpose: How are these external and internal roadblocks keeping you off the path you know you were meant to walk? How can you begin to remove these roadblocks to clear the way forward? It all begins with first identifying and acknowledging the obstacles and getting out of a state of denial or blame. It is your responsibility to move the roadblocks, even though it may not have been your responsibility that put them there.

- Prioritize: This is huge because what you focus on expands and what you prioritize takes the most energy and focus. If you prioritize everything BUT your purpose, you will never find or live it. Make it a top priority because it is more directly linked to your well-being than many of the things you will put on top of it on the list.

- Find your North Star, your inner compass, your personal GPS: Without internal direction and guidance, you will fall prey to the demands and desires of the external world, of others, and of situations and circumstances. Once you have your inner guidance system up and running via intuition and understanding your feelings and emotions, nothing will derail you from your purpose or your journey to fulfill it.

It's Okay to Not Be Okay

One thing that well-being is not is denying our feelings, even the bad ones. It is not a fake, forced attitude of positivity and happiness or pretending we are perfect and never have challenges and difficulties. It is not denying our suffering and pain or refusing to admit we need help when things aren't going well.

It is the acceptance of our humanity and all our feelings as we navigate the human experience. It is being responsible for what we feel and not being afraid to ask for help if we need it. It is also taking downtime and crying if that's what the situation calls for. If we are depressed or anxious, well-being asks that we acknowledge those feelings and seek ways to feel better but allow ourselves to be as we are.

One of the worst things to experience is when you are suffering or feeling bad and you reach out to someone for help, and they respond with "Oh, it'll pass" or, even worse, "Just think about all those who are worse off than you." We tend to negate and diminish our own feelings, and we do it to others often without thinking. It's a form of invalidation that leaves the other person feeling unheard, unseen, and alone.

 One of the worst things to experience is when you are suffering or feeling bad and you reach out to someone for help, and they respond with "Oh, it'll pass" or, even worse, "Just think about all those who are worse off than you."

The push to stay positive, no matter what, is just as damaging to the psyche as it is to always dwell on the negative or wallow in our pain, regret, and grief and never take any steps to work through those uncomfortable feelings. When we push ourselves to stop feeling bad or tell someone who is having a hard time to stop feeling bad, we are denying our, and their, experiences; this is a form of gaslighting: making someone think their reality is false and shaming and guilting them for it.

We need to learn to let ourselves have bad times, to grieve and mourn and cry and scream when we need to, and we need to extend this gift of permission to others, letting them know that we will be there for them if they need us. When someone dies, we don't say, "Get over it already." When someone loses their job, we don't tell them, "Oh, it could be worse … " because to them, right now, nothing could be worse.

Toxic positivity is a real thing. It's a false belief that we must always be positive and smiling, like the Stepford Wives. It is a negation of true emotional pain and the need to process it through to heal. We become trapped in the "put on a happy face" zone to the point where we become numb and robotic, and the sad truth is, those awful feelings will just come back later if they aren't dealt with properly the first time.

Well-being allows us to feel what we feel—the good, the bad, and the ugly—without fear of being shamed, made fun of, or guilted into

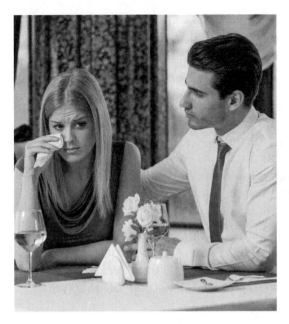

Everyone experiences struggles and sadness in their lives at some point. Even people who seem wealthy and successful on the outside are often struggling with grief, tragedy, and emotional upheaval. Money isn't the way to achieve well-being.

getting over it quickly by those who might feel uncomfortable by our emotions. That is usually a request that is more about how they feel than about how the grieving, sad person feels and is incredibly selfish.

Suppressing bad emotions makes them take root and show up later in behavioral patterns that derail us from our goals and dreams. Just as we don't want to suppress our joy and happiness, we need to feel through the sadness and fear so it doesn't become a black hole within that swallows up everything that comes near from the gravitational pull of its event horizon.

The happiest people on Earth are not free from suffering or pain; they just know how to accept it and process it so that it doesn't become who they are. They get that this, too, shall pass, but they also get that while they are in it, they need to "feel and deal" and not resist it because what you resist persists. They surrender to what is, and once they've felt their way through it, they let it go. Okay, enough of the clichés. If you feel crappy, feel crappy. Don't wallow in the crap. Seek small ways to lift yourself up when you are ready and know that it is all a part of being human.

Part of a well-rounded person includes the ability to feel compassion and empathy for others. When we cut ourselves off from our ability to relate to others and acknowledge every aspect of who they are and what they are experiencing, we are cutting off the flow of connectivity and love that brings about greater well-being. What we do to others we do to ourselves, and that works in reverse, too.

Feel the pain and the fear and the sadness. Have a bad day or a bad week. It's okay. But don't stay there forever. Life is about moving forward on the path you have chosen to walk and will include roadblocks and detours, but it will also include amazing views and incredible new vistas, learning more about who you are and what you are capable of, and meeting up with some awesome fellow travelers along the way.

Diet and Nutrition:
You Are What You Eat

It's impossible to lead a healthy lifestyle with an unhealthy diet. Food is the foundation of our energy, our immunity, our survival, our well-being, and our mental and emotional state, yet for all the technology and access to knowledge we have today, rates of obesity, cancer, heart disease, diabetes, autoimmune disease, and chronic illnesses are rising. Childhood obesity and cancers are on the rise. People, despite more information and access to good-quality foods, are still choosing processed junk foods, high in sugars and white flour, and we, as a nation, are more inflamed than ever.

Half of the adults in the United States alone over the age of 60 suffer from metabolic syndrome, which increases the risk for heart disease, diabetes, cancer, and strokes. This syndrome, which affects many younger people, comes from an unhealthy lifestyle and too many sugar-laden carbs, suppressing the body's ability to use its own fat stores for energy and lose excess weight. If you have a large waist circumference, low levels of HDL cholesterol, high fasting blood sugar, and high blood pressure, chances are good that you fall into this category.

The Important Role of Disease

Disease is a wake-up call and a sign that something is amiss in your body. The role of disease is to allow you to reconsider your actions and behaviors to improve your health and heal the disease. When we are not eating whole, healthy foods; not drinking enough water; or we lack certain minerals or vitamins from a poor diet, our bodies will eventually let us know. It may take awhile, and therein lies the danger. Some diseases like cancer and heart disease may lurk for years waiting to make themselves known, and when we get that diagnosis, we are shocked. Yet, every choice we have made, aside from hereditary and other factors, could have contributed to the disease we are now faced with. The role of a diagnosis is to finally shine a light on what was happening in the dark as we continued with unhealthy habits.

Even a cold or flu is a sign that we are not tending to our immune system as much as we should. Perhaps we are not sleeping well, we are buried in piles of high-stress work, or we are slowly gaining weight and not exercising as much. Then, we get the big boom of illness, and we wonder where it came from. We felt so normal. Meanwhile, so much was going on just below the surface that we were unaware of.

For some people, disease is enough to shake them out of their complacency and change their diet, and their habits, for the better. For others, by the time disease strikes, it may be too late.

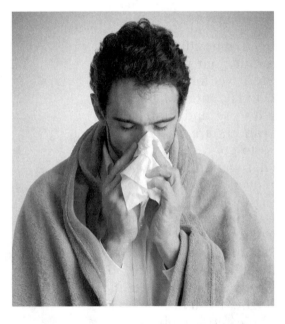

A common cold or flu can be a sign that we are not taking care of ourselves. Stress, not getting enough sleep, and not eating right can weaken our immune systems.

Inflammation Nation

Behind most diseases and illnesses is inflammation. It is pervasive, invasive, and destructive if left to wreak its havoc on the body without any intervention. Inflammation is at the root of most chronic health conditions from allergies to arthritis to immune disorders, heart disease, and cancer. With the modern diet in America and other countries consisting of so many fake and processed foods and the proliferation of drugs and medications prescribed by doctors, plus the amount of stress we deal with daily, it's no wonder that we have become weaker, sicker, and more tired by the day. All these things, and more, contribute to the widespread pandemic of inflammation-related diseases.

Inflammation is not a bad thing. When you suffer a bodily injury, it is the natural response to protect the body from further harm and assist in healing. It is the process by which the body's white blood cells go to work to protect you from infection, bacteria, and viruses. When this protection occurs when no threat is present or continues to occur on a chronic basis, inflammation becomes a problem and, if left unchecked, potentially deadly. Without any invaders for the body's immune system to fight off, it attacks the body's tissues as if they are the problem.

Inflammation is not a bad thing.... It is the process by which the body's white blood cells go to work to protect you from infection, bacteria, and viruses.

Short-lived inflammation is called acute, and longer-lasting inflammation is called chronic. Acute inflammation subsides in a few days, maybe even hours. Chronic inflammation is the baddie because it can continue to do its damage long after the initial trigger or injury, sometimes for months and years. Chronic inflammation is linked to heart disease, cancers, diabetes, asthma, allergies, rheumatoid arthritis, psoriasis and skin conditions, gout, joint and muscle pain, and a host of other ailments. Symptoms can include redness and swelling (a direct result of the body's immune system sending more blood to the affected areas), joint stiffness or warmth to the touch, flulike symptoms, muscle aches and stiffness, clogged sinuses, autoimmune disorders, heart issues, shortness of breath, kidney failure, high blood pressure, and more.

Chances are good that if you are suffering from something that just won't go away, it has to do with inflammation. It affects the body in a host of ways:

- Brain: depression, memory loss, autoimmune disorders, Alzheimer's disease

- Heart: strokes, high blood pressure, anemia, diabetes/high blood sugar, heart attacks

- Liver: fatty liver disease, toxin overload, enlarged liver
- Kidneys: restricted blood flow, edema, hypertension, nephritis, kidney failure
- Lungs: allergies, asthma, COPD, autoimmune reactions to the airway linings
- Thyroid: thyroid disruption and decreased function, reduction in thyroid receptor count
- Skin: rashes, acne, psoriasis, eczema, dermatitis, increased wrinkles and aging
- GI tract: GERD, celiac disease, irritable bowel disease, Crohn's disease
- Muscles: increased pain and soreness, muscle weakness, carpal tunnel syndrome, polymyalgia rheumatica
- Bones: loss of bone density, increased inability to repair bone mass, increased breaks and fractures, osteoporosis

Treating or lessening the impact of inflammation without resorting to chemical, toxic drugs and medications with a list of side effects can be done in many ways. This includes physical therapies to keep muscles and joints in top working order; changing the diet to include more anti-inflammatory foods; using herbs and plant parts known to lessen inflammation; exercise; stress reduction; quitting smoking and excess alcohol intake; keeping weight at a healthy level; supplementation; and looking for ways to remove toxins in the home and office.

Supplements such as omega-3 fatty acids, found in krill or fish oil, curcumin, green tea extract, and white willow bark, work on reducing inflammation. In the section on herbs, we will look at anti-inflammatory "rock stars" that can make a huge difference in healing chronic disease.

Foods to avoid are excessive caffeine; processed foods; anything with trans fats; refined carbohydrates, including breads, pastries, cookies, and chips; fake foods such as margarine (use real butter) and artificial sweeteners; dairy; processed meats such as hot dogs and lunch meat; anything that has chemicals you can't pronounce; food colorings and additives; and preservatives such as BHT and nitrates. In the diet section, we talk more about how to eat healthy, but foods that especially target inflammation include extra virgin olive oil, leafy greens, cruciferous veggies, tomatoes, fruits and berries, and fatty fish such as salmon and sardines. Nuts such as almonds and walnuts, unsalted and raw, are also anti-inflammatory powerhouses, but eat sparingly because they can pack on the pounds.

Severe situations may require medication or surgery, but cleaning up your lifestyle can work wonders at reducing the effects of inflammation and experiencing better health all around.

The Sugar Factor

Our ancestors lived off the land. The land was not made of sugar. Today's diet is so full of obvious and hidden sugars, it is killing us. Americans consume around 156 pounds of sugar per year, about the equivalent of 15 10–pound bags filled with sugar. Excess sugars found in processed and natural foods can cause havoc on the body. This includes:

- Weight gain from insulin resistance and metabolic syndrome
- Liver problems
- Anxiety and depression

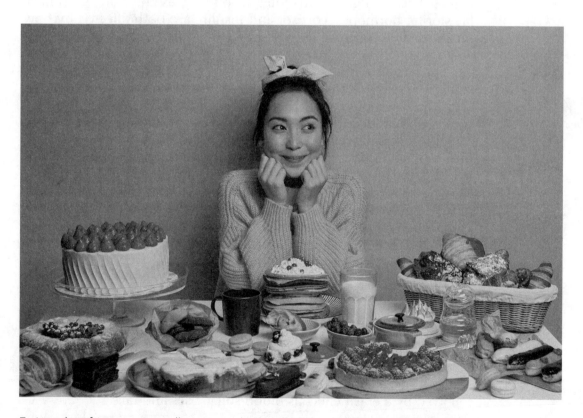

Eating a lot of sugar—especially processed sugar—is not a natural or healthy thing for our bodies. Sugar is readily available these days and is put in almost everything Americans eat and drink.

- Excessive thirst and hunger
- Recurrent headaches
- Sleeplessness and increased insomnia
- Chronic inflammation
- Increased risk of cancer and Type 2 diabetes
- Heart disease
- Cavities and gum disease

Sugar is considered an antinutrient, filled with empty calories. Dozens, if not hundreds, of scientific studies show that a diet high in sugar raises your risk of insulin resistance, diabetes, cancer, and heart disease, but it also does a negative number on your immune system. Sugar decreases your levels of vitamin C and has a similar structure, so it competes with the vitamin C for space in white blood cells, suppressing your immune system's ability to fight off colds and other illnesses. Excess sugar contributes to obesity, as the body's primary fat-storing hormones, cortisol and insulin, are both affected by how much sugar you consume.

Sugars also impact the health of the brain. Even sugars found in fruits, if in excess, can have a negative impact on your health. At the very least, we should avoid the obvious sugars found in cookies, cakes, sweets, and hidden in many processed foods. Sugar addiction is a real thing; in fact, addiction to sugar works on the brain the same way any other addiction does. A team of Harvard Medical School researchers, led by Drs. Laura Holsen, David Ludwig, and their colleagues, published a study in the *Journal of Nutrition* that looked at 72 randomly picked, overweight volunteer subjects over a 20-week period with various percentages of carbohydrates, proteins, and fats in their diets. They found that the highest-carbohydrate group, which ate 60 percent of their calories as bad carbs (note, there are also good carbs, which can be found in fruits and vegetables), had a 43 percent higher level of blood flow in the brain's nucleus accumbens area than the groups with lower levels of carbohydrates did. This part of the brain is associated with reward behaviors, including cravings and addictions. Although further studies are needed, people who are addicted to sugary products know how hard it is to kick them because of the reward response they get after they consume them, even though this is always followed by a crash effect as blood sugar rises and falls.

In the past, we were told that fat was the true enemy of health, not sugar. It might surprise you to know that this was based upon propaganda and paid studies by the sugar industry itself to scientists and re-searchers who downplayed the links between sugar and heart disease back in the 1960s. For five decades, the sugar industry derailed healthy dieting by shaping the world of nutrition with false studies and mislead-ing research, according to internal sugar industry documents published in the American Medical Association's *JAMA Internal Medicine*. This kind of food industry influence peddling, courtesy of a trade group called the Sugar Research Foundation, minimized sugar's detrimental links to heart disease and hand-picked studies to be sent to prestigious journals.

 In the past, we were told that fat was the true enemy of health, not sugar. It might surprise you to know that this was based upon propaganda and paid studies by the sugar industry....

Today, we continue to pay the price of our sugar-laden past with a host of diseases that are all directly related to the inflammatory ef-fects of sugar and highly processed carbohydrates. Fat, which was pre-viously the enemy, now turns out to be far healthier for our body's optimal processes and systems than we thought. Food is fuel, and we've been fooled into thinking that the good fuel is bad and the bad fuel is good for far too long.

Eating a whole- or raw-food diet is the best, but not everyone has the time, inclination, or money to do so. Just making some simple dietary tweaks and understanding the power of food to harm and heal goes a long way toward making better choices and improving health and well-being.

Energy and health bars are supposed to be good for us but con-tain as much sugar as some candy bars, not to mention other shady ingredients like additives and food colors. Eating an energy or power bar as a snack or meal replacement may give you a boost of energy, but it's a sugar high that will end up crashing you later and making you feel worse for it. The American Heart Association states that women should get no more than 25 grams of sugar each day. Consider that a Gatorade whey protein power bar has 29 grams; that alone is a woman's entire day's ration of sugar. Some power bars on the market claim to have low sugar, but check the label for artificial sweeteners that may be just as bad for the bod.

Sugar is in everything, so reading labels is critical to make sure you are not overloading your system with a product that contributes to the worst diseases out there: obesity, cancer, heart disease, and strokes. Often, the word "sugar" never appears, so look for high-fructose corn syrup, sucralose, dextrose, maltodextrin, and fructose, as all are sugars. Even artificial sweeteners can cause problems, as they are often chemical types of sugar with unnatural ingredients and compounds that have been linked to obesity, kidney disease, diabetes, and metabolic syndrome. Just because they don't have calories doesn't mean they are good for you. If you must sweeten something, look at natural alternatives such as monk fruit, molasses, raw honey, cinnamon, and small amounts of stevia. Watch out for things like maple syrup, made from the sap from maple trees, which does contain some nutrients but is high in sugar. Agave nectar is often touted as a sugar alternative, but for someone eating low carb, it is very high in fructose, and, unlike fruit, it doesn't have any healthy fiber.

The stevia plant has been used by Native cultures to sweeten foods and drinks for hundreds of years, and it is safe and inexpensive. Stevia is about 300 times sweeter than table sugar, so use it sparingly. Some people claim it has an aftertaste, too. It is often sold under different brand names, so make sure it is actually derived from the stevia plant.

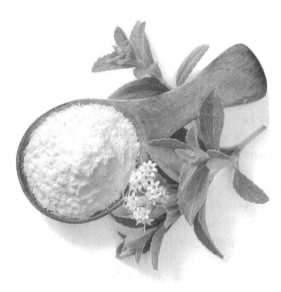

A sweetener can be extracted by the stevia herb that is healthier than regular sugar, although some people complain it has a bitter aftertaste.

Honey in its raw state has over 180 health-promoting substances. It is rich in phytonutrients and has powerful anti-oxidative and anti-inflammatory properties. Make sure it is raw and unfiltered and not the pasteurized generic honey found on most grocery store shelves. Commercially produced honey is heated to destroy bacteria and improve the consistency and flow, but it also kills the living enzymes and good bacteria that honey is known for. The bacteria are a prebiotic with helpful microorganisms that benefit digestion. Raw honey also contains antioxidants called phenolic compounds that prevent cancer and lower the risk of heart disease.

Most of the honey you buy in the grocery store is made in China and sold to the United States. Chinese producers add a step to honey production called ultrafiltration that removes beneficial pollen from the honey. This makes the honey have a longer shelf life and removes any way to identify the country of origin. It can also be mixed at the production site with high-fructose corn syrup and other sweeteners and tainted with pesticides, lead, and antibiotics. Buy local and organic.

Molasses is another wonderful alternative. Blackstrap molasses contains more than one-fourth of our needed daily supply of iron, potassium, magnesium, manganese, and B vitamins. Molasses has much less sugar due to the crystalline-sugar extraction process, and the high antioxidant levels have anticancer properties. Molasses can also help with weight loss. One 2011 study reported in *Science Daily* showed that adding molasses to a high-fat diet reduced body weight and body fat percentages because of decreased calorie absorption. The study concluded that "supplementing food with molasses extract might be a way to address the escalating rates of overweight and obesity."

Molasses is another wonderful alternative. Blackstrap molasses contains more than one-fourth of our needed daily supply of iron, potassium, magnesium, manganese, and B vitamins.

A complete sugar detox will do wonders for your health, but this can be quite intimidating since it is found hidden in so many foods. A good start would be to eliminate high-sugar snacks, products high in processed carbohydrates and check labels carefully to avoid added sugars. The cravings, in time, will go away, and you will find yourself not missing all the sugar. Some people even report that after cutting way back when they do eat something sweet, it repels them. Because sugar acts on the brain's dopamine levels, making you feel great while you are eating it (but not so great later), it is one of the hardest addictions to break, acting on the brain's reward and pleasure centers much like cocaine or tobacco, so start out slow and stick with it. The rewards are worth it.

Fruit sugars, please note, are a different type of sugar called fructose, and when fructose is eaten in the whole fruit and the fiber in it, this supports our blood sugar and reduces the potential for a spike in blood sugar.

Magical Manuka Honey

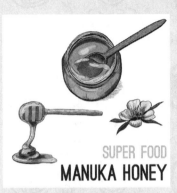

SUPER FOOD
MANUKA HONEY

Manuka honey comes from the manuka tree that is native to Australia and New Zealand. Many people consider the strongly flavored, rich honey to be a superfood.

Bees foraging for nectar in the manuka trees of New Zealand produce one of the highest-quality varieties of honey available. It is considered a monofloral honey because the nectar is derived from a single plant species. Manuka honey trees are original to the Taranaki region of New Zealand and have small, white flowers that bloom during the summer months there. These trees are found in the pristine wilderness, where hives are strategically placed for the bees to produce the fine honey.

Manuka honey has many unique properties and is considered a superfood mainly for its antimicrobial dietary chemical called methylglyoxal (MG). The high amount of MG found in manuka honey makes it a potent medicinal. It has been shown in studies to fight gingivitis and other tooth diseases, heal eye infections, and help heal open wounds and infections on the skin. Manuka honey's MG also fights off viruses and bacteria and can alleviate illnesses, including the flu. These same antiviral properties work to stop sinus blockage and allergies as well as inflammation and irritated airways. Manuka honey has become a popular remedy for allergies and colds for its ability to stop sniffles, reduce sore throat pain, and reduce swollen nasal passages.

Stomach ulcers are also treated with manuka honey. The honey protects the gastric tissues from developing ulcers and heals lesions that have already occurred. Those suffering from cystic fibrosis can also benefit from this amazing wonder honey. A 2019 Swansea University study found that manuka honey used to treat grown bacterial infections on lung tissue was even more effective at killing the resistant antimicrobial bacteria than an antibiotic. The honey could also improve the ability of antibiotics to function better. The combination of honey and antibiotics killed off 90 percent of the bacteria.

One interesting aspect of consuming manuka honey is better sleep. When we sleep, our brains require energy during the night, and a crucial source is glycogen from our livers. Without enough to run on, the brain will cause the body to wake from sleep during the night. Consuming a small amount of honey before bedtime keeps the brain well fed with its favorite energy source so you can sleep better and wake up less often.

Research is ongoing regarding the benefits of manuka honey for fighting cancer, treating diabetic wounds, and reducing the symptoms of inflammatory bowel disease and irritable bowel syndrome. Buying manuka honey as an alternative sweetener to sugar is a huge boost to all-around health markers. It is important to look for pure manuka honey from New Zealand that is raw and minimally processed. It should always be sold in glass jars and carry the New Zealand FernMark license, which certifies the product as native to New Zealand. You might also check the labels or the company website to see if the product originates from the Taranaki region.

Cocoa or Cacao? What's the Difference?

Who doesn't like chocolate? Yet, few chocolate lovers know the difference between cocoa and cacao and what makes one healthier than the other. They are not, as you might have thought, the same thing. They do, however, start from the same place, but it's the processing and destination that creates the big difference between the two and their nutritional benefits.

Both start with the Theobroma cacao tree, which is native to South America. This tree produces seed pods that are cracked open during harvesting and the seeds removed. These seeds are called cacao beans and resemble coffee beans. They can be eaten raw, which provides the most nutrients, but are awfully bitter. They will be fermented and dried before processing occurs.

Raw cacao beans are powerful antioxidants. They also lower blood pressure, improve insulin levels, improve mood, protect the heart, and increase the brain's cognitive abilities. They are chock full of flavonoids and rich in zinc, copper, magnesium, iron, calcium, potassium, and manganese. You can eat them as nibs or cacao butter or use them in cooking and baking. Cacao butter has a white, fatty texture somewhat like lard.

Cocoa comes from harvested seed pods that are heated at high temperatures during processing, which gives them a sweeter flavor and offers different health benefits. Cocoa powder that is dark is called Dutch-processed cocoa and is additionally processed with an alkalized chemical solution to make it richer in taste and less acidic. Natural cocoa powder is more acidic and bitter and is usually what is called for in baking recipes. If buying cocoa, it is best to buy it as a plain powder and look for a high-quality product without added sugars. Cocoa butter and chocolate chips are another way to consume natural cocoa.

The problem with high-heat processing is that it degrades the nutrient content and changes the cacao bean structure molecularly, which means fewer health benefits. Cocoa isn't bad for you; it just doesn't do much good beyond taste. If you truly want the benefits of chocolate, go for the dark chocolate—a higher percentage of cacao (70 percent or higher)—and always look for organically sourced products. Avoid milk chocolate for its high sugar content, dairy, and artificial sweeteners.

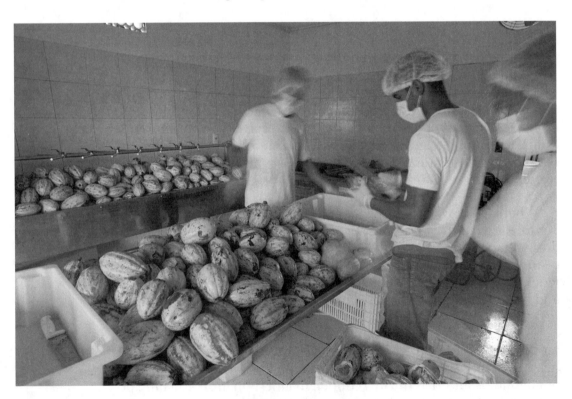

Workers remove seeds from cocoa fruits in this Brazilian processing plant. The seeds are then heated, dried, and turned into cocoa powder. This process removes many of the beneficial nutrients in the seeds, however.

Do know that even many dark chocolate products contain dairy, so if you want to avoid dairy or cannot tolerate it, look for those that contain none. They tend to be a bit pricier and may only be found at health stores but are worth it. Many people say getting used to dark chocolate with a high cacao content is like trying to adapt to drinking black coffee after usually pouring tons of flavored creamer in. It may not be as sweet, but people to learn to like it, especially knowing it is doing something good for their health even as it satisfied that sweet tooth.

The best advice when it comes to diet is to buy most of your food from the outer aisles of the store, where the produce and deli areas are. The processed, boxed, packaged foods tend to be in the inside aisles. Avoid the bakery, too. This may sound simple, but junk foods have been designed with fillers and flavorful additives to get us hooked, especially sugary treats, creating cravings and addictions that lead to greater levels of chronic disease, obesity, cancer, heart disease, strokes, and just about every other ailment. Junk in, junk out.

Perhaps it is our rushed, busy lifestyles that make it all but impossible to slow down and prepare real meals with real foods. We take the easy way out and call for delivery or go through a drive-through, and before we know it, we are in the obese range of body fat, our joints ache, we can no longer sleep well or breathe well, and we find that we are succumbing to more colds, flus, stomach bugs, and down days from poor health.

Building a Healthy Immune System

We eat food to give us energy to function. We also eat food to keep us strong and healthy when faced with illnesses and disease. Our immune system works in conjunction with the nutrients we allow into our body as well as the toxins we consume. One heals us, the other harms us.

Food as Antibiotics

Antibiotic overuse is rampant, leading to more superbugs that defy these drugs. They also harm the immune system and destroy good gut bacteria, especially in children. Here are some powerful natural antibiotics that boost the body's ability to fight off infections and illnesses. Give them a try next time you or your loved ones come down with a nasty bug:

- Garlic
- Apple cider vinegar (always dilute with water or use in a dressing with olive oil to lessen the acidic damage to your teeth)
- Ginger
- Onion
- Raw honey
- Turmeric
- Oregano oil
- Echinacea
- Horseradish root
- Habanero peppers

You can also find more natural antibiotics in the herb list in this book.

Immune Protectors

Several foods strengthen and protect our immune system from external threats such as toxins, viruses, bacteria, mold, and pollution and from internal threats such as chemicals, processed foods, infections, inflammation, parasites, and overall stress to the system. First, we should look at the things we do that harm our immune system:

- Excess consumption of sugars and processed carbohydrates
- Consuming processed meats with preservatives and additives
- Avoiding sunlight
- Chronic lack of sleep and poor sleep quality
- Too many drugs and pharmaceuticals
- Chronic dehydration
- Sedentary lifestyle
- Not enough key nutrients and vitamins

Most people can check off a few, if not all, of the above. When it comes to food, it's all about eating what nature made and avoiding chemical additives and processing. Foods that are considered nutrient dense, low in sugar, in whole or raw form, free from pesticides, and organic are best, including phytonutrient-rich herbs; fruits; leafy, green vegetables; healthy fats; lean protein sources; and fermented foods for gut health. Some of the best choices are garlic, ginger, onions, olive oil and olives, berries, avocadoes, lemons and limes (or the juices), vitamin C-rich fruits, non-starchy veggies (red, green, yellow, purple), mushrooms, green tea, coconut oil and milk (water, too), basil, oregano, thyme, turmeric, wild-caught salmon, grass-fed lean meats, and bone broth.

It is obvious that a good foundation for overall well-being starts with what we eat and drink. Many of the best food choices are, to no surprise, a part of age-old remedies our ancestors used for healing and medicinal purposes. That's because they work for the body and not against it. Choosing foods that heal can keep us from succumbing to the host of autoimmune and immune system disorders now plaguing our world, thanks to quick, fast foods and dinner in a bag or box. These disorders include over 100 different types of diseases of the brain, blood, GI tract, nervous system, thyroid, bones, muscles, skin, lungs, and pancreas plus lupus, eczema, diabetes, Crohn's disease, celiac disease, anemia, multiple sclerosis, epilepsy, Graves' disease, Hashimoto's disorder, fibromyalgia, rheumatoid arthritis, scleroderma … the list goes on and on.

The body's immune system turns on its own cells and tissues with these disorders and destroys healthy cells and tissues, thinking they are foreign substances or dangers. Our bodies then form antibodies to self-antigens, and those antibodies attack our self-antigens, causing inflammation and eventually damage to the tissue or organs. If we had a healthy immune system, our antibodies would remove invading antigens and protect our tissues and organs, keeping us robust and resilient.

Color Yourself Healthy

When it comes to food, nature is a rainbow of fruits and veggies of every color. Each color family offers different benefits, but the most well-rounded meal or salad might include several colorful choices on the plate. Walk through the produce section of your grocery store and marvel at the colors of plant-based foods. Making colorful foods (not any that are synthetically colored or contain toxic food colorings, please) a daily part of your diet goes a long way toward achieving optimal health.

Red

Red fruits and veggies are high in lycopene, which controls blood pressure and reduces cancer and heart attack risks, and high in anthocyanins, which are potent antioxidants that reduce the risk of cancer, diabetes, and Alzheimer's. They include tomato and tomato-

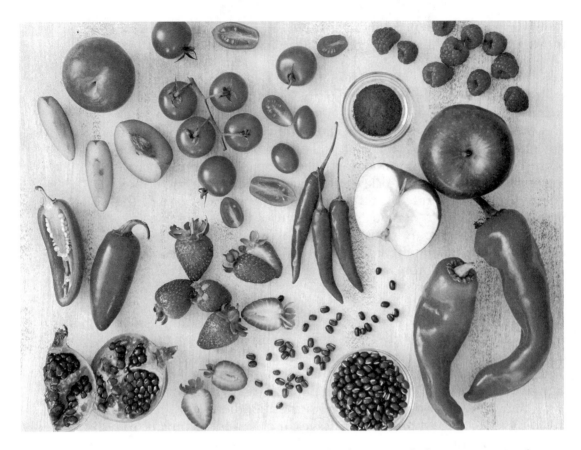

Fruits and veggies with a red color are rich in lycopene, which is a great antioxidant, helping to stave off cancer as well as diabetes and high blood pressure.

based products, red bell peppers, strawberries, raspberries, cherries, apples, papayas, red cabbages, pink grapefruits, watermelons, beets, blood oranges, red grapes, chili peppers, and cranberries.

Yellow

Yellow fruits and veggies contain cryptoxanthin and flavonoids for immune system support. They include yellow bell peppers, lemons, pineapples, nectarines, peaches, apricots, pears, sweet corn, yellow squash, and butternut squash.

Orange

Orange fruits and veggies contain carotenes for eye and skin health, immune system support, healthy bones, and a reduction of cancer and heart disease risks. They include oranges, cantaloupes, tangerines, carrots, ripe peaches, pumpkins, mangoes, persimmons, rutabagas, squash, orange bell peppers, and papayas.

Blue/Purple

Blue and purple fruits and veggies contain anthocyanins and polyphenols, which are powerful antioxidants that slow aging and reduce cancer and heart disease risks. They include blueberries, blackberries, purple grapes, eggplants, prunes, currants, plums, raisins, purple figs, elderberries, and deep-red apples.

Green

Green fruits and veggies contain indoles, lutein, zeaxanthin, and glucosinolates, which maintain good vision and reduce risks of cataracts and some cancers like breast and prostate cancer. They include broccoli, kale, bok choy, lettuce, brussels sprouts, cabbages, spinach, avocadoes, leafy greens, peas, honeydew, celery, okra, green bell peppers, watercress, zucchinis, parsley, and cilantro.

White

White fruits and veggies contain allyl sulfides, which lower blood pressure and high cholesterol and protect against cancers and heart disease. They include pears, onions, leeks, scallions, endive, chives, garlic, celery, white peaches, white nectarines, turnips, potatoes, shallots, and cucumbers.

Water for Life

Aside from the foods you choose to eat, the water you drink to stay hydrated is critical to keeping your immune system working at an optimal level. Water may look clear but be filled with toxins and chemicals that wreak havoc on your immune, endocrine, and nerve systems. Tap water in many American cities contains arsenic, pesticides, nitrates, hormones, lead, aluminum, fluorine compounds, radioactive contaminants, and chromium.

You can buy bottled water but be warned that many brands are just glorified tap water in pretty or convenient bottles. The best choice might be to invest in a great water filtration system, whether a coun-

Foods with Anticancer Chemicals

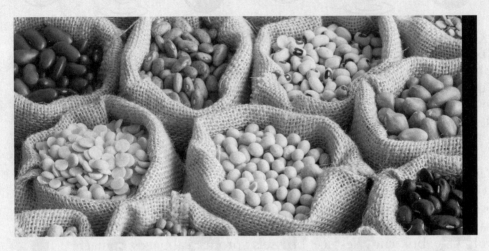

Legumes such as kidney beans, chickpeas, black-eyed peas, black beans, peanuts (not a true nut) and other beans, as well as peas, are high in isoflavones, which destroy cancer gene enzymes.

Nature has provided us with a bounty of foods that protect against cancer, thanks to special chemicals they contain that we may not be aware of when we consume them.

Carotene: Found in carrots, sweet potatoes, squash, yams, pumpkin, cantaloupe, broccoli, and kale. Carotenes neutralize free radicals and single-oxygen radicals and boost the immune system. They can reverse precancerous conditions, and a higher intake of these foods is associated with a lower risk of cancer.

- Capsicum: Found in cayenne pepper and also known as capsaicin, this is a potent antioxidant.
- Isoflavones: Found in legumes, beans, peas, and peanuts. These inhibit estrogen and estrogen receptor function and destroy cancer gene enzymes.
- Ellagic acid: Found in grapes and raspberries, they can remove and block carcinogens.
- Lycopene: Found in tomatoes, a potent antioxidant.
- Polyacetylene: Found in parsley, this chemical inhibits prostaglandins and destroys benzopyrene, a potent carcinogen.

- Terpenes: Found in citrus fruits, these increase the enzymes that break down carcinogens and decrease cholesterol.
- Monoterpenes: Found in carrots, tomatoes, squash, and cruciferous veggies, these are potent antioxidants that remove carcinogens from the liver.
- Lignans: Found in walnuts, fatty fish such as salmon, and flaxseed, these inhibit estrogen activity and prostaglandins and hormones that spread cancer.
- Triterpenoids: Found in licorice, these inhibit estrogens and prostaglandins and slow the rapid division of cancer cells.
- Isothiocyanates: Found in mustard and radishes, these stimulate the elimination of carcinogens from the liver.
- Quinones: Found in rosemary, these inhibit carcinogen and cocarcinogen growth.

Looking at the above list, you can easily combine a number of these foods into a big stew, soup, or salad for a healthy, cancer-fighting lunch or dinner. Most of these items are probably already in your refrigerator or cupboard and are inexpensive alternatives to drugs and pharmaceuticals for empowering your own immune system and body to prevent and fight cancer. Just don't spoil their potent power by adding cheap table salt, sugar and sugary sauces, processed meats or cheeses, and other condiments and flavor enhancers that are filled with pesticides, toxins, and synthetics, or you negate the effects of these cancer fighters.

tertop filter or a large attachment to your pipes or faucet. If you do buy bottled, look for the best spring water you can find, with no added minerals, and be aware of how using plastic bottles is polluting our oceans and landfills. Natural health isn't just about you, as your choices affect the entire ecosystem.

Adding some squeezed lemon or lime juice to water aids in digestion and acts as a gentle detoxifier by tricking the stomach into producing bile that keeps the food moving through the digestive tract. The pectin in lemons also helps your body use more fat and improves your mood and energy levels. Lemons and limes are high in vitamin C, which gives your immune system a boost, and the antioxidants help fight off free radicals and keep skin looking great while boosting the production of collagen to smooth out fine lines.

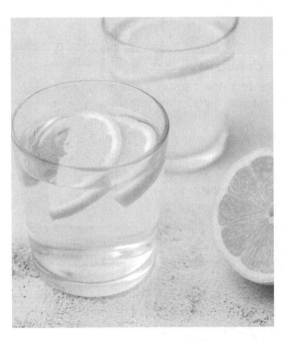

Adding lemon or lime juice to your water can help with digestion as well as act as a detoxifier.

The worst drinks for good health are cow's milk, which is full of antibiotics and bovine growth hormones and cause trouble for those who are lactose intolerant, and sodas and energy drinks, which are loaded with sugar and caffeine. Coconut water and milk, along with almond milks, are good healthy substitutes. Oat milk, hemp milk, cashew milk, and macadamia milk are good choices if, and only if, they do not contain sugars and added flavors.

But nothing does a body good like a big, clear glass of water for avoiding signs of dehydration such as headaches, fatigue, dizziness, bad breath, dark urine, constipation, and low energy, all of which occur when your water intake is too low. The human body is made up of about 60 percent water, and when that level drops as little as 1.5 percent, you are considered mildly dehydrated. If you work out and sweat a lot, it's even more critical to consume water, about 8–12 cups a day for women and 11–15 a day for men. Dehydration is often mistaken for hunger. A recent University of Washington diet study showed that just one glass of water could stop hunger pangs for almost 100 percent of the participants.

The best way to rehydrate is with water close to room temperature. Ice water may be refreshing, but it doesn't make its way out of your stomach until it is adequately warm. Water is a wonder for keeping joints lubricated and removing waste and toxins from the liver and kidneys to be removed from the body and also lessens the urge to drink caffeine or alcohol, improves the brain's memory recall, helps red blood cells carry more oxygen to the muscles and brain, and helps the heart pump more efficiently and with less effort.

If you are trying to lose weight, water can help. A 2013 *Journal of Clinical and Diagnostic Research* study looked at the thermogenic effects of water on body weight, suggesting that drinking water on an empty stomach not only acts as this thermogenic agent but reduces appetite and overeating. Many people who think they are hungry find that a full glass of water does the trick and that their bodies needed hydration, not extra calories. A 2015 randomized, controlled study published in the journal *Obesity* found that people on a diet who drank water before they ate ended up consuming up to 40 percent fewer calories per meal and lost more weight than those who didn't start out with a premeal glass of water. Adding ingredients like lemon, lime, honey, slices of orange or cucumber, or ginger increases the beneficial effect of water by adding in antioxidants.

Did you know that the temperature of the water you shower with can affect your health? Hot and cold water each have their own benefits:

Hot Water

- Opens the pores and cleans skin
- Helps the body remove toxins through the skin as sweat
- Unclogs stuffed nasal passages
- Reduces muscle aches and pain
- Reduces anxiety and promotes calm before bedtime

Cold Water

- Tightens skin
- Gives hair shine
- Increases alertness and wakes you up in the morning
- Decreases inflammation and swelling
- Stimulates the immune system
- Boosts metabolism
- Stimulates antidepression hormones

Not All Oils Are Created Equal

When it comes to oils, vegetable or processed seed oils are the worst for your health. These industrially processed oils are toxic and contain omega–6 polyunsaturated fatty acids (PUFAs) that cause a radical increase in oxidative free radicals and mitochondrial dysfunction. Among these bad oils are soybean, cottonseed, sunflower, rapeseed/canola, safflower, and corn oil. Omega–6 heavy oils contain the inflammatory linoleic acid. Yes, it's true that the healthier oils have linoleic acid, too, but not in the high levels of the seed oils.

Many chronic illnesses have too much omega–6 and seed oils at their foundation, including age–related macular degeneration, according to Dr. Chris Knobbe, president of the Cure AMD Foundation. These toxic fats create a cascade of negative effects on the lipids in the body that can lead to damage in the mitochondrial membrane and cause dysfunction to the mitochondria. This can then lead to insulin resistance, fatty liver disease, metabolic syndrome, and Type 2 diabetes because your body is unable to burn fats for fuel the right way.

Omega-6 in excess is linked to obesity, heart disease, and nonalcoholic fatty liver disease and creates an imbalance with the good omega-3, which often is not consumed enough.

Too much omega–6 in your diet can also increase inflammation, thanks to the presence of arachidonic acid, which increases the production of these compounds. Omega–6 in excess is linked to obesity, heart disease, and nonalcoholic fatty liver disease and creates an imbalance with the good omega–3, which often is not consumed enough. The ideal ratio is near 1:1, but instead of increasing omega–3, you should focus on less omega–6.

Your best bet is a good olive oil or coconut oil. Look for organic brands that contain no other ingredients. Some olive oil brands are not 100 percent olive oil but a mix of oils, so check labels and do some online research to find the purest brands.

Food Allergies and Sensitivities

With all the chemicals in our food and the processing it goes through, it's no wonder that food sensitivities and allergies are skyrocketing and are behind many autoimmune conditions. Add to this vaccine ingredients and pharmaceuticals in our water and soil, and it is easy to understand why our children today suffer from more food allergies than older generations ever did.

Food allergies often develop in infancy and affect children more than adults. A food allergy reaction usually appears within two hours or less of exposure to the food and can be life–threatening if not immediately treated. Problems usually manifest in skin rashes, breathing issues, and digestive troubles. The most common food allergies are peanuts, milk, shellfish, and eggs.

Food sensitivities are not deadly and can happen at any age and affect a larger segment of the population. A delayed response to a sensitivity can occur, up to 72 hours later, which usually manifests in skin rashes, joint pain, digestive issues, bloating, eczema, headaches, irritability, and weight gain. The most common sensitivities are to sugar, gluten, milk products, corn products, and eggs.

It may be hard to pinpoint which food is the culprit and can require removing one food per week, then introducing it back into the diet to see if any reaction occurs. Children are often directed to have food allergy blood tests if their parents are concerned for their well-being at school, where they may not be able to control what they eat.

Gluten sensitivity or intolerance is rampant in society, but gluten allergies are not as common. Celiac disease is gluten intolerance and is a type of autoimmune disorder, meaning your immune system responds poorly to gluten products such as bread. A gluten allergy will have more severe symptoms, but both require a diet free of most, if not all, gluten. Some of the symptoms include bloating, gas, abdominal pain, fatigue, nausea, cramping, and possibly anemia, which is often caused by celiac disease.

If you have these symptoms, try doing without gluten products, but watch labels carefully. If the symptoms are severe, work with your doctor to pinpoint problem foods and how to eliminate them completely from your diet.

Fear of Fat

Thanks to a well-financed sugar industry of the past, fat has gotten a bad rap when it comes to a healthy diet. The sugar industry deflected blame for obesity and disease increases onto fats. Undoubtedly, trans fats are not good for you, but healthy fats are, and we are not getting enough of them in the average American diet. We are afraid of fat.

Our bodies need some healthy fats to get the essential fatty acids needed for

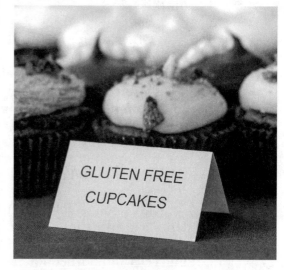

Grocery stores and bakeries in the United States are increasingly offering gluten-free choices in baked goods for those who have a sensitivity to it.

healthy nervous systems, eyes, hair, skin, brains, and cell membranes. Without enough fat, we can gain weight because fat satiates us sooner and stops us from overeating. Increasing our fat intake can not only kick our weight loss into gear because we eat less but also improve our appearance and give our skin, hair, and nails a more healthy, youthful appearance.

Healthy fats include avocadoes, coconuts and coconut oil, olives and olive oil, real butter, whole cream, and cheeses. We don't need to gorge on fats, but they should be a part of our diet. Instead of covering vegetables with margarine, which is a fake and manufactured food, a pat of butter is a better choice. Instead of pancakes full of wheat and flour, covered in sugary syrup, a two–egg omelet filled with veggies is a better choice. Instead of pouring chemical–laden, flavored creamer into our coffee, a touch of stevia with a spoonful of heavy whipping cream or half–and–half is a better choice.

Our bodies need fat. Our brain needs fat. Our skin and hair need fat. We assume our bodies run on carbs and glucose, but that's only because most of us feed ourselves only those sources of fuel and energy. Our bodies can run just as efficiently on fats and, when our glucose levels are depleted, even start burning our own stored fat, which leads to weight loss. You can also get plenty of fat eating grass–fed meats without cutting out the fat or taking off the skin.

Other sources of healthy fats are nuts and seeds, but these can be high in calories, so only a handful a day goes a long, long way to– ward good health. When balanced with plenty of nonstarchy veggies (for those concerned with having too many carbs in their diet) and some lean protein sources, healthy fats are a mandatory part of giving our bodies what they need to run at an optimal level.

MCT Oil: The Fantastic Fat

MCT stands for medium–chain triglycerides, a form of saturated fatty acid sometimes called medium–chain fatty acids. Triglycerides get a bad rap from our fears of cholesterol, but they are transported into cells and burned for energy or stored as body fat if we don't burn them off. MCT is made up of caproic acid, caprylic acid, capric acid, and lauric acid. MCTs go to the liver, and the body absorbs them more effectively than long–chain fatty acids.

MCT is considered one of the healthiest fats. They stimulate digestion, feed the brain with healthy energy, and have a direct benefit to positive gut bacteria. MCT oil, derived from coconut oil, is a big part of a ketogenic lifestyle, which encourages the body to burn its own fat for fuel by reducing carbohydrate intake enough to stimulate it. This metabolic process produces ketones when the body goes from burning glucose to burning fat.

MCT oil helps the body get into ketosis quicker and provides a healthy source of fuel when you cut down carb intake. The best MCT oil is pure, organic, cold pressed, and coconut based and can be used in salad dressings, coffee, smoothies, shakes, sauces, teas, and for baking. It helps with weight loss by pushing the body into fat-burning mode and keeping you feeling satiated more consistently so you won't continuously snack the way you do when your diet is heavy in carbs (blood sugar rises and dips, causing cravings).

Our bodies need fat. Our brain needs fat. Our skin and hair need fat. We assume our bodies run on carbs and glucose, but that's only because most of us feed ourselves only those sources of fuel and energy.

Other than coconuts, sources of MCT, albeit in smaller amounts, include grass-fed butter, whole-fat dairy like milk and yogurt, and palm oil. The richest source is coconut oil and is usually tasteless, even in coffee or tea. One of the greatest benefits of using MCT oil is the ongoing source of energy and brain clarity reported by those who use it daily because it provides the brain with the most optimal form of fuel: healthy fat.

Speaking of Coffee ...

Coffee is a mainstay for millions of Americans who swear they cannot live without it. A good cup (or more!) of coffee has multiple benefits, including lowering the risk of overall mortality. An abundance of scientific research has proven that coffee contains antioxidants and active substances known to reduce inflammation and protect against many diseases, including colorectal cancer, heart disease, and Alzheimer's. Dark-roasted coffee specifically reduces the breakage of DNA strands that occur naturally and can lead to cancerous tumors if not repaired on the cellular level. Coffee improves brain and cognitive functioning and gives you more antioxidants than most vitamins do to strengthen your immune system.

One cup of coffee contains riboflavin/vitamin B2 (11 percent RDI), pantothenic acid/vitamin B5 (6 percent RDI), potassium (3 percent RDI), manganese (3 percent RDI), magnesium (2 percent RDI), and niacin/vitamin B3 (2 percent RDI). Along with antioxidants, these vitamins and minerals protect your body from oxidative stress and fend off many age-related diseases. In the traditional Western diet, coffee is the number-one source of antioxidants for many consumers. You get even more benefits when you drink coffee along with eating a food high in antioxidants. The American Institute for Cancer Research includes coffee on its anticancer food list. The high antioxidant content protects the body at a cellular level, and numerous studies show that coffee drinkers have marked decreases in colorectal and liver cancers.

Doctors safely recommend drinking up to four cups a day unless you have high blood pressure or a sensitivity to caffeine, in which case that amount should be dropped back down to one or two cups a day. Caffeine does stimulate your nervous system, but the boost to blood pressure is a small one and the benefits of coffee may outweigh the concerns.

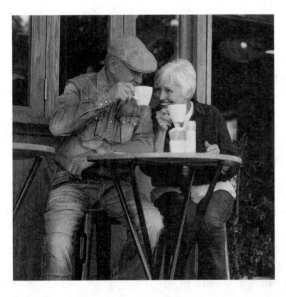

Some research has shown that modest amounts of coffee in your diet can reduce the rise of certain types of cancers and may even prolong your life.

Several larger studies, such as the June 17, 2008, article "The Relationship of Coffee Consumption with Mortality" published on the *PubMed* website, found that regular coffee consumption was associated with a "modest" reduced risk of all-cause mortality, as high as 20 percent for men and 26 percent for women. Multiple studies also show that coffee drinkers consistently have a 23–50 percent lower risk of developing diabetes. Drinking 3–6 cups (or more) a day seems to have the greatest effect. Another study determined a 7 percent drop in diabetes risk with just one cup of coffee per day.

Additional studies prove a strong connection between coffee consumption and a lower risk of neurodegenerative diseases such as Alzheimer's and dementia. Caffeine has protective properties against these and other diseases of the brain, including Parkinson's. Coffee boosts cognitive brain functioning and increases focus. It even improves mood. Coffee also reduces the risk of liver problems such as cirrhosis, nonalcoholic fatty liver disease, and liver fibrosis, and coffee drinkers are more likely to have healthy levels of liver enzymes. Decaf coffee has the same effect, so it's not the caffeine here but the coffee bean itself that offers such protection to the liver.

Those seeking to lose weight also benefit from daily coffee consumption. About 100 milligrams of caffeine, the equivalent of about two cups of coffee per day, boosts your metabolic rate by 8–11 percent and increases the body's fat-burning ability by 10–29 percent. Just don't pour in sugary creamers as this can offset the benefits of coffee to battle the bulge. If caffeine jitters bother you too much but you want a little bump in your energy level, you can even buy half-caffeinated coffee nowadays and get the pleasures of drinking coffee with half the caffeine intake.

The key is to only buy coffee that is organically grown, non-GMO, pesticide-free, and vacuum-packed in bags for better protection against contaminants.

However, take note: the kind of coffee you buy is critical because the mass-produced, highly processed coffee that is most found on the marketplace is contaminated with pesticides, molds, and mycotoxins, all of which can wreak havoc on your overall health. Mycotoxins are molds that occur naturally inside and outside of coffee beans and can cause symptoms from overall pain from inflammation to allergies, kidney disease, and chronic fatigue syndrome.

Mass-produced coffee is loaded with chemicals and additives, and many of them can also diminish the robust flavor. These chemicals can also trigger stomachaches and digestive issues. A lot of coffees sold at grocery stores are mixed with beans from plants from different countries, some of which may have been under- or overdried or covered in pesticides, which tends to be your lighter roasts.

The key is to only buy coffee that is organically grown, non-GMO, pesticide-free, and vacuum-packed in bags for better protection against contaminants. Look for single-country-origin coffee that comes from the same farm and has the same roasting profile. The best-tasting coffee is shade grown because the beans have a more mature and complex flavor, yet a very small percentage of coffee is grown in the shade. You may also want to look for coffee grown at higher elevations and in mountainous regions for exceptional taste and quality. Also, check that the coffee is labeled "fair trade," which means that it is grown and produced in a sustainable environment and that the growers, usually farmers, get a fair wage for producing the coffee. Your morning cup of joe may be more expensive following this advice, but it will be far healthier and help to rid your body of excessive toxins while also promoting fair-trade practices for a better environment. It's worth the extra cost.

Farm Fresh

Eating healthy is not rocket science. You can do wonders simply by avoiding the center aisles at your local grocery store and staying

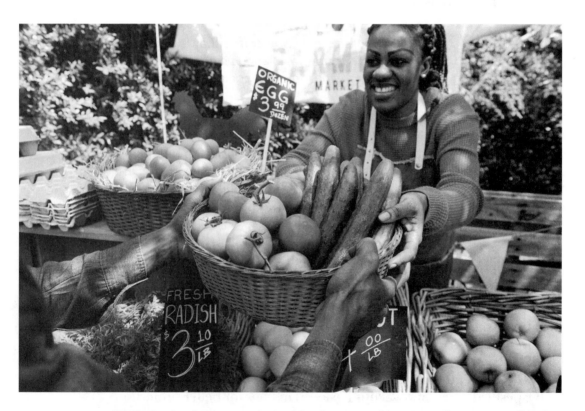

Purchasing locally grown and raised foods at, say, a farmers' market, is an excellent way of obtaining healthier foods while also boosting the local economy.

away from the bakery section, but you can also find local farms and ranches, or farmer's markets, to discover great sources of eggs, meat, dairy, fruits, and veggies, all grown in your area by people who are a part of your community. Locally grown foods are less likely to have added antibiotics and growth hormones, pesticides, and other chemicals, but always ask. If they claim they are "organic," make sure that means something. The great thing about local food sources is that you can ask questions and often tour the farms or facilities to see how they operate. If you like honey, find local apiaries that sell their products in health food stores or at farmer's markets. The same goes for jams, nut butters, teas, desserts and pastries, ethnic foods, herbs, and more. It's fun to find awesome local companies with cool brands you can put your money and support behind and give less to those big-box stores, factory farms (and their cruel treatment of animals), and big agriculture operations.

The farmer's market in your town or city can become your best friend when it comes to eating for well-being. Yes, the prices may be a tad higher, but it's worth it, isn't it? Grocery stores do offer some organic products, but rarely are they locally grown. Why not eat right and help your community at the same time? Building relationships with local growers often means you are the first to find out about a new product, a big sale, or even some freebies for loyal customers.

Fake Meat? No Way!

With all the talk of genetically modified organisms (GMOs) that are being added into our foods, seeds, and animals to increase growth and produce more, more, more, we have seen the rise of "Franken-foods" that barely resemble real food, except for their ability to be consumed. Spliced together, genetically altered, edited, changed, and manufactured, many of the things we eat barely qualify as edible. In the last five years, with increasing numbers of people going vegetarian and vegan, fake meats have become the new rage.

Beyond Meats and Impossible Foods are two of several companies flooding the market with plant-based burgers and meat products. These companies call their products healthy and better for the environment because they don't require giant factory farms overcrowded with animals that are fed gruel and shot up with growth hormones and antibiotics, which eventually make their way onto our dinner plates and into our bloodstreams.

Yet, one of the hallmarks of a healthy food is the number of ingredients it contains: the fewer, the better. Beyond Burgers contain 22 ingredients and are ultraprocessed foods that are filled with chemicals. These food formulations are made mostly, if not entirely, from substances extracted from food such as oils, fats, and sugars as well as modified starches, hydrogenated fats, flavor enhancers, colors, additives, and other chemicals, all to make this plant–based burger taste good. The process by which this happens is the ultraprocessing to make them look like a burger patty. Don't be fooled by their marketing campaigns and advertising. You'd be far better off eating grass-fed meats from local farms and ranches.

Impossible Foods include nothing found in nature and hold 14 different patents, with more to come. Do you patent healthy foods like fruits and veggies? No. These patents show just how unnatural these fake foods are and that they are created entirely in a lab setting where numerous extractions, compositions, and methods occur to make the product consumable. Nothing is healthy about any of these foods, so vegetarians and vegans thinking they are being offered a great alternative to meat should look elsewhere. Even the aroma is added into these fake meats during the processing.

These product manufacturers also may be fudging the truth a bit on their claims of helping the environment. They compare their operations to those of huge factory farms, also known as concentrated animal feeding operations (CAFOs), which are notorious gross polluters. They cannot compare with the much more pro–environment nature of nature itself on small– and medium–sized farms where animals roam free and feed on grass out in a pasture. This is false advertising as fake as the food itself.

Do yourself a favor and buy whole foods, preferably local. Don't be swayed or fooled by commercials and ads. Avoid the inside aisles of the store unless you're buying nonfood products, and always, always check the labels for additives and extra ingredients. You are what you eat. Don't eat fake foods.

Apple Cider Vinegar: The Science behind the Superfood

One natural product has been all the rage lately for those seeking to detox and lose weight. Apple cider vinegar does wonders for the body in several ways, with science backing up its claims. Made through a special fermentation process, this vinegar contains acetic acid, which is what gives it its potent taste and smell. The higher-quality vinegar will always contain "the Mother," the *Mycoderma aceti* made of acetic acid bacteria, enzymes, and strands of proteins that develop on fermenting alcoholic liquids. The Mother is the stuff that makes it look cloudy. Clear apple cider vinegar is not anywhere near as effective. Most organic brands such as Bragg always contain the Mother.

Apple cider vinegar helps lower blood sugar levels in those with insulin resistance and diabetes. In a 2007 research study for the journal *Diabetes*, Andrea W. White and Carol S. Johnston found that diabetic patients who ingested 2 tablespoons of apple cider vinegar with 1 ounce of cheese before bedtime had a reduction in their fasting glucose levels the next morning. Another study showed improvement in insulin sensitivity. When you lose your sensitivity to insulin, you put on weight, run the risk of developing diabetes, and have higher blood sugar levels. This study, published in the 2015 *Journal of Diabetes Research*, showed that people with Type 2 diabetes who drank 30 milliliters of the vinegar mixed in 20 milliliters of water within five minutes of a meal had a significant increase in glucose uptake.

Apple cider vinegar (ACV) reduces belly fat by reducing visceral adipose fat and lowers cardiovascular risks such as heart attacks and strokes. It also lowers LDL cholesterol and triglyceride levels when 30 milliliters were taken twice a day for eight weeks. The reductions were significant, too, proving the many benefits of including this powerhouse in your diet. By reducing fat-storing hormones, thanks to the acetic acid, your body will not hold on to as much excess fat, helping your weight-loss goals. At 3 calories per tablespoon, it won't add to your calorie count much.

Vinegar also fights off harmful bacteria and viruses that can lead to food poisoning, such as *E. coli*. ACV has a history of being a potent disinfectant and a natural preservative. Used topically on the skin, ACV improves conditions like eczema and dry skin by rebalancing the natural pH of the skin and strengthening the protective skin barrier and also prevents skin infections and dark spots. It can be diluted with skin toner or a face wash if it's too harsh on the skin.

The caveat is the taste. The best way to take ACV, to avoid too much acid coming into contact with tooth enamel that could be broken down or cause stomachaches, is to dilute 30 milliliters with

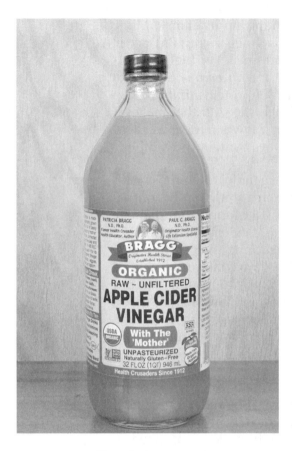

Bragg is a good brand of organic cider vinegar to buy. Cloudy-looking vinegar is better to buy than clear because the cloudiness indicates it contains healthy enzymes and bacteria.

water and take before a big meal once or twice a day. You can also use this amount as part of a salad dressing and add spices to dilute the potent acidic taste, or you can take quality supplements without fillers, although not many studies show that pill supplementation is as good as the real deal, so for more punch, take it in its natural form. Some people swear by diluting it with a glass of water and adding a few squirts of lemon juice for a great morning detox.

Apple cider vinegar gummies have become all the rage as a way of taking ACV without the acidic taste, but no studies confirm that these gummies have enough of the ACV to work. You are far better off taking it in liquid form, as the average gummy on the market contains about 500–600 milligrams and the beneficial amount you need is 1–2 tablespoons a day, which is about 15–30 milliliters respectively. If 1 milliliter is the equivalent of 1,000 milligrams, you can see how many gummies you'd need to pop each day to hit the recommended amount, which is not only difficult but cost prohibitive. Gummies may also contain sugars and other fillers your body can do without. Until gummies and supplements can catch up to the amount needed to be of benefit, stick to finding ways to use the liquid ACV to get the highest benefits.

Recipe for ACV Mini Detox Drink

Drink this upon waking up and right before dinnertime.

1 tbsp. ACV

12 oz. water, preferably room temperature

1 tbsp. lemon juice

3–5 drops liquid stevia

Cruciferous Cancer Crusaders

By the year 2030, cancer diagnoses are expected to rise to over 23 million per year. After heart disease, cancer is the leading cause of death despite billions upon billions of dollars being poured into research to find cures. Cancer is still so mysterious, and theories abound as to what it is, what causes it, and how to treat it. Conventional treatments like surgery, radiation, and chemotherapy have their downsides and often do more damage than good to the body's innate ability to fight the cancer by weakening the immune system.

We know that the foods we eat have great impact on our health, and it's common sense to eat fewer fake and processed foods and more raw, natural, organic foods to ward off what cancers we can (that are not hereditary or a product of environmental toxins). The herb section contains dozens of cancer-fighting plants, but one of the biggest crusaders against the Big C are cruciferous veggies in the Brassica family, which includes broccoli, kale, broccoli sprouts, cauliflower, radishes, turnips, watercress, cabbages, rutabagas, and many others. These crusaders contain antioxidants and anti-inflammatories, compounds that work so well to fight off cancer that they have been labeled anticancerous.

Cruciferous veggies contain sulforaphane, an anticancer compound that has been widely studied for preventing cancers of the stomach, bladder, colon, lung, skin, breast, and prostate.

Cruciferous veggies contain sulforaphane, an anticancer compound that has been widely studied for preventing cancers of the stomach, bladder, colon, lung, skin, breast, and prostate. This compound has the capacity to act as a signaling molecule that inside of the cell switches on more than 200 genes that are dormant because of the presence of toxins and poor health habits. Once these genes are switched back on, they produce enzymes that detoxify. One antioxidant that is turned on by the switch is glutathione, which adds to sulforaphane's ability to promote cancer death and reduce the expression of estrogen receptors that could lead to breast cancer.

Broccoli and broccoli sprouts contain sulforaphane, with the sprouts boasting 100 times more of the potent compound. Broccoli also contains a powerhouse flavanol called quercetin, which goes after cancer stem cells and is also found in abundance in onions. Quercetin is one of cancer's biggest enemies and can be taken in supplement form if you cannot stand broccoli or onions.

A 2014 French study found that people who consume cauliflower and other cruciferous veggies have a lower risk of developing cancer because of a special anticancer compound called PEITC. PEITC is known for killing mesothelioma cells. Cauliflower also contains glucosinolates, another potent anticancer compound. Cutting or chewing cauliflower releases compounds called isothiocyanates (ITCs), which are known to inhibit cancer growth. These compounds also protect against DNA damage.

A great snacking habit would be eating a bowl of mixed cruciferous veggies with a homemade ranch or blue cheese dip instead of the usual go-to potato chips or cookies. Dips made with whole cream and organic cheeses sprinkled with healthy herbs also add some good fats into the mix, or you can make guacamole with avocado and salsa (with onions) for a great snack that can push cancer back in its tracks.

Fasting for Health and Weight Loss

Ever notice how many hours of the day you spend eating? One of the oldest therapies for health and well-being, including weight loss, involves hours spent doing just the opposite: not eating. Fasting has been around for thousands of years as an important part of the prevention and healing of diseases. Hippocrates, the father of Western medicine, wrote that fasting allowed the body time to heal itself. Another great figure in the history of medicine, Paracelsus, wrote that fasting is the "greatest remedy, the physician within."

Fasting has been a part of religious traditions and Ayurvedic medicine. The Bible speaks of fasting many times. Muslims fast regularly during Ramadan. Fasting is part of Judaism, too, as one aspect of Yom Kippur. In ancient Greece, even the father of numbers and mathematics, Pythagoras, celebrated the virtues of going without food for specific amounts of time. Though fasting was often included as part of a spiritual belief or ritual, it has some heavy-duty modern science behind it as a way for the body to reset and renew the immune system and give new life to cells and organs.

Fasting as a therapeutic modality became more popular in the nineteenth century. One pioneer, Dr. Herbert Shelton, claimed to have helped over 40,000 people with water-fasting at his school of health in San Antonio, Texas, which he started in 1928. Dr. Otto Buchinger helped popularize fasting in Germany, and many German hospitals offer fasting weeks to patients. In the Western world, fasting is seeing a huge revival, introducing both long fasts and intermittent fasts into health and weight-loss programs. Hundreds, if not thousands, of books on the subject are available along with fasting apps for cell phones, podcasts, and video channels offering instructions on how to incorporate not eating into daily life.

Scientific studies abound showing that a 72-hour fast totally renews the body's immune system. At around the 18–20–hour mark of fasting, a process called autophagy takes place, which is the death and clearing out of dead cells to be replaced by new ones. Autophagy is like cleaning out the pipes of the body's system so everything flows better and is one of the benefits of going beyond just the usual overnight "fast" until morning breakfast. It also boosts your body's defenses against bacteria. Short-term fasting assists mitochondrial networks to work more efficiently. Mitochondria are the cells' powerhouses, so healthy mitochondria mean healthy cells.

For some people, doing a three–day water–only fast is terrifying to consider. Even doing 24 hours with only noncaloric liquids can be intimidating. The results of longer fasts, nothing beyond three days, are tremendously beneficial, but shorter fasting periods, known as intermittent fasting, also have plenty of benefits. Intermittent fasting is exactly as it sounds. You spend a specific amount of time refraining or restricting from eating, usually 12 hours or more, then eat your caloric intake in a window of time. This allows your body time to digest the food and lower blood sugar levels back down from the insulin spikes that come with eating, and hopefully, if you can go on long enough, begin to use your stored fat for fuel, aiding weight loss.

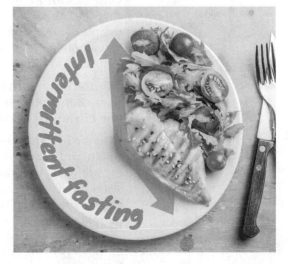

The logic behind intermittent fasting is that not eating for periods of about 12 hours allows your body the time to properly digest foods and keep blood sugar levels from spiking.

The different types of intermittent fasting are:

- Time-restricted Eating: This method allows you a specific number of hours you can eat within your "eating window," and the rest is for fasting. During your fasting state, you can consume water, noncaloric drinks, or black coffee. You "break the fast" usually the next day with breakfast or an early lunch. Some people love the 16:8 fasting period. This would be 16 hours of fasting and eight hours of eating from your first to last meal. Keep in mind that most of your fasting hours would be while you are asleep, and you would always, no matter the fasting protocol, stop eating three hours before bedtime. Other time breakdowns include 14:10, 18:6, 20:4, and 23:1, which is often called one meal a day (OMAD). This style works best if you fast for at least 16 hours, but you can ease your way in. Also, once you enter your eating window, you don't pig out on whatever you want. You eat healthily and keep calorie counts low enough to not undo the good the fast did.

• The 5:2 Fast Cycle: This allows you to eat normally for five days and then for two days, you drastically cut caloric intake to 500–800 calories, depending on if you are a woman or man. You get to eat every day, but on two of those days, your body is shocked into a much lower caloric intake.

• Alternate-day Fasting: This means you fast one day for the full 24 hours, then eat the next day, then fast, then eat. This is hard for beginners, and it might be easier and just as effective to stick to a 24-hour fast once or twice a week while eating normally or doing 16:8 on the off days.

• OMAD: This involves sticking to a fasting window of 23 hours, then eating all your necessary calories within one hour. Some people cannot stomach such a big feast and prefer their calories spread out a bit more, but doing OMAD every now and then after a junk-food binge won't hurt you.

• Warrior Fasting: This involves not eating for 20 hours and fitting your eating into a four-hour window. You can have two meals or one big meal, but don't eat outside that window.

• Extended Fasting: This involves longer fasts of at least 24 hours. Again, only water, black coffee, and noncaloric liquids like teas are allowed. Any fast over 72 hours is discouraged, and plenty of scientific data is available to show that longer fasts are not necessary. The human body can go without food for weeks, but most people wouldn't want to try it!

People who do this regularly become fat adapted and begin to burn off their own fat stores and store less food intake as excess fat. They become fat-burning machines and have reported better sleep, more energy, clearer skin, sharper brainpower, better sex lives, and weight loss of mainly fat after initial water loss.

Fasting is healing, and maybe once or twice a year, a good three-day fast will totally rejuvenate your immune system. When starting out, it is best to check with your doctor to see if fasting has any dangers, as it does with children and pregnant women who need full caloric intake on a steadier basis, but if you want to try intermittent fasting, tons of resources exist online and off. A good rule of thumb is to try one week doing 12 hours fasting, 12 hours eating, then the next week, increase the fasting window by an hour, and do that until you have reached the sweet spot of 18:6. However, if you can only go 16:8, you will still see many benefits if you stay consistent, don't eat tons of junk and excess calories during your eating window, and remember to drink a lot of water to stay hydrated and avoid fasting headaches and fatigue.

Fasting does allow you to eat all the foods you crave if you don't go overboard. If you want weight loss, though, you must also be sure that what you eat is as important as when you eat. No matter what fasting type you choose, you do get the added benefit of not having to buy as much food, and you spend much less time thinking about what you will be eating next.

A 2010 research study published in *Cell Cycle* showed that fasting produced much fewer side effects in cancer patients going through chemotherapy. Their nausea, fatigue, diarrhea, and vomiting lessened during fasting. Fasting also helps inhibit the growth of IGF–1, insulin–like growth factor 1, which is linked to the growth of cancerous tumors and Type 2 diabetes.

A 2018 animal study showed that fasting protected against metabolic changes associated with and caused by Alzheimer's disease, including insulin resistance, fat gain, and poor cognition levels. Other studies have shown that fasting improves health markers such as blood sugar levels, blood pressure, cholesterol levels, and inflammation. A 2014 review in *Translational Research* showed that intermittent fasting improved insulin resistance on a dramatic level and helped it function optimally, resulting in a lower risk of developing diabetes.

We put so much time and effort into what we eat to the point where we have become obsessed with food and the "next meal." It is ironic that so many health benefits come when we go for certain lengths of time not eating.

Vitamins, Minerals, and Supplements

Thanks to a decrease in the nutrient levels of our soil along with added toxins and chemicals that create disease and illness and processing of foodstuffs that removes most of their nutritional value, the vitamin and supplement industry has become a billion-dollar one filled with products that promise to make up for what has been taken away from nature. Though the first line of defense against disease and lack of well-being should be a better diet, that is not always possible, as more and more of our foods lack the nutrients that our bodies need. We are not all able to buy a piece of farmland and grow our own food, so we turn instead to the supplement market to make up for it. In an article for the April 2020 issue of *Health Magazine* called "The Scoop on Supplements" by Jennifer King Lindley, many people believe that everyone should be taking a supplement. According to JoAnn Manson, M.D., chief of preventative medicine at Brigham and Women's Hospital in Boston, "It's preferable to get vitamins and minerals from food. They are better absorbed, and you get the other health benefits like fiber and antioxidants." But unless you shop regularly from local farmers and meat providers or visit farmer's markets looking for the best organic produce available, this has become more difficult with more factory farming and big agribusiness.

A vitamin is an organic substance that is classified as either fat soluble or water soluble. Fat-soluble vitamins include vitamins A, D, E, and K and dissolve in fat. They can accumulate in the body in excess amounts. Water-soluble vitamins include C and B-complex, including B6, B12, and folic acid (B9), which must be dissolved in water before the body absorbs them for use. They are not accumulated in the body and exit via our urine. The word "vitamin" was coined in 1912 by biochemist Casimir Funk, considered the father of vitamin therapy, who wrote in a research publication about them. *Vita* means "life," and *amine* refers to a nitrogenous substance essential for life. All vitamins were discovered by 1948.

Minerals are inorganic substances that are found in soil and water. They are consumed by animals or absorbed into plants and then consumed by people. Among them are calcium, sodium, and potassium and trace minerals such as copper, iodine, manganese, and zinc. Minerals play a critical role, even those found in tiny amounts, in the processes and systems of our bodies, including immunity, thyroid function, antioxidant defense, oxygenation, regulating blood sugar, digestion, detoxing poisons, building strong bones, and regulating lipids.

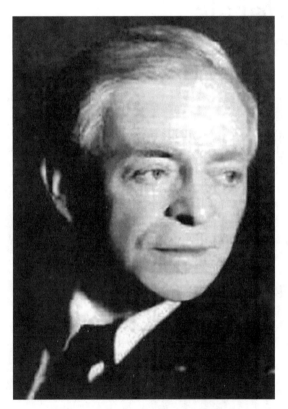

Born Kasimierz Funk in Warsaw, Polish biochemist Casimir Funk (1884–1967) figured out that vitamins are organic molecules that are essential for synthesizing nutrients.

Some groups of people, such as pregnant women, need certain vitamins that cannot always be found in food. Mark Moyad, M.D., says in the same article, "In specific situations, supplements have a profound ability to make people healthier." One might add that today, most people are deficient in several critical vitamins and minerals, including vitamin D, which is leading to a sicker society than ever before. So, it may be wise to investigate adding that extra boost, and you can get blood tests from your doctor to help determine if you are low and in need of extra supplementation.

Sadly, when we go see a doctor, we are rarely told to improve our diet, exercise, and take a good–quality vitamin or supplement. Instead, we are given a prescription for pharmaceuticals with dozens of side effects that treat the symptoms and ignore the cause. This is because most medical schools lack training on anything alternative or natural, focusing instead on allopathic treatments. According to Melinda Ring, M.D., director of the Osher Center for Integrative Medicine, "Most medical schools are not providing training on dietary supplements, even though so many of their patients are taking them. Your doctor may be fabulous and still not have a background in this topic."

Though taking a vitamin or mineral supplement should always require research into the quality of the product, what it does, what medications you may be on that can cause issues, and whether or not it contains fillers and additives, everyone should know some basics about supplementing their diet to boost health and well–being.

Before we look at the vitamins and minerals and how they can help, it's important to look for safety standards. Not all vitamins and minerals are made in America or tested for quality. The Food and Drug Administration is lax to safety test these products, as it is more indebted to the pharmaceutical industry that helps fund it. So, you may be on your own finding quality research studies and information. Always check who funds a research study and be wary of any that are funded by the product manufacturers. This goes for anything you put into your body, natural or synthetic.

You may be paying less for a product that is more mass produced and more for a product with huge overhead and marketing budgets attacked.

The USP label seen on many vitamins and supplements pertains to the U.S. Pharmacopeia, an independent source that does quality tests and presents the accepted standards most supplements adhere to. NSF International is another nonprofit organization that sets safety standards. But this doesn't mean that you are limited to products approved by these organizations; many doctors and physicians are creating their own product lines that should be considered, as they are on the front lines of treating patients. Just do your due diligence and check labels for fillers that you don't need to be consuming.

Another thing to remember is that cheap is not always bad and expensive is not always higher quality. You may be paying less for a product that is more mass produced and more for a product with huge overhead and marketing budgets attacked. Always read reviews, keeping in mind that some are planted for or against the product, but you can often glean important details from the experiences of others. Buy a one-month supply first to see if you have any negative reactions and check with your doctor if you take pharmaceuticals (your local pharmacist is often even more educated on vitamin and supplement interactions, so ask them, too). Some vitamins and minerals may increase blood flow, something you need to be wary of if on a blood thinner. Others may cause some bloating and gas, something to be aware of if you already suffer from IBS or other digestive disorders. Some supplements may have a sedative effect, something to be aware of if you are on an antidepressant.

Multivitamins are the most widely purchased form of supplementation, as they contain most of the recommended vitamins and minerals in one bottle, but buyer beware because you may react badly to one ingredient, and good luck trying to isolate it. They also work well for people who don't have the most ideal diets and need extra supplementation across the board. Unless you need a lot of one vitamin or mineral, which would require purchasing individually, the only caveat is looking closely at labels and checking the recommended dietary allowances (RDA) since many multis fall short, especially with minerals. Also, be aware of multis with iron. Check with your doctor or pharmacist about how iron might interact with medications or if you really need the extra amount to begin with.

Women will need different daily allowances than men, too. Pregnant and breastfeeding women also have special needs when it comes to supplementation as well as some dangers to avoid. The RDA listed on the label is a good starting point, but don't take too much more than that unless you know you have a deficiency or know you do not consume enough foods on the lists below.

Iron Issues

Iron is critically important because it feeds the blood, and blood is our conduit to supply oxygen to the body and brain. If you are vegan or vegetarian, getting enough iron and the right kind is critical, as you will need twice the amount of plant-based iron to meet your needs. When we don't have enough iron, this is a condition called anemia where blood lacks an adequate amount of healthy red blood cells, which carry oxygen to the body's tissues.

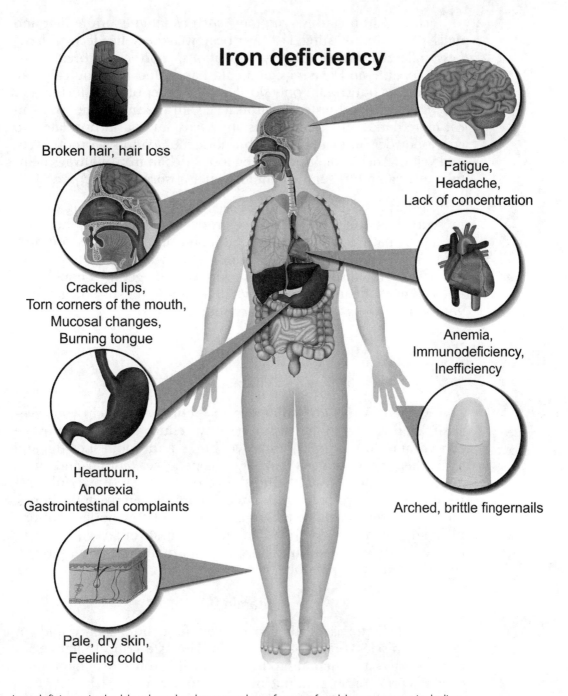

Iron deficiency

Broken hair, hair loss

Fatigue,
Headache,
Lack of concentration

Cracked lips,
Torn corners of the mouth,
Mucosal changes,
Burning tongue

Anemia,
Immunodeficiency,
Inefficiency

Heartburn,
Anorexia
Gastrointestinal complaints

Arched, brittle fingernails

Pale, dry skin,
Feeling cold

Iron deficiency in the blood can lead to a number of uncomfortable symptoms, including headaches, dizziness, fatigue, heart paliptations, shortness of breath, and more.

Lack of iron causes symptoms such as fatigue, brittle hair and nails, pale skin, sweating, fast heartbeat, weakness, headaches, dizziness, inflamed or sore tongue, palpitations, shortness of breath, unusual appetite and cravings, and cold hands and feet. You can take supplements but should only do so on the order of your doctor after having your blood tested for iron levels. In the meantime, you can eat more dark, leafy greens; nuts and seeds; and dark chocolate and cocoa powder. You can also try burdock root, dandelion root, beets, and yellow dock root. When eating foods rich in iron, it always helps to take a vitamin C supplement for better absorptions.

Just as you would hopefully research any synthetic drug you are prescribed, do the same with these products. Even though they may be called "natural," that doesn't automatically mean they are processed and manufactured that way or that they are completely free of side effects. You also want to make sure you are getting enough, but not too much, in addition to the vitamins and minerals you get from your food (always the best primary source).

Vitamins

Vitamin A

Vitamin A includes carotenes and retinols that help your eyesight, keep your skin and tissue healthy, reduce the risk of prostate cancer and lung cancer, improve bone and tooth health, and strengthen the immune system. The lycopene, zeaxanthin, and lutein are beneficial for eyesight, and the carotenoids are powerful for a healthy immune response. Too much vitamin A can harm the bones. Most people get adequate amounts in food and may not need a supplement. Vitamin A is found in beef liver, shrimp, eggs, carrots, cheeses, fortified milk, pumpkins, squash, mangoes, turnip greens, spinach, and sweet potatoes.

Vitamin Bs

B1: Thiamin is needed to convert food into energy and for healthy muscles, brain, hair, and skin. This is a critical vitamin for nervous system functioning. It is found in brown rice, ham, pork chops, acorn squash, watermelons, tomatoes, and spinach.

B2: Riboflavin converts food into energy and promotes a healthy brain, skin, hair, and blood. It is found in milk, eggs, cheese, yogurt, meats, leafy greens, enriched grains and cereals, whole grains, and oysters.

B3: Niacin converts food into energy and is essential for a healthy brain, nervous system, blood cells, and skin and helps lower cholesterol levels. It is found in poultry, fish, meat, potatoes, peanut butter, mushrooms, whole grains, fortified foods, avocadoes, peanuts, squash, and tomatoes.

B5: Pantothenic acid converts food into energy and helps to make neurotransmitters, hemoglobin, lipids, and steroid hormones. It is found in egg yolks, chicken, whole grains, avocadoes, tomatoes, broccoli, and mushrooms.

B6: Pyridoxine makes red blood cells; improves sleep, mood, and appetite; and strengthens cognitive abilities and the immune system. It is found in bananas, chicken, tofu, watermelons, legumes, fish, and potatoes.

B7: Biotin converts to energy and breaks down glucose for energy. It makes and breaks down fatty acids and contributes to healthy hair and nails. It is found in eggs, almonds, whole grains, fish, soybeans, and organ meats.

B9: Folate is vital for the creation of new cells and DNA synthesis. It prevents fetal brain and spine birth defects when taken by pregnant women, reduces heart disease and colon cancer risk, and offsets breast cancer risks in women who consume alcohol. It is found in spinach, legumes, tomatoes, leafy greens, chickpeas, fortified grains, okra, orange juice, tomato juice, turnips, broccoli, fortified cereals, and asparagus.

B12: Cobalamin breaks down fatty acids and amino acids and helps make red blood cells. It lowers homocysteine levels and reduces heart disease risk, protects nerve cells, and makes DNA. It is found in meat, fish, poultry, eggs, fortified cereals, fortified soy milk, and dairy products. If you use a lot of antacids, it's a good idea to supplement with B12, as antacids interfere with the vitamin's absorption. If you feel fatigued a lot and don't consume much animal protein or are vegan or vegetarian, you may benefit from supplementation. Brain fog and fatigue are classic symptoms of low B12.

Vitamin C

Also called ascorbic acid, vitamin C lowers the risk of many cancers, including breast, stomach, and mouth cancers. It protects the eyes against cataracts and makes collagen, the connective tissue that keeps skin youthful and supports blood vessel walls. Vitamin C protects the immune system and neutralizes unstable molecules that can dam–

age cells. It also helps battle allergy symptoms. Vitamin C deficiency is associated with gingivitis and tooth loss. Getting enough in your diet or through supplements makes for better teeth and builds strong and healthy gums. It is found in yellow bell peppers, guavas, lemons and limes, brussels sprouts, spinach, papayas, strawberries, broccoli, kale, grapefruits, oranges, and kiwis, among other fruits and veggies.

Vitamin C protects the immune system and neutralizes unstable molecules that can damage cells.

Vitamin D

Also known as calciferol, vitamin D helps form teeth and bones and keeps them strong, boosts the immune system, and maintains normal blood levels of calcium and phosphorus; it also treats allergies, asthma, and allergic rhinitis. Vitamin D deficiency is often seen in people, especially children, who suffer from allergies. Deficiency is also linked to gingivitis and gum disease as well as high blood pressure. Optimal levels of vitamin D contribute to decreases in cancers and diabetes when at optimal levels. It is found in grass–fed butter and meats, grass–fed raw cheeses, mushrooms, fortified milk and cereals, fortified juices, fatty fish such as salmon, egg yolks, and liver; the best way of all to get vitamin D is getting about 20 minutes of sunlight exposure on large amounts of skin without sunscreen two to three times per week. One of the most likely vitamins you are deficient in and need supplementation for, it behooves you to get your levels checked by your doctor. It should also always be taken with fat in foods or an omega–3 supplement. Vitamin D3 is far superior to vitamin D2, and studies show that vitamin D3 reduces mortality rates and rates of cancer, MS, diabetes, and other major diseases. It is always taken in conjunction with vitamin K for absorption and proper synthesis so that it doesn't drive excess calcium into the arteries and increase hardening of the arteries. Dozens of research studies point to vitamin D's role in fighting cancer and that higher levels at the start of a diet can promote weight loss. It truly is one of the wonder vitamins for health and well-being.

Vitamin E

Also known as alpha–tocopherol, vitamin E is a potent antioxidant that neutralizes unstable molecules that can cause cellular damage. It also protects lipids and vitamin A from damage and protects

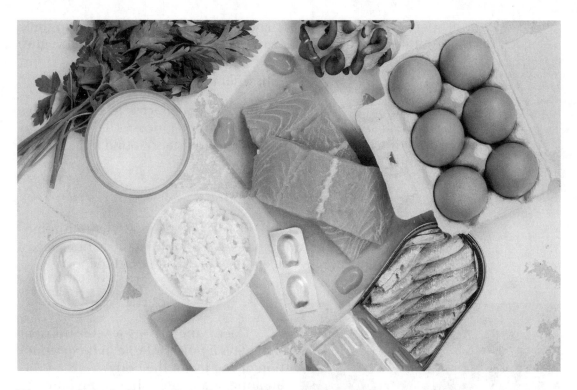

When people think of vitamin D, it often brings to mind milk and milk products, but this essential vitamin can also be found in fatty fish, cereals, mushrooms, egg yolk, liver, and grass-fed meats.

against Alzheimer's disease. It is found in avocadoes, nuts, whole grains, seeds, tofu, wheat germ, leafy greens, and many vegetables.

Vitamin K

Also called phylloquinone or menadione, vitamin K works in conjunction with vitamin D3 for optimal absorption and synthesis. It helps prevent hip fractures, activates proteins, and regulates blood levels of calcium to help blood properly clot. It is found in cabbage, eggs, liver, spinach, milk, broccoli, green veggies, kale, and sprouts.

Minerals and Other Supplements

Calcium

Known for its bone–building properties, calcium is a necessity for strong teeth, too, and it aids weight loss. You need enough to prevent osteoporosis and bone breaks and injuries. Calcium is found in milk; dairy; fortified cereals; leafy, green vegetables; sardines; tofu; and yogurt.

Chromium

Chromium helps regulate normal blood glucose levels, enhances activity of insulin, and frees energy from glucose. It is found in brewer's yeast, which is the best source, but is also found in meat, fish, eggs, poultry, potatoes, nuts, and cheese.

Copper

Copper helps make red blood cells and plays a role in iron metabolism and a strong immune system. It is found in liver, nuts, seeds, shellfish, beans, prunes, whole grains, cocoa, and black pepper.

CoQ10

Coenzyme Q10 is a vital nutrient that plays a powerful role in the production of energy for the body's cells and, as an antioxidant, helps boost the immune system. It also lowers the risk of heart disease and cholesterol levels and prevents periodontal disease and gingivitis. If you take statins for high cholesterol, it is imperative that you supplement with CoQ10, as statins strip the body of this important nutrient.

Glutathione

Considered the body's master antioxidant, glutathione is made from the amino acids glycine, cysteine, and glutamic acid. It reduces inflammation and the risk of chronic diseases, reduces oxidative stress in the body, improves insulin sensitivity, promotes liver health and fights fatty liver disease, and supports healthy cell growth and repair. It also detoxifies the body, and some say it increases metabolism to aid weight loss.

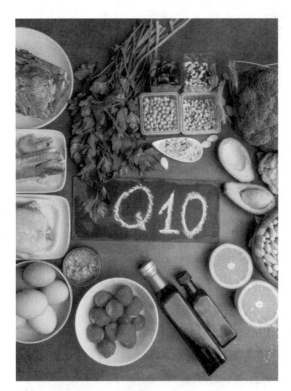

CoQ10 can be found in such foods as organ meats, fatty fish, soybeans, lentils, peanuts, oranges, strawberries, pistachios, sesame seeds, canola and soybean oils, pork, beef, chicken, spinach, broccoli, and cauliflower.

Iodine

Iodine helps the thyroid to set body temperature; assists nerve and muscle function, growth, and reproduction; and prevents congenital thyroid disorder. It is found in iodized salt and seafood. Do not take extra iodine if you don't need it. Some countries automatically add iodine to food, salt, and drinking water, so beware if you are traveling and already get enough in your diet.

Iron

Iron is critical to help hemoglobin in red blood cells and myoglobin in muscle cells and to move oxygen throughout the body. It is necessary for chemical reactions that make collagen, amino acids, hormones, and neurotransmitters. Iron is usually only supplemented if tests show you are low. Women of child-bearing age and menopause, or anyone with a history of anemia, should check to see if they need iron. Iron is hard to absorb through vegetables, so vegetarians and vegans might have to eat twice the amount of iron-rich foods to make up for not eating meat. It is found in red meats, poultry, eggs, some fruits, green veggies, fortified breads, grain products, and cereals.

Magnesium

Magnesium is one of the most important minerals needed for many of the chemical reactions in the body. It works with calcium for muscle contraction, blood clotting, and to regulate blood pressure levels. It is important to build strong bones and teeth. It can have a calming effect for those who are stressed or anxious and is good for the brain. Most of the magnesium in the body is found in your bones, so if you have low blood levels, your body will take the magnesium out of the bones. It's important to maintain optimum levels to sleep well, battle stress, keep your brain functioning with clarity and sharpness, regulate your mood, give you more energy, lower blood pressure, and keep hormone levels in check. It is found in green vegetables such as spinach (cook it to bring out more magnesium levels than raw spinach provides), broccoli, nuts, legumes, sunflower and other seeds, milk, halibut, cocoa and cacao, and whole-wheat bread. Several types of magnesium supplements exist, each with their own benefits (calming, increasing clarity and energy, good for the brain, etc.), so do some research to see which is best for your needs. Coffee is the best liquid source of magnesium, higher than any food source with around 1,000 milligrams per 8-ounce cup, but keep in mind that adding milk with its calcium and sugar sweeteners to your coffee will diminish the absorption level of the magnesium, so opt for black coffee with honey.

Manganese

Manganese metabolizes amino acids, helps form strong bones, and metabolizes carbohydrates and cholesterol. It is found in fish, nuts, legumes, and whole grains. Some manganese may be found in your tap water, so be careful to not go above recommended levels, especially if you have liver disease.

Molybdenum

Molybdenum is a part of enzymes that ward off a form of neurological damage in infants that leads to early death. It is found in legumes, nuts, milk, and grains. It is rare for adults to be deficient, so no need to worry about supplementing.

Omega-3

Essential fatty acids are part of the brain's building blocks. Without enough in the diet, the brain doesn't function as well, and memory suffers. Omega-3 is also good for lowering triglycerides, LDL cholesterol, improving joint health, lessening inflammation in the body, and strengthening the heart. It is important to maintain the proper balance between omega-3 and omega-6 fatty acids. We don't get enough of the beneficial omega-3s and usually too much of the omega-6s. Increasing our intake of omega-3 fatty acids with fish such as salmon, walnuts, flaxseed, or omega-3 supplements can do wonders for good health, and studies show that around 1,200–1,400 milligrams can lower inflammation and lessen joint pain on par with aspirin or ibuprofen. Fish oil has been the most popular supplement but is often filled with contaminants and fillers, so be careful when buying. A better option is Arctic krill oil, which is often purer and more potent. (If you have a shellfish allergy, talk to your doctor before taking a krill oil supplement.)

Phosphorus

Phosphorus builds and protects bones and teeth, converts food into energy, carries lipids into the blood, and moves nutrients in and out of cells. It is found in dairy, meat, fish, poultry, eggs, liver, broccoli, almonds, peas, and potatoes. One usually does not require supple-

mentation of phosphorus if they are getting enough of these foods.

Potassium

Potassium balances fluids in the
body, maintains a steady heartbeat, and
helps send impulses to and from nerves.
It is needed for muscle contractions and
helps alleviate restless leg movements. It
also contributes to lowering high blood
pressure levels. Too little potassium can
cause you to crash or faint from weakness, but too much of it is not beneficial
either, especially for your heart. It is
found in meat, milk, grains, legumes,
fruits, and vegetables. You rarely need to
supplement with potassium unless your
levels are extremely low or if you are
taking a diuretic for high blood pressure,
which often depletes potassium levels.

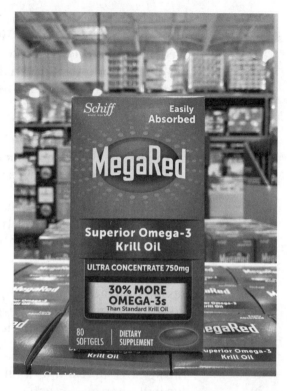

If you have an allergic reaction to shellfish, talk to
your doctor first before taking a krill oil
supplement for its omega-3 benefits.

Probiotics

Did you know that your body contains far more bacteria than it does cells?
The right number of good bacteria is a huge contributor to overall
health and contributes about 80 percent to the working order of your
immune system, yet nutrition, diet, drugs, lifestyle, and the overuse
of antibiotics have contributed to imbalances in our systems between
the good stuff and the bad stuff.

Probiotics are made of good live bacteria and/or yeasts that live
in your body. Good and bad bacteria are naturally found in your
body. When you get an infection, the bad bacteria are more populous
and your immune system is out of balance, which is restored as the
good bacteria destroy the bad bacteria. Your body's bacterial system
is called your microbiome, which is a community of diverse organisms
that keep you healthy. Trillions of microbes are inside of you, including bacteria, fungi such as yeast, viruses, and protozoa. A probiotic
must have the additional characteristics of being isolated from a
human, surviving in the intestines after being ingested, being a
proven benefit to your microbiome, and being safe to consume.

We mainly think of probiotics as the domain of the gut, but they are found in your mouth, vagina, skin, lungs, and urinary tract. A well-balanced diet with a lot of fiber does wonders to keep your microbiome working at optimal levels, but often, life gets in the way. Bad diets, drugs and medications, stress, and exposure to toxins all contribute to the imbalances.

The best probiotics you can look for in stores contain Lactobacillus, Bifidobacterium, *and possibly the yeast* Saccharomyces boulardii.

The best probiotics you can look for in stores contain *Lactobacillus, Bifidobacterium,* and possibly the yeast *Saccharomyces boulardii.* Many types of bacteria fall under the probiotic label. Supplementing comes down to finding the right amounts of different types of bacteria and not just buying something over the counter at a supermarket. Do your research first to pinpoint the best types of probiotics and how much you need. For example, for good oral health, you would look for *S. salivarius* and *Bacillus* coagulants.

Major allergies are linked to microbiome imbalances, as are a host of digestive and immune disorders, yeast infections, urinary tract infections, diarrhea, eczema, irritable bowel syndrome, sepsis, and upper respiratory infections. Probiotics can also change the environment of the mouth to make it harder for plaque and gum disease to take root. One of the best ways to get high amounts of probiotics in your diet is by eating fermented foods such as kimchi, sauerkraut, pickles, kombucha, kefir, buttermilk, sourdough bread, tempeh, miso soup, cottage cheese, and high-quality yogurts. It is better to get your probiotics via food and drinks than supplements because so many products on the market fail to include the right types of bacteria in the right amounts.

Fermented foods have been around for thousands of years to preserve the freshness of foods without refrigeration. The fermentation process occurs when natural bacteria create lactic acid by feeding on sugars and starch. Fermented foods contain important enzymes, fatty acids, and strains of probiotics needed for thriving and healthy gut flora. They can aid in weight loss, too, as they reduce inflammation in the body and better metabolize sugars.

Quercetin

Known as the "king of flavonoids," quercetin has powerful antioxidant properties and fights inflammation, lowers the risk of heart disease, lowers the risk of cancer, provides defense against neurological disorders, and defends the body against infections. It is part of what makes certain foods richly colored and is widely used for its antihistamine effect and ability to lessen allergy symptoms, which it does even better when coupled with vitamin C. Scientific studies abound showing that this supplement works wonders for fighting respiratory diseases such as asthma, bronchitis, and sinus blockages. Quercetin also contains phytonutrients, plant-based compounds that are beneficial to a variety of health issues. It is found in red onions; cherries; kale; tomatoes; apples; capers; dill; cilantro; watercress; dark berries and grapes; olive oil; green, leafy vegetables; and radicchio.

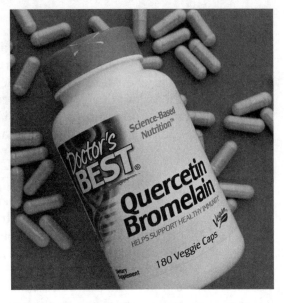

Quercetin is a powerful antioxidant that aids in heart health and also lowers your risk for cancer.

Resveratrol

A glass of red wine a day can keep the doctor away, or at least at bay, thanks to a plant compound found in wine that acts like a powerful antioxidant. Resveratrol has been studied and shown to reduce cholesterol, improve heart health, protect brain function, and lower blood pressure. You can get it in grapes, some berries, peanuts, and wine. The compound is concentrated mainly in the skin of grapes and seeds of berries. A 2015 study review showed a marked decrease in systolic blood pressure with high doses of resveratrol, which may be from its ability to assist the production of nitric oxide, which relaxes blood vessels and allows blood to flow with greater ease. Animal studies show that it also helps decrease body weight in mice by working on the fats in blood. Resveratrol also decreases oxidation of LDL cholesterol and keeps plaque buildup on artery walls at bay.

While supplementing may not make sense, a handful of berries or red grapes might be enough or a glass of red wine. This is one supplement that has many positive animal studies behind it but not many human studies.

Selenium

Selenium is an antioxidant that neutralizes unstable molecules that can damage cells. It is also necessary for regulating thyroid activity. Some research studies suggest it may play a role in reducing the risk of developing cancer. It is found in organ meats, seafood, walnuts, and grain products. Plant foods contain some selenium, but because of depleted soil, it may not be much.

Zinc

Zinc is a critical nutrient for balancing the immune system and reducing immunological stress. It forms many of the body's needed enzymes and proteins, helps create new cells, frees the vitamin A stored in the liver for use, boosts the immune system, helps heal wounds, and can delay age-related macular degeneration. It is found in red meat, poultry, seafood, oysters, beans, nuts, and fortified cereals and grains. Vegetarians and vegans absorb less of the zinc in food, so they must consume twice as much nonmeat food or take a supplement. Today, zinc is one of the most common nutrient deficiencies in modern countries.

The threat of too much salt causing high blood pressure and heart disease is real when we go way over the recommended amounts.... Too little salt, however, can wreak havoc on our bodies, and we don't make salt ourselves if we don't have enough in our diet.

Let's Talk about Salt

Salt, or sodium chloride, has been vilified in mainstream media and by many doctors who haven't caught up with the research, but it is essential to so many bodily processes. Salt is known to assist hydration, affect blood pressure, and balance electrolytes, but its wonders go far beyond that.

Getting too much salt and getting too little salt both lead to problems, but the body will excrete excess salt in the urine. The threat of too much salt causing high blood pressure and heart disease is real when we go way over the recommended amounts and, in our highly processed and junk-food-laden diet mentality, that is easy to do. Too little salt, however, can wreak havoc on our bodies, and we don't make salt ourselves if we don't have enough in our diet.

Salt is a necessity for fluid balance in the body and to properly transmit nerve impulses. It also assists in the contraction and relaxation of muscles. Our kidneys will balance the amount of salt (sodium) in our body, and if it is too low, the kidneys hold on to it. If it's too high, the kidneys excrete it up to a certain point. Here is where too much salt becomes a problem. Too much salt builds up in the blood and attracts water, which leads to water retention and higher blood pressure, both of which can become chronic because the heart must work a lot harder to get blood through the arteries. If you have kidney disease already, excess salt will be harder to get rid of, and a proper balance will be harder to achieve.

Here are other essential ways salt plays a role in our bodies:

- Supports digestion and the absorption of nutrients
- Eliminates pathogens through stomach acid
- Transports iodine into the thyroid gland to produce thyroid hormones
- Produces stomach acid
- Helps us absorb vitamin C and deliver vitamin C and glutathione into our organs
- Improves sleep
- Assists the movement of neurotransmitters
- Balances magnesium and calcium levels
- Lowers stress hormones and LDL cholesterol
- Reduces the viscosity of blood for healthier blood flow

So, how much is too much? One teaspoon of table salt is about 2,325–3,500 milligrams of sodium, which is over the daily recommendation of 2,300 milligrams by the Dietary Guidelines for Americans; 1,500 milligrams is the amount most often prescribed to heart patients by cardiologists.

We get salt in our diets via natural sources and processed foods. Many of the foods we eat contain sodium even before we sprinkle table salt on them. Always check labels to add in the natural levels before considering additional salt. Processed foods are notorious for their high sodium content, including many labeled "health foods," as the added salt serves to make the foods more palatable. Some of the

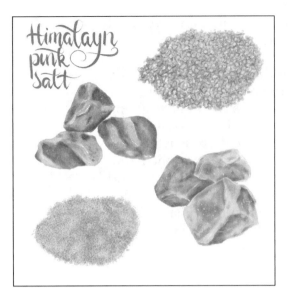

Himalayan salt has a pink hue and is often found in rock salt or coarsely ground forms. It contains, in addition to sodium, calcium, iron, potassium, and magnesium.

worst offenders are frozen dinners, snack foods, processed meats and cheeses, bacon, soups, and fast foods.

Basic table salt, which we habitually put on everything, adds even more as well as being in other condiments for flavoring. One tablespoon of soy sauce packs about 1,000 milligrams of sodium. Imagine putting that on an already salty meal on a continuous basis.

Higher-quality sea salt and Himalayan salt are always a better choice than the average cheap table salt, which has been found to contain plastic particulate matter. It's perfectly fine to add salt to foods, but perhaps start out with whole and fresh food choices to begin with. If you do go for condiments and other products, look for lower-sodium versions. You can taper your taste buds off a salt addiction quickly when you cut out the chips and fast foods and lessen the amount you add on top of what the foods contain; soon, you will find that you are somewhat repulsed by high-sodium products. An abundance of herbs and spices can add flavor and jazz up a meal without resorting to using the saltshaker until your wrist aches. Try replacing salt in recipes with different herbs to taste, but when buying herbs at the grocery store, wait for it … check the label for added salt.

As always with manufacturers' labels, look for sneaky ways they get salt as sodium into their products without telling you. Sodium-containing products that add to your overall salt intake daily include baking powder, MSG, baking soda (sometimes listed as sodium bicarbonate), sodium citrate, sodium nitrite, and sodium alginate. Even lower-sodium products can deceive, as they can claim to have only half the sodium of similar products but still be sky high. An example would be a lower-sodium chicken noodle soup with half of what other soups contain, yet they still claim 750 milligrams of sodium for a single serving. Imagine having the whole two-serving can! That would leave you little wiggle room for your other daily meals.

Don't cut salt down too drastically, as this upsets the balance of electrolytes and incapacitates the many ways sodium works for your benefit. Be sensible, read labels, replace with herbs and spices, wean yourself off of fast and processed foods (easier said than done but so worth it for your health), and let your body tell you when it is getting too much (water retention, persistent thirst, increased urination, head-aches, intense cravings for salty foods, higher blood pressure readings) or not enough (weakness, lack of energy, muscle twitches and cramps, headaches, nausea, vomiting). As an experiment, write down all your salt intake for one week to see exactly how much you consume. You can look on the labels, and for fresh foods and produce, look online for sodium levels. Add it up and get an average daily intake. It may shock you to see just how much, or how little, you consume.

How Do You Know When You're Low?

When our bodies are lacking in something they need for optimal health, they let us know through symptoms and repeated illnesses. It then becomes a challenge of trying to decipher the messages we are getting and making adjustments and improvements where needed. Sometimes it's as simple as improving our diet and getting more sleep and exercise, but other times, the origins of those symptoms may be more subtle.

Some of the most common reasons for micronutrient defi-ciencies are:

- Leaky gut syndrome
- Metabolic syndrome
- Poor diet
- Lack of quality sleep
- Sedentary lifestyle
- Blood sugar imbalance
- Thyroid issues
- Chronic stress

Vitamin and mineral deficiencies do leave clues. Common signs can be looked out for, and a good blood panel will confirm defi-ciencies once other things have been ruled out. These are some of the signs that you may need more of a particular vitamin or mineral.

Hair, Skin, and Nails

Brittle nails, dull and dry hair, and skin that is breaking out in rashes or acne are signs of not getting enough biotin or B7, which helps convert food into energy. Biotin deficiencies are rare, but they do manifest in noticeable external symptoms in the hair, skin, and nails. You might try eating more biotin-rich foods such as fish, meats, organ meats, egg yolks, spinach, nuts, dairy, seeds, bananas, broccoli, cauliflower, and whole grains to see if that helps before considering a pill form.

Hair issues such as dryness and lack of body that are not addressed by a change in shampoo products or diet and hair loss may also be a sign of poor sleep; autoimmune disorders; iron deficiency; lack of adequate protein intake; hormonal imbalances, especially during pregnancy and menopause; lack of good fats in the diet; dehydration; stress; and thyroid issues.

Scaly skin patches and dandruff can be a problem pointing to a lack of zinc, niacin (B3), riboflavin (B2), and pyridoxine (B6). Eating more nuts, seeds, seafood, legumes, dairy, whole grains, fish, eggs, poultry, and organ meats could help alleviate the problems. Bruising and unusual nosebleeds benefit from increased vitamin C, and vitamins A and E work wonders for dry and bumpy skin on the back of the arms. Zinc helps with red stretch marks, and B2 and biotin are great for healing dermatitis.

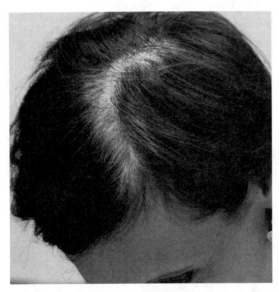

Hair loss is not just a male phenomenon. Women can get thinning hair, too, and when they do it can be an indication of a deficiency in certain vitamins and minerals.

Hair loss is specifically associated with not getting enough iron, zinc, niacin, or biotin. Linoleic acid and alpha-linolenic acid (ALA) are also associated with hair loss, as they are essential fatty acids needed for hair growth. Many hair-loss supplements are on the market but check first with your dermatologist to see if a dietary deficiency is the real cause. You can also take in more meat, eggs, flaxseed, chia seeds, dairy, organ meats, legumes, dark leafy greens, seeds, nuts, and whole grains to see if the condition improves.

Fatigue and Low Energy

This can be attributed to so many deficiencies, but fatigue and low energy are mainly caused by a lack of vitamin B12. When the body is not given enough foods and nutrients for energy production or is burnt out from over-exercise, stress, and lack of sleep, fatigue will occur, so see your doctor for a blood test to pinpoint a nutrient deficient cause. Lack of iron can cause anemia, which leads to extreme tiredness. So many things manifest as low energy, so this may be one of the hardest culprits to identify.

Mood and emotions are also affected by deficiencies. Depression can be helped with increased B1, B5, and biotin. Dizziness may require more iron, B2, and B12. Anxiety is assisted with more B1, B5, and B6. Taking extra vitamin D and B3 together plus B5 and B6 can help with insomnia. Trying to increase food and supplementation to alleviate mood and emotional issues is far safer than turning to pharmaceuticals that have dangerous side effects.

Getting Sick Too Much

Ever get three colds in a month? Two flu bugs in a year? Are you always feeling out of sorts? Like fatigue, being sick all the time is a great indicator that something is off. Before you look to more extreme possibilities, it could be a lack of vitamin C or D, both of which are critical for powerful immune function. It might also be a mineral deficiency that is harder to pinpoint, thus the need for a good blood panel. You can eat more vitamin C- and D-rich foods, supplement, and get more exercise and sunshine to boost immunity.

Eyes, Teeth, and Gums

Bleeding gums may be a sign of not enough vitamin C and/or folate. Teeth also need adequate calcium and vitamins D, A, and K to strengthen tooth enamel and keep gingivitis at bay. Canker sores can be a deficiency of vitamin B3 or B12, calcium, or folate. A sore tongue might need more of vitamin B2 or B3.

Eye health is related to vitamin A intake, and poor vision at night may mean that you are not getting enough. Vitamin D can improve nearsightedness, along with zinc, and vitamin C helps heal ruptured blood vessels in the eye. Low vitamin A levels can also cause tiny growths on the whites of the eyes.

Muscle Health

Our muscles may cramp, twitch, and be sore enough to keep us from doing the things we love. A vitamin or supplement may help before turning to aspirin, Tylenol, or pharmaceuticals. For cramping, try magnesium or vitamin B1, B2, or B6. For twitchy, restless legs, eat a banana or avocado for the potassium boost or try increasing magnesium, calcium, and vitamins D and B–complex. Swelling or edema can be aided with more potassium and vitamins B1 and B6. If you experience clicking joints, try increasing your intake of manganese. Vitamins B12 and B5 can reduce numbness and tingling sensations.

Antibiotics can do a number on the stomach and digestive system and cause fatigue and weakness.

The takeaway here is that by improving your diet overall, finding ways to live a healthier lifestyle, or adding vitamins and minerals, you can often take care of many symptoms and issues. If these symptoms persist or are debilitating, it may then require a good intervention with a holistic approach or a doctor visit to get a blood panel to identify specific problems. Be sure to talk to your doctor or practitioner about any medications or antibiotics you are taking, as they can be culprits in these symptoms and problems as well. Antibiotics can do a number on the stomach and digestive system and cause fatigue and weakness. Side effects of medications, even over–the–counter ones, must be taken into consideration when trying to identify the cause of any given problem, but improving your diet and lifestyle changes for the better sure won't hurt.

Herbs and Plants as Good Medicine

For every ailment, nature provides a plant that can cure it. This author did not make that up, it's an old saying that has many origins; all of them speak to the incredible healing power to be found in plants. Mother Nature truly is the original doctor and pharmacy rolled into one. The use of herbs and plants as medicinals goes back thousands of years and is the foundation of not only ancient Chinese medicine and Ayurvedic medicine but of all healing. Long before we built factories and processing plants to make the drugs of today, we knew how to grow and gather up the greenery and turn it into remedies for health and well-being. Chances are that your older relatives remember using herbal remedies and ingredients not just to make food taste better but to heal whatever ailment they suffered from. This included both internal and external issues from a sore throat or cold to skin rashes to irritable bowel syndrome to gout and everything in between.

Because these ancient, and sometimes primitive, remedies don't have the same advertising dollars behind them as synthetic pharmaceuticals and over-the-counter drugs, we don't see commercials on television urging us to use them more often, which is very sad. One can easily look around and see the rises in heart disease, cancer, diabetes, obesity, and immune disorders to see that perhaps we have been paying too much attention to the modern ways of dealing with sickness and disease and not enough to what our ancestors once utilized. Old is not always bad, and new is not always better.

Herbal remedies also offer the added benefit of not being synthetic, not having extra coloring and additives, and being nontoxic to the body (give or take a few toxic mushrooms and herbs!). They truly speak to the power of our beneficial relationship with nature and how we should be doing everything we can to continue to protect her gifts, not destroy them.

Many healing herbs and plants can be found in your grocery store, your backyard, your garden, and certainly out in nature herself. In a later chapter, we will get into healing remedies that include these wonderful items, but first, it helps to get to know what they are and what they are capable of; see the appendix for a complete list.

Herbs exist in five types, according to taste:

- Salty: High in minerals such as sodium. Plantain is a salty herb.
- Sweet: Astragalus is a sweet-tasting herb that is often used in tea form.
- Bitter: Oregano is a perfect example of a bitter-tasting herb.
- Sour: Elderberries or cranberries are tart or sour.
- Pungent: Strong odor and flavor and can be warming and spicy, such as cayenne pepper.

Good Weeds

Not every weed is a stubborn, useless annoyance that requires you pull it out from the root to save your yard or garden. Some weeds are beneficial and have many medicinal properties. When harvesting weeds to eat or use, never pick any close to the curb or street in order to avoid pollutants from cars and exhaust or near sidewalks, where dogs are more likely to urinate. Wash and allow the weeds to dry completely before using in salves, balms, and infused oils.

- Dandelion: This common weed grows everywhere and is easy to pull up by the root or with a small trowel. You can eat dandelion flowers, which have a slightly tangy taste, or make tea out of the plant parts.

- Plantain: This medicinal weed is a powerful healing agent for skin and epithelial tissue. You can find it everywhere in parks, play-grounds, hiking paths, and in the woods, and the two different types, identifiable by the thickness of their leaves, can be easily har-vested by hand.

- Pokeweed: This weed grows throughout the United States but mainly in the South on undis-turbed earth. The tall plant, with broad leaves and dark-purple berries, is often found growing just on the edge of a field or near runoff streams. It is tough to pull from the ground, so you will need a shovel.

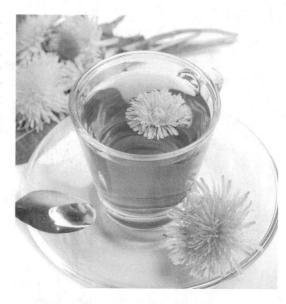

Most people think of dandelions as a bothersome weed invading their grass lawns, but did you know every part of this plant is edible?

- Purslane: This plant has thick, teardrop-shaped leaves and a succulent, mucilaginous texture similar to okra. It can be consumed in salads and balances out the flavor of stronger greens.

- Sheep sorrel: This weed has a tangy taste and is used in gourmet dishes. The leaves are shaped like arrows and are smaller than French sorrel but with a similar taste. It makes a great addition to a salad along with other greens and is best chopped finely, as it can have a slight bitterness.

- Curly dock: Also related to French sorrel, this weed is slightly tangy with tougher leaves, so it should be used sparingly in a salad.

- Wood sorrel: It is not related to other sorrels–go figure–but it does have a slightly tangy flavor. Its leaves are softer and more succu-lent in texture.

- Lamb's quarters: One of the most common garden weeds, it is also one of the most palatable as a substitute for spinach. It is a very tall plant with tender leaves, but the shorter plants tend to be the most tender.

- Chickweed: This tiny, sprawling weed has a natural texture and fla-vor similar to baby lettuce and can be harvested by the handful.

- Garlic mustard: Similar in taste to mustard greens, this weed has a hint of garlic to its flavor. Harvest when young; this is when the leaves are the most tender.

Sassy Soursop: The Superstar Healer

The leaves of the soursop plant are a healing superpower, minus the cape. They contain compounds that fight infections and cancer; boost immunity and kidney and liver health; treat diabetes, blood disorders, fevers, diarrhea, and rheumatism; lower blood pressure; promote healthy skin and hair; assist in better sleep; alleviate gout and osteoporosis; stop back pain; improve eye health; enhance gastrointestinal health; and relieve stress.

All these benefits are packed into the leaves of just one plant. Mother Nature rocks. However, soursop is not safe in large amounts. If you choose to drink it as a tea or take it in supplements, follow the dosages carefully. Too much of a great thing is not always a great thing and, sometimes, less is more. You can also use the soursop fruit in a dessert or put it in the juicer, but limit your intake to a half a cup two or three times per week.

Nature's Pain Relievers

Put away the aspirin and try one of these natural herbs and plants for pain relief. They can be consumed in food, teas, or supplement form:

- Garlic: earaches and sore throats
- Cloves: toothaches and swollen gums
- Cherries: headaches and joint aches
- Turmeric: overall chronic pain
- Horseradish: sinus pain
- Peppermint: sore muscles and joints
- Ginger: muscle pain, cramping
- Pineapple: stomach pain, gas
- Blueberries: bladder/urinary infections
- Cranberries: urinary infections
- Peppermint: sore throats
- Menthol: sore throats and stuffed nasal passages

Herbs for a Better Sex Life

Sex is important to a healthy lifestyle and sense of well-being. All too often, it gets relegated to the back burner on the stovetop of life, and we don't realize how much we miss it until we are rarely having it! Many factors are involved in a diminishing sex drive, including stress, diet, exercise, time, and how we feel about ourselves, but all of that is under our control, which is the good thing. The bad thing is that all of that requires some attention and effort to make more productive choices that help get us back on track sexually.

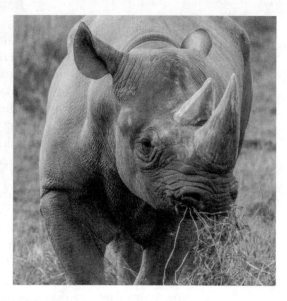

Your sex life can be improved in a number of ways with herbal remedies and supplements. In the past, people would turn to strange things like ground-up rhinoceros horns or buffalo testicles to increase libido, cure erectile dysfunction, or bring about sensual pleasure. Sexual issues can be dealt with in many natural ways without resorting to bringing about the extinction of a species or killing animals, and they often have fewer side effects than pharmaceutical drugs.

Unfortunately, in some countries people believe that ground-up rhino horn helps with libido. But rhino horn is just compressed hair and has no benefits. Sadly, a lot of rhinos are killed each year for the horn trade.

Erectile Dysfunction

A number of herbs have successfully treated erectile dysfunction (ED), including panax ginseng, maca, ginkgo, and yohimbine. These herbs work to deal with anxiety over performance and increase blood flow and stamina.

Panax ginseng is an herb that has been used in China and Korea for over 2,000 years as a tonic. The roots are used in teas and supplement form to boost stamina and concentration, and some clinical studies show that it improves penile rigidity, girth, and erection duration. As an antioxidant, it releases nitric oxide (NO) into the blood, which can help with ED, and some use a cream version to stop premature ejaculation. Supplement dosage is about 900 milligrams three times a day for eight weeks as per human clinal trials and is a short-term solution; always do your research and check with your doctor before taking it.

Maca is a Peruvian root vegetable that is rich in iron, magnesium, iodine, and amino acids. Maca exists in three types: red, black, and yellow. Black maca is often used to improve memory and alleviate stress. In animal trials, maca improved sexual performance in rats, but this is not really evident in humans. Perhaps it is a placebo effect, or perhaps by dealing with stress, it allows the man to relax and enjoy sex. It is generally safe to take about 3 grams per day in supplement form for a few weeks to improve libido, but it does show an increase in blood pressure at 0.6 grams a day, so do not take it if you have hypertension.

Yohimbine comes from the bark of the West African evergreen tree and has been used to treat ED for decades, as it activates increased NO to the nerves of the penis, widens penile blood vessels to increase blood flow, and prolongs the duration of erections. It also increases libido in men and has been studied in several clinical trials that showed erection improvement and greater ability to achieve orgasm. Combining yohimbine with L-arginine showed significant effects on erectile function, as L-arginine is an amino acid that expands blood vessels. The people in clinical trials took about 20 milligrams per day, spreading it out throughout the day, but side effects include nausea, stomach cramps, indigestion, and diarrhea. If you have high blood pressure (BP) or take any BP meds, this is not the combo for you, as it does raise BP levels. Yohimbine alone boosts adrenaline and can cause headaches, jitters, insomnia, and sweating. Talk to your doctor first before taking.

Ginkgo biloba (also known as maidenhair) is an herb from a Chinese tree that has been studied quite a bit for its ability to enhance sexual performance and function as well as boost memory and brain sharpness.

Ginkgo biloba (also known as maidenhair) is an herb from a Chinese tree that has been studied quite a bit for its ability to enhance sexual performance and function as well as boost memory and brain sharpness. One research trial saw sexual function improvement in 76 percent of participants in men who were on antidepressant medications, making this an effective herb for ED caused by medication side effects. However, other studies showed little improvement, positing that ginkgo is not a cure for ED but one potential treatment. Ginkgo has been taken in supplement form for decades, and in the study above, the dosage was about 40–60-milligram capsules twice daily for a period of four weeks, but this herb can cause problems if you take blood thinners, so check with your doctor first.

Another herb that has not been researched much yet but shows potential in anecdotal use is tongkat ali, which grows in the Malaysian rain forest and has been used for centuries to enhance libido, increase levels of testosterone in men (which increases fertility), and improve sexual performance. It also helps alleviate ED and has gotten the nickname "Malaysia's home-grown Viagra." It also increases muscle mass, strength, and mental clarity; reduces stress and anxiety; and lowers blood sugar levels. It can be taken in supplement form.

Women's Sexual Function

For women, sexual function and libido may take a nosedive when they become mothers or caretakers and so much of their energy is taken up by the needs of others. Maca works to boost female libido without side effects unless you are not supposed to take increased iron, but it could be the increase of nutrients that are responsible. Maca has a lot of vitamins C and B6 and copper, so it naturally boosts energy and mental clarity. Anytime you feel and think better, you enjoy sex more.

Age and hormonal fluctuations must also be taken into consideration. Many women, after menopause, lose their libido and can benefit from a legume like red clover, which is known to increase sex drive because of its high amount of isoflavones that are similar to estrogen. It is often taken to relieve menopausal symptoms, and a study in the journal *Obstetrics and Gynecology International* found that women who were postmenopausal and took 80 milligrams of red clover isoflavones over a 90-day period had a marked improvement in mood, sleep, energy, and libido. Some research shows that red clover also strengthens bones and improves cardiovascular functioning.

Some small studies show that panax ginseng helps women almost as much as it does men. It boosts immunity, improves cardiovascular function, and improves sexual desire in clinical studies, but more research is needed to show just how effective it can be for sex drive. It is a part of Ayurvedic medicine and has been around for a long time, but check with your doctor on dosage for supplements, or try a ginseng tea or extract first to see how you feel and if any side effects arise.

Another herb with roots in Ayurvedic medicine that may help women is fenugreek, a plant cultivated all over the world. The seeds have been used for centuries for their anti-inflammatory and libido-

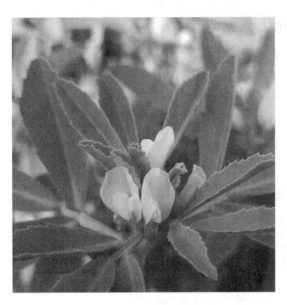

Fenugreek is a common, flowering plant with seeds that are valued for their anti-inflammatory and libido-enhancing properties.

boosting properties, and some studies show that fenugreek seeds increase the activity of testosterone and estrogen. One study that showed improvement had 80 women take 600 milligrams of fenugreek in supplement form daily and, compared to the placebo group, showed a significant increase in sexual desire and arousal after eight weeks. Fenugreek is well tolerated, but it can cause digestive issues and should not be taken if you are pregnant. The herb does interfere with certain prescription medications, so check with your doctor or pharmacist first.

For women, body image and energy levels are directly tied to how they feel about sex and how much they prioritize sexual activity. Working on improving diet, cutting out toxins and processed foods, sleeping more, alleviating stress with exercise or meditation, and dealing with financial and relational stressors in a proactive way can all help increase the desire for physical touch and sexual contact.

More Sexy Herbs to Try

Other herbs that boost libido, increase energy, move more blood flow to the genitals, and make you feel good and randy all over are listed below. The concept of aphrodisiacs is an ancient one, as our ancestors worked with the natural world to find plants and foods that turned them on. These herbs can be used in many forms, including teas, infusions, or in supplement form, and many also relieve anxiety, depression, and stress and improve well-being, which is paramount to feeling sexy and attractive.

- Ginger
- Ginkgo
- Damiana
- Yohimbe
- Ginseng
- Rhodiola

- Maca
- Ashwagandha
- Licorice
- Astragalus
- Guarana

If you want to indulge the senses, try:

- Coriander
- Cloves
- Nutmeg
- Cinnamon
- Vanilla bean
- Star anise
- Orange peel
- Peppermint
- Rose
- Cacao
- Red clover
- Red raspberry
- Angelica
- Dong quai

These herbs can be used alone or in blends, with honey for an added aphrodisiac boost.

For natural ways to improve sexual function for both men and women, try the following:

- Eat aphrodisiac fruits such as figs, bananas, and avocadoes.
- Eat more chocolate.
- Limit the amount of alcohol you drink.
- Eat a healthier diet with foods that are less processed.
- Reduce stress and find ways to improve sleep.
- Get more exercise to increase blood flow and body confidence.

The above may seem obvious, but sometimes, the most common-sense causes can be at the heart of sexual problems, including how we feel about ourselves and relate to others, body image, outside stresses and job performance at work, dealing with raising children or caring for elderly parents, and current events that are scary and stressful, all of which tap us out energetically and leave us with little desire for sex, let alone time.

For women, stress often means they don't want to even think about sex, yet men might want to use sex as a way to relieve stress, causing problems in your relationship. Something as simple as removing processed, chemically derived food products from your diet, which can lead to weight gain, lower testosterone levels, hormonal dysfunction, and feeling tired and sick all the time, can do wonders to improve libido and sexual desire. While supplements and herbs can help boost sexual function, it all begins with taking good care of yourself in body, mind, and spirit.

Anti-inflammatory Rock Stars

Herbs and spices that fight inflammation abound, but a few stand out as the rock stars:

- Ginger: Along with turmeric, ginger belongs to the rhizome family. These plants have underground stems that grow horizontally with roots that grow downward and stems and leaves that sprout above the ground. This powerful herb has been a mainstay in ancient Chinese and Indian medicine and became popular in Europe when the Roman Empire began trading it. It has over 100 different compounds, with gingerol as the active compound providing most of its health benefits. It reduces inflammation and can prevent colon cancer, lower obesity, lower inflammation from osteoarthritis, relieve muscle pain, and help heal metabolic syndrome to aid in weight loss. It also stops nausea and motion sickness.

- Turmeric: This staple of Indian cuisine is one of the most potent anti-inflammatory herbs around. It is used to add flavor and color to curry powder, mustard, butter, and some cheeses and has been a part of both traditional Indian and Chinese herbal medicine for thousands of years. It is now one of the most scientifically researched herbs, with over 12,000 peer-reviewed and published biomedical studies backing up claims of its benefits to health. The U.S. National Center for Biotechnology alone includes over 6,000 studies of turmeric and curcumin, its active compound, which reduces pain and inflammation equal to ibuprofen but with no nasty side effects. It also improves conditions for those suffering from ulcerative colitis, osteoarthritis, lupus, and diabetes. Turmeric has been shown in studies to be as effective as several pharmaceuticals, many with dangerous side effects. Some of these studies compared it to Lipitor/Atorvastatin (cholesterol medications), corticosteroids, Metformin (diabetes drug), Oxaliplatin (chemotherapy drug), Amoxicillin (antibiotic), Pro–zac/Fluoxetine (antidepressants), aspirin/ibuprofen/naproxen (anti–inflammatory medications), and aspirin for blood thinning. In all the above cases, turmeric was found to be as effective as these conventional medications.

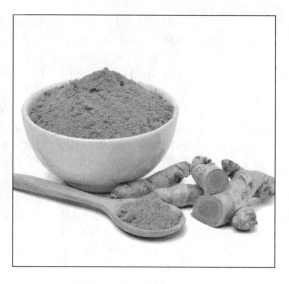

- Boswellia: Also known as Indian frankincense, this herbal extract from the *Boswellia serrata* tree has been used as an anti–inflammatory in Asian and African cultures. It can be utilized in a supplement pill form but also as a resin or cream. It has been studied widely and found to reduce inflammation from arthritis and inhibit cancer growth with no side effects.

Ginger root and turmeric (the latter is a key ingredient in curry) are popular, flavorful spices that also have the side benefit of being anti-inflammatories.

- Rosemary: Native to the Mediterranean area, this fragrant herb is popular in cooking meals and salads. It's from the same family as thyme, basil, and oregano and is a rich source of anti–inflammatory agents with many medicinal uses. Rosemary oil used in massage has been found to reduce pain and inflammation in those with rheumatoid arthritis by 50 percent.

Other potent anti–inflammatory rock stars include cinnamon, cloves, cayenne pepper, bioflavonoids such as quercetin and rutin, black pepper, and white willow. Several herbs on the master list in this book do help with inflammation, but these are the ones you will benefit the most from including in your diet or supplement program. Because inflammation is such a big part of so many chronic and major diseases from allergies to cancer to lupus, using these herbs can have a far–reaching effect for better health overall.

Ashwa-who? The Super Root

One of the most popular wonder herbs today is ashwagandha, a staple of Indian Ayurvedic medicine. For 5,000 years, Indians have used this herb to benefit the body's immune, neurological, endocrinal, and reproductive systems. Used in supplement and oil form, it is considered a broad–spectrum remedy for physical and mental health known for its anti–inflammatory and antioxidant properties and its ability to slow the aging process, assist weight loss, and promote calmness and a sense of well–being.

> *Used in supplement and oil form, it [ashwagandha] is considered a broad-spectrum remedy for physical and mental health known for its anti-inflammatory and antioxidant properties....*

The root and leaves of this plant are commonly used as medicinals and are sometimes referred to as Indian ginseng, winter cherry, or somnifera root. It is the presence of withanolides, which are steroidal lactones, that make this herb such a powerhouse ingredient for overall health and well–being. The name "ashwagandha" means "smell of horse" because the herb is alleged to give you the strength of a horse. Oh, it also smells like a horse, too. It is one of the most heavily studied herbs of recent times, with over 200 current studies examining its ability to do the following:

- Improve thyroid function
- Reduce anxiety and depression
- Assist in weight loss
- Reduce stress
- Stabilize blood sugar levels
- Lower cholesterol
- Prevent cancer and treat existing cancer
- Increase energy, stamina, and endurance
- Improve libido
- Boost immunity
- Relieve insomnia and promote better sleep

A 2017 study in the *Journal of Alternative and Complementary Medicine* found it beneficial for normalizing thyroid levels, and another study in the *Journal of Ayurveda and Integrative Medicine* found it improved cognitive function in patients with bipolar disorder. When it comes to treating anxiety, a 2009 study in *PLOS One* showed that the herb was comparable to the pharmaceuticals lorazepam and imipramine but without the side effects. It is also a powerful adaptogen, an herb that can help the body and mind adapt to stress. It does this by helping the body to maintain homeostasis during emotional and physical

stress. In fact, it is the most widely studied and commonly used adaptogen herb.

Other Adaptogen Herbs

Herbal adaptogens have a beneficial impact on our ability to handle
stress. A lot of research has been done on
adaptogens and how they work to lower
levels of our fight–or–flight hormone,
cortisol. It's good for cortisol to be released into the bloodstream during times
of acute stress or danger, but elevated
levels that never go down become
chronic stress, which then leads to many
chronic illnesses. This can result in adrenal system burnout, digestive tract issues,
rapid aging, and increased blood pressure and heart rate. Adaptogens are a
class of plants that heal by balancing and
restoring the body's normal stress response and increase tolerance to the ongoing stressors we deal with daily.

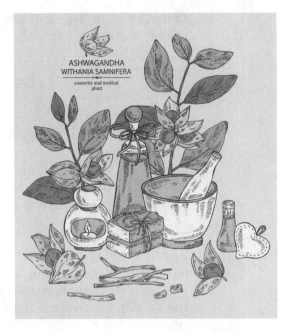

All parts of the ashwagandha plant can be used,
including the fruit, seeds, leaves, and roots.
Leaves can produce a narcotic, the roots are used
to stabilize mood, the fruit helps with skin
infections and eye diseases, and the seeds
coagulate milk.

Some of the best adaptogens include Asian or panax ginseng,
a potent herb that affects various stress–response systems in the
body, improves mood, and brings clarity and better mental performance; holy basil or *tulsi*, which promotes calm, battles stress, sharpens
cognition, lowers blood pressure, reduces seizures, reduces pain
levels, and lowers blood corticosterone, a stress hormone, along with
its other many medicinal benefits; astragalus root, used in ancient
Chinese medicine to boost immunity and strengthen the body
against stress; licorice root to increase energy, boost endurance, and
boost the immune system along with regulating stress hormones
such as cortisol; rhodiola, a potent root that exerts an antifatigue effect while sharpening mental performance and concentration and
decreasing cortisol levels; and cordycep mushrooms, which are nutrient rich and full of antioxidants that lessen oxidative stress and
regulate cortisol levels.

These and any other adaptogens you may want to try could be
harmful if you have preexisting conditions, so check with your doctor

first. Always be aware of any countereffects with pharmaceuticals you are taking, too.

Herbs for Heart Health

Heart disease is the number–one killer in America and now is estimated to kill over 31 percent of people worldwide. Heart health is all about healthy diet, exercise, stress reduction, and being aware of family history, but some herbs specifically work to protect and strengthen the heart, reduce blood pressure, and lower the risk of death from cardiac arrest and other cardiovascular diseases.

Hawthorn is one of the most powerful herbs for reducing blood pressure and reducing cardiac mortality in people with compromised left ventricular function. A study in the *European Journal of Heart Failure* with 2,600 adult subjects showed that 900 milligrams of hawthorn extract a day on patients with class–II and –III heart failure and compromised left ventricular ejection fractions saw a reduction in death by over 37 percent. Hawthorn extract strengthens and tones the heart muscle and enhances a strong heartbeat while also dilating coronary arteries to assure better blood flow and lower blood pressure. It also regulates cardiac rhythm and reduces angina, a type of chest pain caused by exertion.

Hawthorn is one of the most powerful herbs for reducing blood pressure and reducing cardiac mortality in people with compromised left ventricular function.

Other studies have shown that the extract from hawthorn berry reduces shortness of breath and fatigue and increases tolerance to exercise. The berries are rich in antioxidants and anti–inflammatory compounds that reduce the oxidative damage that triggers heart disease. The best place to find quality hawthorn berries is not a supermarket but rather a farmer's market or health food store. They can be eaten as is, dried, ground into powder, in a tea form, or as a liquid or pill supplement.

Celery juice is cheap and easy to make in a juicer or blender and contains phytochemicals and magnesium, both of which lower blood pressure. It also contains potassium, which helps rid the body of excess fluids. The potassium can also balance out levels if you are taking a water pill already, so you don't lose too much of the important trolytes. Celery juice has the added benefits of getting rid of acid reflux, bloating, constipation, and digestive issues.

Hibiscus is a colorful, red blossom and common garden plant in subtropical and tropical regions. Like hawthorn, it is a traditional medicinal for lowering blood pressure and supporting a healthy heart and is even known to fight obesity and promote a healthy weight. A lot of scientific research is behind the use of hibiscus as a natural way to lower blood pressure on par with some pharmaceuticals such as Captopril and without the pesky side effects.

Hibiscus extracts contain compounds that lower bad LDL cholesterol and triglycerides and help prevent atherosclerosis, thanks to their natural plant pigment, called anthocyanins, which are potent antioxidants also found in berries. Anthocyanins work to inhibit oxidation of fats, which can be harmful. Hibiscus is a tasty and relaxing tea that can be purchased in stores or made with ½ teaspoon of dried, ground flowers in 8 ounces of water. It is tart, like cherries, but can be sweetened to taste with a natural sweetener.

Other heart–healthy herbal rock stars include cayenne pepper for its powerful capsaicin; garlic, which is a potent treatment for diabetes, heart disease, and high blood pressure by increasing the body's natural levels of nitric oxide, which widen and relax blood vessels; ginger, which reduces high blood pressure and the risk of stroke by inhibiting the actions of pro–inflammatory molecules in the body, neutralizing free radicals, and reducing oxidative damage to tissues and cells; and curcumin, which in studies by the Cleveland Heart Lab was shown to prevent blood clots, reduce the inflammation that leads to heart attacks and strokes, reduce the stickiness of blood platelets that could lead to blood clots, and improve the health of the heart's fragile arteries. Of these, only curcumin works best in supplement form, and one 2017 meta–analysis for *Nutrition Journal* showed that 1,000 milligrams of curcumin taken for one month protected patients from heart disease by improving levels of bad LDL cholesterol and reducing levels of fats found in the blood.

Okey Dokey, Artichokey

Artichokes look like big, green, spiny balls, but they are a delicious vegetable to cook, steam, or pickle. The fact that they are jam-packed with antioxidants like rutin, quercetin, cynarin, and gallic acid,

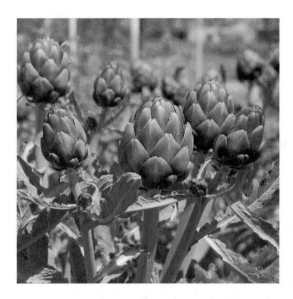

Did you know that the artichoke is just a type of thistle plant? But in addition to being a tasty food, it is also full of antioxidants.

all of which protect the heart and reduce your risk of developing liver disease and diabetes, makes them a must–have in your natural health diet.

A 2020 study published in *Cellular and Molecular Biology* put artichokes at the top of a list of vegetables rich in antioxidants, thanks to their high levels of phytonutrients. These plant compounds have been studied for decades for their ability to lower cholesterol levels and improve heart health. An older study done in 2008 using 1,280 milligrams of standardized artichoke leaf extract was shown to cause a moderate reduction in the cholesterol levels of 75 patients when taken over a three–month period. Another study in 2013 used 1,800 milligrams and showed a larger decrease in cholesterol, up to 18.5 percent compared to the placebo group.

Artichoke leaves interfere with the production of cholesterol in the body. The phytonutrients may play a role in preventing excess buildup of cholesterol by inhibiting the action of enzymes in the liver and assisting increased bile production and elimination. Cholesterol is a good thing and a necessity for good health, but if your bad LDL levels are too high, this may be a great alternative to taking side–effect–riddled statins.

If you can't stand cooking them or eating them (try steaming and scooping mayo or a homemade dressing with the "petals"), you can take an artichoke leaf extract in a supplement form, but make sure it is high quality and contains no fillers.

Right-in-Your-Pantry Rock Stars

Many of these herbs require a little effort to find, but one powerhouse exists in most pantries right now: black pepper. Thought of as nothing more than a condiment to add to salads and meals, this "king of spices" does a body good in a myriad of ways.

Native to India, black pepper, or *Piper nigrum*, was traded widely and eventually made its way west to become a staple of American cuisine. It was traditionally used as a carminative agent to relieve gas, vomiting, diarrhea, and abdominal pain, but newer research revealed a plethora of other benefits. The main active ingredient in black pepper is piperine. This is where pepper gets its heat and flavor but is a powerful antioxidant and anti–inflammatory that can prevent cancer tumor growth, protect against chronic illnesses such as liver disease, and slow the aging process. Black pepper essential oil contains phenolics, which are flavonoids and proanthocyanidins, both anti–inflammatory.

Black pepper also has a protective influence on the heart, regulates lipid metabolism and oxidation, and can prevent and treat cardiovascular disease. It also prevents uptake of the bad LDL cholesterol and improves the lipid profile. Piperine also protects the liver from damage induced by tertiary butyl hydroperoxide and can stimulate the regeneration of the liver by restricting fibrosis. That same piperine has been shown in scientific studies to be antimutagenic, and pepper extract can inhibit development of solid tumors in mice and has antitumor effects in MCF–7 breast cancer cells, which induce oxidative stress.

Black pepper regulates blood sugars and allows nutrients to be better absorbed into the body.

It doesn't end there. Black pepper's piperine has been shown in animal studies to significantly improve memory in rats with an Alzheimer's–type disease, and it can restore mitochondrial functioning in cells that have been exposed to toxic insecticides. Black pepper regulates blood sugars and allows nutrients to be better absorbed into the body. Piperine helps increase the absorption rates of other powerful anti–inflammatories such as curcumin and resveratrol.

In addition, a great reason to add quality ground black pepper to every meal possible is that piperine is known to block fat cell formation and has many benefits for weight loss and obesity. Other potent compounds and agents in black pepper have also proved successful in ancient Indian medicine and in modern times to treat chronic bronchitis, asthma, cholera, malaria, viral hepatitis, and diseases of the spleen. In addition, black pepper has antidepressant, antifungal, larvicidal, analgesic, and antimicrobial properties.

Black pepper is proof that nature contains everything necessary for optimum health, and in this case, it's probably already lurking in your pantry or cabinet, but beware of the finely ground product that might contain fillers and microplastics. Instead, buy whole pepper-corns and a good grinder and grind it fresh as needed.

Cannabis

As more states legalize the use of marijuana, or pot, as a medicinal or for recreational use, cannabis has been included in most lists of herbs and plants that are of benefit to human health. Cannabis is an herbal drug made from the *Cannabis* plant, an annual flowering plant. Cannabis has three "source plants": *Cannabis sativa, Cannabis indica,* and *Cannabis ruderalis.* Cannabis has its geographic origins in central Asia and India. It is now grown and produced all over the world as a recreational and/or medicinal drug.

This plant contains unique terpeno-phenolic compounds called cannabinoids that affect the central nervous system and have a relaxing and calming effect and are found in the leaves and flowers of the *Cannabis* plant. Other compounds such as terpenoids are secreted by glandular trichomes, which occur mainly on the floral calyxes and bracts of the female plants. Once dried, cannabis is often called buds or marijuana, and the resin of the plant is called hashish. Other extracts are usually referred to as hashish oil.

Over 480 identifiable chemical constituents can be found in the *Cannabis* plant, and approximately 85 of them have been categorized as cannabinoids. The two most abundant are CBD and THC. Most people refer to the popular form of cannabis as CBD, which stands for cannabidiol, which is a noneuphoric, nonintoxicating cannabinoid that can be used to prevent and treat nausea, seizures, anxiety, migraine headaches, and general pain. CBD also treats epilepsy and, in the States, where it is legal, can be found in a broad range of products from edibles to salves and balms.

CBD oil is known to treat a variety of ailments and is legally sold in most states, as it does not contain THC. It is used to do everything from heal acne and skin issues to alleviate depression and anxiety. The oil can be consumed orally or massaged into the skin. Oral sprays have been approved in a number of countries to reduce pain and muscle spasms in people with multiple sclerosis and have also been used to reduce pain from chemo treatments for cancer patients and to alleviate nausea and vomiting. A 300-milligram dose of CBD oil was found in one study to reduce anxiety in men and seemed to be

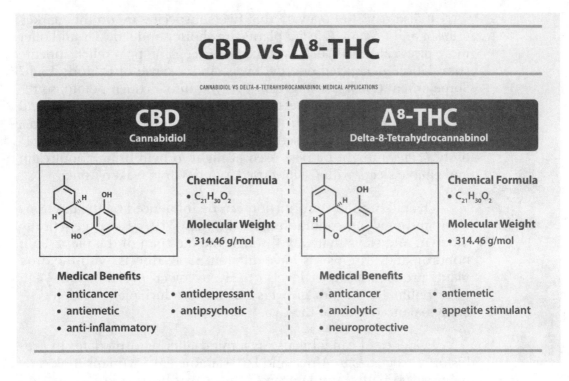

CBD vs Δ⁸-THC

CANNABIDIOL VS DELTA-8-TETRAHYDROCANNABINOL MEDICAL APPLICATIONS

CBD
Cannabidiol

Chemical Formula
- $C_{21}H_{30}O_2$

Molecular Weight
- 314.46 g/mol

Medical Benefits
- anticancer
- antiemetic
- anti-inflammatory
- antidepressant
- antipsychotic

Δ⁸-THC
Delta-8-Tetrahydrocannabinol

Chemical Formula
- $C_{21}H_{30}O_2$

Molecular Weight
- 314.46 g/mol

Medical Benefits
- anticancer
- anxiolytic
- neuroprotective
- antiemetic
- appetite stimulant

Two chemicals found in marijuana are CBD and THC. Both of these have health benefits, but only the THC will get you high. This is why many people prefer CBD oils as a safe way to get a number of benefits.

the sweet–spot dosage, as any more or less was not as effective. CBD has shown antidepressant effects in several animal studies.

The main psychoactive compound in cannabis is THC, which stands for tetrahydrocannabinol and is what gives the user the "high" of pot smoking or consumption. THC offers far fewer benefits and far more side effects than CBD, but some people like to use both in a blend for their respective properties. Products higher in THC may cause more side effects like anxiety, hallucinations, paranoia, a decrease in blood pressure, nausea, lethargy, and delayed reaction times. Some in the scientific community are concerned that long–term use can lead to memory and cognitive issues, but studies are needed. It behooves anyone considering using cannabis in any form to first check with their doctor to see if they have existing health issues or take medications that could countereffect the CBD or THC and to always start out with smaller amounts to acclimate the body and mind to the effects.

It also pays to be aware that two subspecies are on the market, *C. indica* and *C. sativa. C. indica* plants are shorter and stockier and offer more physical effects such as relaxation, sleep and pain relief, appetite stimulation, decreased energy levels, and a sense of a "body high." Some potent *C. indica* strains can turn you into a couch potato, so relaxed you can barely move. *C. sativa* plants are taller and longer and offer a cerebral "head high" with more alertness, possible euphoria, uplifting emotions, increased productivity, higher energy, and creativity. *C. indica* might be best used at night to help bring about calm and enable sleep, with *C. sativa* used as a daytime waker–upper.

Overall cannabis production can be influenced by the environment and growing conditions, but the CBD–THC ratio is genetically inherent and stays that way through the life span of the plant. Both nondrug and drug plants have different ratio aspects, with the drug plants producing higher levels of THC to lower levels of CBD. With cross–pollination tactics, growers can also produce plants with a generally balanced ratio of the two.

Evidence of cannabis use as a mind–altering drug dates to prehistorical societies in Africa and Eurasia. Ancient Scythians took cannabis steam baths, and later in China, it was burned in incense and inhaled for its psychoactive effects. The hemp form is used to make clothing, textiles, rope, paper, and other products.

Smoking cannabis is just as much of a problem for the lungs and airways as smoking tobacco, so be aware of the potential for increased bronchitis, inflammation and irritation of the airways....

Though not a lot of scientific research has been done on the long–term effects of smoking or using cannabis, in the short term, it can be a great way to alleviate pain, bring about calm and better sleep, and stop potential seizures. Smoking cannabis is just as much of a problem for the lungs and airways as smoking tobacco, so be aware of the potential for increased bronchitis, inflammation and irritation of the airways, and possibly chronic obstructive pulmonary disease (COPD). It might be a better choice to consume in edibles, which can range from cookies and brownies to gummy bears. Cannabis ranks just behind alcohol, tobacco, and caffeine in global use as a recreational drug and became hugely popular during the 1960s as a mindopening way to relax and get high.

Two extracts, dronabinol and nabilone, are FDA-approved for treating the side effects of AIDS and chemotherapy. A 2017 National Academies of Sciences, Engineering, and Medicine report did a review of hundreds of studies on cannabis and did find substantial evidence of its success as a pain reliever and for relief of nausea and vomiting for those undergoing chemotherapy. It also found moderate evidence of success at treating sleep apnea and pain from fibromyalgia and MS. Older respondents claimed it worked well on joint pain, too, and a 2020 research letter featured in *JAMA Internal Medicine* stated that marijuana use doubled in those aged 65 and older. CBD is believed to act as an anti-inflammatory agent specifically in molecules called cytokines and brain cells called microglia, which both lead to inflammatory responses in the body.

Mushrooms and Cordyceps

Mushrooms are not plants but fungi. Many are delicious to eat and contain powerful medicinal properties. Here is an interesting factoid: in evolutionary terms, mushrooms are closer to humans than plants. They have been used for thousands of years as a staple of Chinese medicine and in ancient Egypt and Rome for their longevity properties, and over 2,000 species are edible as a great low-calorie source of fiber, protein, and antioxidants.

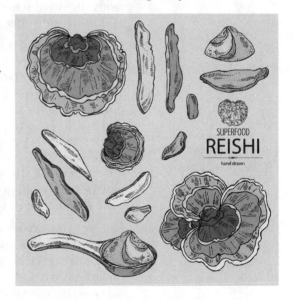

Mushrooms can mitigate the risk of developing a variety of diseases including cancer, diabetes, heart disease, and Alzheimer's. They contain selenium, copper, thiamin, magnesium, zinc, potassium, phosphorous, and other vitamins and minerals, and they taste great, too. Mushrooms have been shown in many studies to boost the immune system by stimulating microphages that enhance the body's ability to fight off foreign bodies. They are linked to weight loss and improvement of body mass index, and because of their high antioxidants such as beta glucans, they reduce hypertension, balance blood sugar levels, and heal metabolic disorders.

Reishi mushrooms are favored in Chinese medicine, where they are known as the "spirit plant" and used to fend off many types of diseases.

The most popular mushrooms are:

- Crimini: Used in salads and cooking, easy to find. Native to North America and Europe. They come in white and brown colors and have the telltale rounded cap. Along with button and portobello, crimini mushrooms are the most widely used.

- Chaga: The king of medicinal mushrooms, chock full of antioxidants that fight cancer, heart disease, stomach issues, and more. Polysaccharides boost the immune system and fight off infections. A single cup of chaga tea has the same antioxidants as 30 carrots.

- Cordyceps: Long, squiggly mushrooms that boost strength, increase stamina, support balanced blood sugar levels, increase energy and vitality, and lessen symptoms of bronchitis and breathing problems. These are parasitic fungi, but don't let that creep you out. They also reduce triglyceride levels and promote heart health as anti–inflammatories, and their beta glucans increase the amount of adenosine triphosphate (ATP) in the blood, which gives energy and provides optimal cell function.

- Lion's Mane: They look like cauliflower or pom–poms but pack a punch to improve mood and memory, stimulate new neuron growth, reverse aging's effects on cognitive thinking, and may even fight off cancerous tumors. This lesser–known species also heals digestive issues and protects the nervous system, all with no known side effects.

- Reishi: A staple of traditional Chinese medicine, these mushrooms have an ancient record of healing and preventing disease and are called "the spirit plant" because they relax the body and the mind. They also fight off viruses, boost the immune system, heal skin disorders, fight cancers, fight diabetes, kill bacteria and parasites, and battle HIV, hepatitis, and heart and liver disease. Reishi's properties create a sense of well–being and reduce anxiety and depression. They are bitter to eat but great in a tea or ground into a protein drink. They also contain antihistamines that can eliminate or reduce allergy symptoms, and they fight free radicals with their abundance of vitamins A, C, beta carotene, and selenium.

- Shitake: This savory mushroom is eaten the world over and contains immune–boosting compounds that also fight off heart problems and cancer. Native to East Asia, they come in colors from tan to dark brown and have their trademark large caps. They are great in meals because they are low in calories with high fiber and nutrients, including the same amount of important amino acids found in meat. The sterols, lipids, terpenoids, and polysaccharides all serve to boost the immune system and fight tumors, and the lentinan inhibits the growth of leukemia cells. These compounds also lower bad cholesterol, reduce artery wall plaque that can lead to a stroke or heart attack, and, in Chinese medicine, the shitake is known to increase longevity.

Some mushrooms are poisonous, so if you decide to go foraging for them out in the woods, be sure to know which can be safely consumed. Never guess. Also check with your doctor or pharmacist for possible countereffects with any medications you are taking. Some people find it hard to stomach mushrooms in their food, but they are also available in tea and supplement forms.

Magical Mystical Mushrooms

A growing body of research and scientists encourages the legalization of psychedelics, including mushrooms, for treating depression, anxiety, and mental disorders. In a February 12, 2019, article for *Healthline* titled "Mushrooms as Medicine? Psychedelics May Be Next Breakthrough Treatment," Gigen Mammoser looks at the growing use of magic mushrooms to treat depression, anxiety disorders, and alcoholism as part of a potential treatment plan that includes "psilocybin therapy sessions." Other studies have been conducted at Harvard, Stanford, King's College, Imperial College, Mount Sinai, the University of California at Berkeley, and the University of Zurich among other notable university research centers. Psychedelics are shown to improve the following:

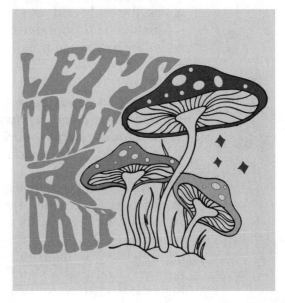

- Anxiety
- Depression
- Obsessive-compulsive disorder
- PTSD
- Addiction
- Eating disorders
- Dementia

Research studies have been looking at and continue to look at the use of these mushrooms as part of therapies that could benefit from the active ingredient, psilocybin, which accounts for the psychedelic properties that include feelings of euphoria, altered states of percep-

The psychedelic properties of some mushrooms that contain psilocybins first gained popularity in the hippie culture of the 1960s.

tion and sense of time and space, hallucinations, and mystical experiences. Researchers seek FDA approval for these medicinal mushrooms, still considered a Schedule 1 drug, that affect the mind and spirit and create a sense of connection and openness that harkens back to the 1960s hippie era.

Several studies have used psilocybin therapy for depression, enough to give it a "breakthrough therapy" designation to fast-track current research and inspire more to come. Trials have been ongoing at the Usona Institute, a psychedelic research center, and Johns Hopkins University School of Medicine has conducted its own pilot study that showed psilocybin therapy can help stop smoking. The head of that study, Matthew Johnson, Ph.D., also stated that psilocybin could potentially treat alcohol and cocaine addiction. Another study done by Dr. Charles Grob of the UCLA David Geffen School of Medicine found promising preliminary results using psilocybin to treat anxiety of people with cancer or at the end-of-life stage.

Aside from medical uses, psilocybin can also help the spirit by increasing perception and a sense of openness and connection. They can also increase creativity and inspiration while dissolving ego and a sense of separation from others. This kind of profound spiritual shift can be important for improving overall well-being because if the spirit is sick, the body and mind will follow. Psychedelics have been known to dissolve ego boundaries and create a oneness with all, which is why they became so popular during the Woodstock era of peace, love, and understanding.

Psychedelics have been known to dissolve ego boundaries and create a oneness with all, which is why they became so popular during the Woodstock era of peace, love, and understanding.

A study in the *Journal of Psychopharmacology* in 2011 titled "Mystical Experiences Occasioned by the Hallucinogen Psilocybin Lead to Increases in the Personality Domain of Openness" found that subjects were affected by psylocibins in five broad domains of the personality: neuroticism, extroversion, openness, agreeableness, and conscientiousness and that a significant increase in openness occurred with higher doses. All were suggested to lead to mystical-type experiences.

Today, many seek out these experiences and use small or micro-doses of psilocybin, while others are braver in consuming larger amounts, but under no circumstances does this book promote any use without first doing your research and talking with your doctor, as preexisting conditions or medications could be countereffective. Another issue arises in finding a quality product if you don't look for it yourself and make sure that what you are taking is what you think you are taking. As the body of research grows, the FDA approval of these products may be right around the corner, opening up the mind and spirit to a whole new level of well-being. Microdosing exposes you to a subperceptual dose of the psychedelic to see how your body and nervous system respond and how well you can still function with daily activities. Most people who start with these tiny amounts find that it is just enough to help them focus better, reduce anxiety levels, improve mood, and impart a sense of expansiveness, clarity, and unity, which is why microdosing is being researched as a treatment for ADHD.

People who have experienced these psychedelics report greater capacities for empathy, compassion, connection to nature and the planet, lower incidents of domestic violence and crime, more interest and engagement in spiritual practices, and a higher level of concern for the environment and fellow human beings.

Weight-loss Wonders

Some of the best herbs to consider for weight loss work to boost metabolism, assist in fat burning, and accelerate the body's own ability to get rid of body fat and prevent storing more of it in the cells. Remember, no herb will help you shed pounds if it isn't part of a healthy lifestyle of eating right and moving your body.

- Turmeric supports healthy blood sugar levels and prevents excess body fat gain.
- Cayenne pepper boosts metabolism, thanks to the capsaicin, to burn more calories while cutting cravings for fats, salt, and sweets.
- *Hoodia gordonii* can suppress the appetite and reduce caloric intake.
- *Gymnema* balances blood sugar levels and blocks sugar absorption.
- Cumin may help decrease body fat and works on lowering triglycerides and LDL cholesterol (the bad one).
- Dandelion contains chicoric acid, an effective weight-loss compound, and breaks down fat in the blood.
- Cinnamon contains cinnamaldehyde, which normalizes blood sugar and reduces belly fat.

The Amazing Benefits of Hawthorn Berries

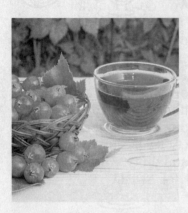

Hawthorn berries are excellent for lowering blood pressure and treating heart disease. They can be eaten as is, made into jams and jellies, fermented in wine or vinegar, or steeped in a tea.

As far back as 659 C.E., China has records of hawthorn berries used to support the health of the heart and, in the 1800s, these berries were widely used to treat high blood pressure, heart failure, and heart disease.

An abundance of new research shows how this amazing berry extract has anti-inflammatory and anti-atherosclerotic effects. It is also a potent antioxidant and works to heal digestive issues, including constipation, and improve liver function. The high polyphenol content has been demonstrated to improve skin elasticity and density, and the berries include properties that fight aging.

It is the rich flavonoids found in these berries that can reverse heart disease, support a healthy liver and digestive system, and improve the look of your skin. The extract from the berries also acts as a vasodilator to raise nitric oxide levels in the blood and increase the heart's working capacity as well as reduce lipid retention and vascular plaque formation. The berries also contain fiber, which acts as a probiotic to improve healthy gut bacteria, and even have protective properties on the stomach lining.

The flavonoids found in hawthorn leaves are so potent that they have been shown to improve liver health even in cases of nonalcoholic fatty liver disease.

Studies have also shown that these berries reduce blood pressure and have no side effects like many popular blood pressure medications do. Specific flavonoids in the berry extract benefit the body's connective tissue, increase local circulation, boost collagen building, and make skin look and feel better with fewer wrinkles.

Hawthorn plants grow throughout North America in the wild and in many gardens and have thorns and an applelike fruit that can be red or black. It is a member of the rose family and has white and pink flowers. The plants grow well in most garden conditions if you want to cultivate your own supply. Hawthorn can be also consumed in teas made with the leaves and/or berries or supplements if the berries are hard to find. Studies have shown that supplementation can take about six to eight weeks to see the best benefits. The *Journal of the American College of Cardiology* reported, according to a paper published titled "Foundation Task Force on Clinical Expert Consensus Documents," that the ideally effective dosage should be 300 milligrams per day. Make sure to look for any unnecessary fillers, too.

Keep in mind that the seeds of the plant are toxic and can be lethal to a small child. Never consume them!

- Ginger stimulates metabolism and promotes a flat belly.
- Milk thistle promotes improved blood glucose levels, improves body mass index, and flushes toxins from the body.
- Ginseng elevates energy levels and promotes the oxidation of fat.
- Yerba mate increases thermogenesis, boosts metabolism, and suppresses appetite.
- Green coffee beans promote metabolism and help reduce storage of body fat.

Always check with your doctor before taking any of these for weight loss, especially if you are taking pharmaceuticals that may have a countereffect. Many of the above ingredients come in tea form, a good starting point to see if they work for you.

In addition to the above herbs, current scientific studies are finding the importance of probiotics and gut health for weight loss. Without a healthy gut, it will be almost impossible to lose excess weight. It is also critical to detox the body from chemicals and toxins as much as possible. The latest science shows that an increasing toxic load from the environment, food, and water are getting in the way of our natural detox pathways, leading to unwanted weight gain, hormone imbalances, fatigue, and brain fog. Many of the above herbs have detoxing properties that can aid weight loss from that standpoint as well.

Live a Longer Life with These Herbs

Nature is filled with plants and herbs that increase longevity and fight the signs of aging in humans. You might say that much of what ages us comes from our overly processed diets and consuming toxins as well as the exposure we get in the air, our water, and the medications we take. Staying youthful and healthy becomes a tougher fight as we are exposed to more aging chemicals, foods, products, and stressors.

What follows are some top youth-extending herbs that can be consumed in foods or as supplements, extracts, or essential oils:

- Turmeric is a powerhouse yellow spice that seems to show up on every list of herb benefits. That's because it has antioxidant and anti-inflammatory properties that inhibit the expression of pro-inflammatory genes, which are behind many age-related diseases. This includes cancer, heart disease, Alzheimer's, and metabolic disorders causing obesity and diabetes. The natural compound in turmeric, curcumin, is known for its ability to slow aging and postpone the onset of these diseases. It's difficult to consume enough of it to do this, so a supplement works best to get the advantages of this amazing herb.

- Also known for promoting youthful vitality and health is the Ayurvedic mainstay Ashwagandha, which because of its adaptogen properties helps the body ward off stress, protect the cells against damage, and improve the function of nerves and the brain. The endcaps of our chromosomes, known as telomeres, have a lot to do with how our cells age. The shorter these telomeres become, the more we age internally and externally. Ashwagandha's antioxidant properties not only increase the beneficial telomerase activity but also stop the shortening of telomeres to increase life span.

- Cinnamon not only makes foods and drinks delicious, but the extract also promotes expression of collagen to make skin more elastic and youthful. It promotes systemic good health, which is of benefit to increasing longevity, thanks to its antioxidants and anti-inflammatories and also its ability to heal wounds, protect the liver and heart, lower blood sugar and blood pressure, and inhibit the markers known to cause Alzheimer's disease. Cloves also have these properties, and both have been shown to extend the life span of roundworms by modulating multiple longevity genes involved in stress response and insulin signaling. Cloves contain eugenol, which inhibits oxidative stress and age-related diseases.

- Ginger has several active compounds that are antiaging, including 6-gingerol and 6-shogaol. Both prevent oxidative stress and the types of inflammation that lead to age-related disease. These compounds fight high blood pressure, diabetes, atherosclerosis, Parkinson's disease, and Alzheimer's disease and can be consumed as food or in teas and supplements.

- Cilantro adds a kick of color to any meal, and the seeds, known as coriander, have many age-fighting properties. The leaf extract protects the skin against aging caused by too much sun exposure. Cilantro protects the body from neurotoxins such as mercury found in dental fillings, and the leaves have been used in many detox formulas to protect the liver from heavy metals.

- Ginseng has a beneficial effect on the human brain and improves learning and memory in the elderly. It includes three different species: Korean, Chinese, and American. Ginseng is chock full of hundreds of phytochemicals that are antiaging and prevent oxidative stress, inflammation, aging skin, declining immune system, tumor growth, and neurological disorders. It also protects the skin from UV radiation sun damage.

Cilantro protects the body from neurotoxins such as mercury found in dental fillings, and the leaves have been used in many detox formulas to protect the liver from heavy metals.

Other antiaging, longevity-promoting herbs and plants include *Ginkgo biloba*, which prevents mitochondrial dysfunction that can lead to neurological cell death; milk thistle, which contains active components that reduce damage in the liver from free radicals; Gotu kola, used as the "elixir of life" in ancient Chinese medicine for its active compounds that revitalize the brain and nervous system and improve wound healing and growth of new skin cells; resveratrol, found primarily in red grape skins and wine and strengthens the heart, lowers bad cholesterol levels, fights cancer, and stimulates production of SIRT 1, which benefits mitochondrial function; blueberries, with their life-expanding polyphenols that prevent cancer, obesity, and degenerative diseases; grapeseed extract, which has more powerful antioxidant effects than vitamins C and E and beta-carotene and assists in the synthesis of collagen and elastin for more youthful skin; and the perennial herb bacopa, a mainstay in Ayurvedic medicine that improves brain health as you age as well as memory and cognitive abilities.

With the many expensive antiaging skin products on the market that contain allergens and fillers or are way too cost-prohibitive and with the various injections and surgeries available to tighten skin for a more youthful appearance, it's good to know that nature has some cheaper and less dangerous equivalents:

- Pycnogenol, or pine bark, in its extract form of supplementation has been shown to improve the hydration and elasticity of skin. It can also speed up wound healing and reduce scarring.
- Astaxanthin, obtained from marine algae, is not an herb per se, but it is a potent oral and topical antioxidant and antiaging nat-

ural alternative. The reddish pigment that belongs to a group of chemicals called carotenoids is what gives color to salmon, shrimp, lobster, and trout. It not only can be applied topically to the skin but can also be taken as a supplement. Its many effects include fewer wrinkles, more skin elasticity, reduced redness from UV rays and sun exposure, reduction of undereye puffiness, and a reduction of wrinkle depth.

- Boswellia's gum resin contains compounds including boswellic acids that in skin creams can significantly improve sun damage, fine lines, and skin elasticity.

- Camu-camu berries contain compounds that prevent aging and have a high content of vitamin C, all of which stimulate the production of collagen and prevent sun exposure damage.

- Aloe vera can provide antiaging benefits when applied topically or taken orally. It heals burns and wounds, and the gel is so rich in vitamins and enzymes that it can soothe acne and sunburn. Taken orally, it offers significant improvement in skin elasticity and increased production of collagen. The sterols found in the plant reduce facial wrinkles and produce more collagen and hyaluronic acid, which is found in many expensive face creams.

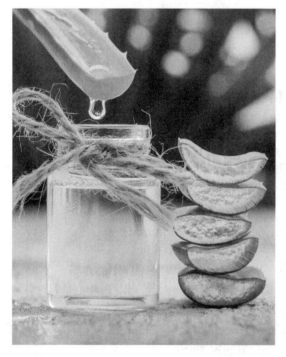

The succulent plant aloe vera is well known for how it can treat burns and cuts, and it is also found in many face creams.

- Maple leaf extract, like Botox injections, tightens the skin and makes it smoother but without the high cost and potentially dangerous side effects. The red leaves contain over 100 phenolic compounds that maintain skin elasticity, lighten age spots, and reduce skin inflammation.

Using natural extracts and supplementation is far less expensive than purchasing products that often contain ingredients that can trigger allergies, rashes, and a sore wallet or pocketbook. Nature has provided everything needed for battling the effects of aging, both internally and externally.

Does Collagen Really Improve Skin?

Collagen is a protein that is naturally produced in the body. It helps improve the elasticity of and increase blood flow to the skin and reduces visible wrinkles and fine lines. It is one of the building blocks for bones, skin, hair, muscles, tendons, and ligaments and helps us look more youthful.

In our twenties, we start to lose collagen. During menopause, women lose up to 30 percent of normal collagen production, which is why older skin starts to sag and wrinkle. Many women–and men, too–turn to collagen powders, supplements, and creams to restore some of that lost skin elasticity and plumpness. It can be thought of as the glue holding blood vessels, corneas, and teeth together, too, as it is a building block of these things.

The body contains 16 different types of collagen, with four main types that focus on supporting skin, bones, organs, tissues, tendons, teeth, and joints. Some dermatologists and experts feel that collagen supplementation is beneficial; others don't quite agree. Dermatologist Dr. Ohara Alvaz was interviewed for Cedars-Sinai's health blog and states that evidence of collagen supplements being of benefit is not definitive. She says the issue is how we ingest things and how they are broken down and absorbed into the bloodstream, and it is not clear on how ingested collagen does enter the bloodstream. "I tell patients the jury is still out on taking collagen," she says, adding that if they pick a safe collagen product, it won't do much harm. She suggests focusing on products made with retinol and vitamin C, which have been demonstrated to work to improve skin.

Collagen peptide powder can be mixed into smoothies, foods, juices, soups, and even baked goods without changing their texture.

Other research shows that taking collagen supplements as collagen peptides can play a protective role against disease development and progression and improve the appearance of the skin by minimizing wrinkles. Supplements may also increase muscle mass. It all comes down to doing research into what collagen supplements are best and of the highest quality. Collagen peptide powder can be mixed into smoothies, foods, juices, soups, and even baked goods without changing their texture. Marine collagen made from fish skin is a good option.

When choosing a supplement, it is important to look for collagen that comes in a hydrolyzed form, which means it has been broken down to promote better digestion and absorption when consumed.

Look for collagen peptides marked as Type I and Type III to get the best collagen proteins, and make sure they are not derived from GMO cows. Look for grass-fed derived collagen powders, which can come in different flavors, and watch out for fillers and additives.

You can also eat foods high in antioxidants to help prevent the breakdown of your own natural collagen. Getting adequate levels of copper and vitamin C help the body make procollagen, which contains the amino acids glycine and proline, so foods such as fruits, bell peppers, strawberries, egg whites, cabbage, mushrooms, dairy, organ meats, sesame seeds, cashews, lentils, and cocoa powder all boost natural production. Eating too much sugar and processed food destroys the actions of collagen in the body.

The Powerhouse Seed

Growing throughout Eastern Europe, the Middle East, and the western part of Asia is a small shrub with purple or white flowers called *Nigella sativa*. The fruit of this shrub contains tiny, black seeds that have been a part of natural medicinal remedies for thousands of years and were even found in the tomb of King Tut. These seeds have been used for healing and protection and have also gone by the names of black cumin, black caraway seed, and black onion seed. What makes these seeds stand out as one of nature's powerhouses is the oil made from them and the health benefits it imparts.

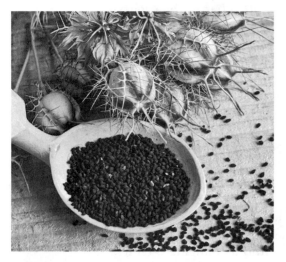

Nigella sativa is also known as black caraway seed, black cumin, and black onion seed. The oil has many uses ranging from controlling high blood pressure and inflammation to treating psoriasis and acne.

Black seed oil has been used to treat everything from asthma to high blood pressure, skin issues, high cholesterol, rheumatoid arthritis, stomach upset and cramps, acne, psoriasis, and more. It has antibacterial, antifungal, and anti-inflammatory properties. The part of the oil called thymoquinone has been shown in studies to reduce tumor growth in rats, and the oil has also been shown to reduce damage caused by radiation to kill cancerous cells. It also enhances natural killer T cells, which fight viral infections and improve the immune system.

Studies at the Indian Council of Medical Research found that black seed oil causes a partial regeneration of pancreatic cells, lowers elevated serum glucose levels, and lowers serum insulin concentrations. It also protects against liver damage from hepatic ischemia reperfusion injury and protects the liver tissue from toxic metals, including radioactive chemicals such as cadmium. The oil also promotes skin health and softness, and research has found the oil beneficial in fighting obesity by reducing inflammation, increasing liver health, improving glucose intolerance, and regulating glucose levels.

You can take a quality supplement; grind the seeds to sprinkle on salads, soups, curries, flatbreads, or toasted bagels; or add them into other seasonings such as cumin seeds, mustard, and fennel. The oil can be taken orally or applied to the skin and hair.

The Power of Carminative Herbs

When it comes to digestion, carminative herbs and plants do wonders to aid the digestive tract, stopping gas, bloating, and nausea. These herbs contain volatile compounds traditionally used in natural healing. The phytonutrients provide therapeutic support to the digestive system. Many of these herbs are already in the average diet, such as garlic, onions, ginger, fennel, peppermint, mint, and cinnamon.

Carminative herbs work in several ways. They modulate intestinal contractions and stimulate the flow of bile in the digestive tract. They also reduce surface tension inside the intestines, which decreases abdominal pain and bloating. They also have an antifoaming property, which lowers the number of CO_2 bubbles and helps expel gas pockets more easily, which reduces discomfort. They are antimicrobial and heal good gut microflora while destroying bad gut bacteria. The high levels of antioxidants found in these herbs fight cancer and repair tissue. Certain spices can also relieve menstrual cramps, such as cardamom and peppermint, which also work to alleviate stomach cramps in general.

Carminative herbs include peppermint, spearmint, basil, black pepper, ginger, garlic, onion, oregano, myrtle, tarragon, saffron, holy basil, chamomile, caraway seed, fennel, avocado, lemon verbena, dill, rosemary, celery seed, catnip, sesame, cayenne pepper, cumin, escarole, hyssop, angelica root, and parsley. You can use these herbs in a variety of ways: as herbal teas, in the form of essential oils, consumed as foods, juiced with greens and veggies, or included in fermented foods and drinks. Many can be used as fresh herbs and seasonings on salads and meals.

Herbs You Can Grow in a Jar of Water

You can grow many herbs at home, but some only require a glass or jar of water, and the first two just need a sprig or stem with leaves to get started. The next three should have the root intact; you can buy the plants first, then replant a couple of roots and stems in a glass or jar. No soil or dirt needed! Try the following in a mason jar or large glass:

- Mint (grows from a sprig)
- Oregano (grows from a sprig)
- Basil (grows from a root)
- Thyme (grows from a root)
- Rosemary (grows from a root)

Other herbs can be grown around the house or outdoors from seeds purchased at the store but will require pots and dirt. Once your water-grown plants begin to take root, replant them traditionally as well as in your garden or in a pot with nourishing soil. No need to run to the store next time you're out of fresh basil for your salad or sauce.

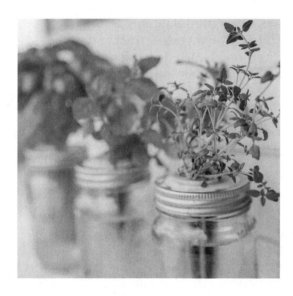

Herbs such as basil, mint, and thyme are easily grown at home using jars filled with water.

Plants as Natural Air Purifiers and Cleaners

Indoor air is typically more polluted than outdoor air, and we are exposed to it for hours and hours at a time every day of the week. Items such as furniture, upholstery, cleaning products, and synthetic building materials emit toxic chemicals such as benzene and formaldehyde into your home or office. Nature has provided us with many indoor plants known to reduce chemicals and volatile organic compounds (VOCs) as an alternative to fans and machines for purifying the air in your home or at work.

NASA was one of the first organizations to research the use of houseplants as air cleaners back in the 1980s when it teamed with the Associated Landscape Contractors of America to figure out ways to purify air at space facilities. NASA determined that plants were a great choice to get rid of toxins and improve air quality both in the space-craft and in your home. Here are the top choices:

NASA determined that plants were a great choice to get rid of toxins and improve air quality both in the spacecraft and in your home.

- Aloe vera: This succulent plant has been around for thousands of years. It is known for the gel it produces to aid in the healing of cuts and burns. It also cleans the air of formaldehyde and ben-zene, which are emitted by some paints and chemical-based cleaners used in the home or office. It is easy to grow yourself and easy to maintain.

- Areca palm: This small, cluster-forming palm plant comes from Madagascar and requires bright, filtered light with shade from the sun. It cleans the air of benzene, carbon monoxide, formaldehyde, trichloroethylene, and xylene and was rated the most efficient air-purifying plant by NASA and the Associated Landscape Contrac-tors of America.

- Azalea: A colorful, flowering shrub that reduces the amount of formaldehyde throughout your home; it grows best in cool tem-peratures with some sunlight. The flowers come in a variety of colors, but the nectar and leaves can be toxic to small children and pets, so keep on high shelves.

- Bamboo palm: Also known as the reed palm, the bamboo palm needs a location in the house or office with full sun or bright light. It is pet friendly and cleans the air of benzene, trichloroethylene, and formaldehyde.

- Chinese evergreen: This perennial comes from the tropical forests of China and produces blooms and berries that clean the air of benzene, carbon monoxide, formaldehyde, and trichloroethylene.

- Chrysanthemum: A popular household plant with bright flowers that clean the air of benzene. The plant needs plenty of bright light and sun for full-blooming flowers and comes in many colors that will go with any home or office décor, but pick the floral va-riety and not the garden variety.

- English ivy: English ivy thrives in less light and needs to be wa-tered often. It cleans the air of benzene, carbon monoxide, for-maldehyde, trichloroethylene, and mold allergens.

- Gerbera daisy: This colorful flower filters out benzene and trichloroethylene and needs plenty of sunlight and well-drained soil. You can find a variety of colors at the local nursery.

- Golden pothos: Golden pothos is a vine, so it works great in a hanging basket and any light but direct sunlight. It is easy to care for and cleans the air of formaldehyde, xylene, toluene, benzene, and carbon monoxide.

- Peace lily: This is a smaller plant, but it works just as well as larger plants to clean the air of formaldehyde, benzene, and trichloroethylene. The peace lily was at the top of NASA's list for removing formaldehyde, benzene, and trichloroethylene: the three most common VOCs. This plant needs shade and weekly watering in order to flower for most of the summer months.

- Red-edged dracaena: With more than 40 varieties available, this shrub can grow as tall as your ceiling. Do not have around pets, as it can be toxic. It cleans the air of xylene, trichloroethylene, and formaldehyde.

- Snake plant: This plant likes dry weather and a little sun and cleans the air of benzene and formaldehyde, common in cleaning products, toilet paper, tissues, and personal-care products. It is one of the hardest houseplants to kill. These plants are typically used in bathrooms because they thrive in low light and humidity. Snake plants absorb carbon dioxide and release oxygen at night, the opposite of most plants, so they work wonders in your bedroom to boost oxygen and improve sleep.

- Spider plant: This is a resilient plant with little, white flowers and doesn't need to be watered a lot. It is also fine for children and pets to be around. It cleans the air of formaldehyde, carbon dioxide, and xylene and loves cool to average temperatures and bright, indirect sunlight. The flowers will turn into baby spider plants called "spiderettes."

- Weeping fig/ficus: Ficus plants are more high maintenance, requiring bright, indirect light. You must allow the soil to dry between watering, but when cared for well, they last years and years and clean the air of formaldehyde, benzene, and trichloroethylene. Because these chemicals are found in carpeting and furniture, place these plants in bedrooms and living rooms.

The Power of Movement

Well-being begins with a healthy body. Diet is only one part of the equation. It is just as important to get adequate exercise and daily movement to avoid the many diseases associated with a sedentary lifestyle, including heart disease, stroke, cancer, diabetes, and many others. Obesity is skyrocketing, in all age groups, as we adapt to a society that shuns being outdoors doing things, playing, and moving around in favor of sitting in front of computer and phone screens.

Movement is critical to feeling your best, but it doesn't have to mean hours of grueling work at the gym on monstrous machines or running for hours at a time to the point of exhaustion. We all know that getting enough exercise is important. We have the DVD programs, the YouTube videos, the exercise bikes, the hand weights, the home machines, and the expensive gym memberships, yet rarely do we feel at our best. Exercise has become a chore rather than a way to connect body, mind, and spirit. It focuses way too much on just the physical and not enough on embracing a more holistic perspective, one that takes every aspect of who we are into account.

Hundreds of books, DVDs, and programs about aerobics and weightlifting are out there; you don't need another. We have exercise bikes and treadmills today that talk back to you and show you gorgeous landscapes from all over the world as you huff and sweat. We don't need anything else. When it comes to moving more, we have apps and smart watches that count our steps and bracelets that time us as we walk or run. We have so much technology linked to exercise you'd think everyone would be incredibly healthy.

We know that exercise not only helps us look better, but it also boosts heart health, improves oxygen flow to the organs and brains, boosts the release of human growth hormone (HGH), which is necessary to stay youthful in every way, lowers levels of stress and anxiety, lowers the risk of dying of several diseases, keeps blood pressure levels regulated, burns excess body fat, and a host of other great things. We are told by our doctors, government, and public health agencies to get more exercise. We know that the healthiest people are those who exercise on a regular basis, but too many of us still don't feel motivated enough to get up off our butts and do it.

We know that the healthiest people are those who exercise on a regular basis, but too many of us still don't feel motivated enough to get up off our butts and do it.

Something seems to be missing, and it's not another "program." What you may need instead are suggestions for making movement a more integrated, beneficial, and natural part of your day that keeps you in shape while also destressing your mind, harmonizing your emotions, and bringing you back to the present moment. Movement that means something. Movement that matters.

All over the world, cultures recognize that staying healthy is more than just running a marathon a week. It's about finding balance and harmony between the external and internal, between the physical, mental, and spiritual. We may think our bodies are just a mass of bone, tissue, and blood, but they are a vehicle through which we live our lives. Therefore, the ways we ask our bodies to move are paramount to total well-being. If we run them into the ground, our mind follows, and vice versa. Finding ways to incorporate movement into everyday life that serves all our needs on every level is key. Yes, you can still use the equipment and go to the gym and run that marathon, but also take the time to breathe into a yoga pose, do a nature walk while you chant silently, or dance your way across the living room floor, whether or not someone is watching.

Dangers of the Sedentary Lifestyle

Leading a sedentary or inactive lifestyle leads to as many diseases and conditions as a terrible diet. The two together can be your ticket to dying sooner or living with some major conditions that are like a ticking time bomb. Hundreds of studies exist documenting the results of sitting too much:

- Obesity
- Heart disease and stroke
- Cancer
- High blood pressure
- High cholesterol
- Low immunity
- Low metabolism
- Insulin resistance
- Poor blood and body fluid circulation
- Muscle loss
- Loss of bone density and minerals
- Hormonal imbalance
- Accelerated aging
- Osteoporosis
- Type 2 diabetes

Although experts say that exercise only contributes 15 percent to weight loss, with diet contributing 85 percent, exercise does assist in burning excess body fat and keeping one's metabolism working optimally. It also helps to strengthen the heart and lungs and improve circulation, so weight loss is not the only benefit one should consider when taking up an exercise program. Limited activity packs on pounds because the body never gets around to burning off those excess calories, not to mention that if all you do is eat and sit, your body will always burn fat from food and never tap into your own fat stores, so you stay fat.

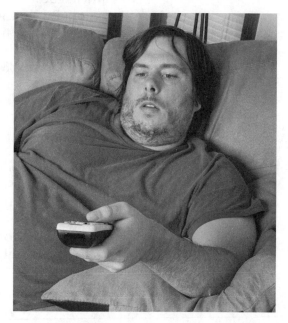

Being sedentary doesn't just make you fat and weak, it can lead to high cholesterol, high blood pressure, diabetes, and osteoporosis.

The heart needs movement because sitting around all day allows blood flow in the lower extremities to slow or stagnate, according to cardiologist Robert Greenfield, M.D., in "8 Biggest Health Risks Associated with a Sedentary Lifestyle" by Elizabeth Blasi for the *Aaptiv* website. This increases the chances of the formation of blood clots that can travel up to the heart and lung areas. Exercising consistently also raises the good HDL cholesterol and lowers the bad LDL and triglycerides, which also protects you against heart disease and strokes. It also lowers blood sugar levels and increases insulin sensitivity to help you avoid Type 2 diabetes. This can be accomplished with a few brisk walks per week or other regular aerobic exercise.

Inactivity is a precursor to chronic diseases that can often be turned around with an exercise program or getting up and moving on a regular basis. No matter your age, getting into action can improve health markers tremendously, and obviously, the sooner you start, the better. Coupled with a healthier diet, it can mean the difference between being overweight, tired, sick, and miserable all the time and feeling younger than your age; being fit, healthy, and up for any challenge; and having a sense of overall well-being.

Blasi's article goes on to show how a sedentary lifestyle contributes to depression. Psychotherapist Kevon Owen is quoted as saying, "The body likes to move. It likes it so much that it responds to activity by producing dopamine, the brain's chemical that signals enjoyment." Not getting enough exercise feeds depression and makes it harder to deal with everyday challenges. You've heard of the runner's high, achieved after a certain amount of running, and this high is available to anyone who exercises. No, you don't have to run 20 miles to get the benefits of that burst of dopamine.

With our children indoors more often, glued to their gadgets and electronics, childhood obesity and chronic illnesses are skyrocketing, even childhood cancers. Previous generations grew up playing outside, but too many of today's kids rarely go walking, hiking, bike riding, swimming, or do outdoor sports. They are going to pay the price for it in their adult years unless parents encourage them to get up and get out and move.

Exercise Basics

Before we look at some of the different types of exercise programs available, let's look at how we can all incorporate more activity in our day–to–day lives. Doing housework, cleaning out the garage, gardening and mowing the lawn, standing while talking on the phone, taking stretching and movement breaks for every hour or so that you sit at your desk, walking to a colleague's office rather than emailing, taking the stairs instead of the elevator, having walking meetings with colleagues, getting a standing or treadmill desk, setting up a home gym, buying an exercise video or program if you can't join a gym, buying a medicine ball or set of dumbbells … the list goes on and on.

Making exercise and movement as pleasurable as possible is the key. The more you move throughout the day, the better....

You can even do exercises while watching television instead of sitting on the couch. Put down a yoga mat or a pair of weights in front of the TV or buy a treadmill or exercise bike that you can use while watching your favorite show. It makes the time go by faster and allows you to binge watch a few episodes of your favorite series while working out. This way, you get to have your cake and eat it, too, only you don't really eat cake. Making exercise and movement as pleasurable as possible is the key. The more you move throughout the day, the better, as you are not only burning extra calories but keeping your body active beyond the times you choose for your more structured exercise program. It all counts.

Always start out slow if you have any medical issues and build up to more activity when you can do so safely. It is our default setting to do things the easy way, so this may require some discipline and maybe a phone app to remind you to move, but it will soon become habit, one of the healthiest habits you can ever take on for yourself and for those who want you to be healthy.

Aerobics

Exercise can be categorized in two ways, both of which are beneficial for their own reasons. Most people are familiar with aerobic activity. The word aerobic means "with oxygen," which exemplifies this type of exercise. The intense, often repetitive and rhythmic activities that make up aerobics get the heart to pump oxygenated blood to working muscles so they can burn fuel and move the body. The body must have oxygen present to be able to burn carbohydrates or fat as fuel.

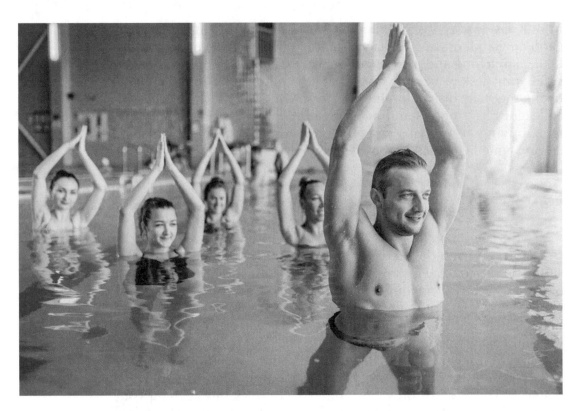

Doing aerobics in a pool is a great way to get exercise that has a low impact on your joints. Also, the water provides extra resistence.

Hundreds of studies show the benefits of aerobics, often called cardio because of the benefits to the cardiovascular system. The *World Journal of Cardiology* reported in multiple studies that aerobics improves cardiovascular health and especially lessens the risk of heart disease. It also reduces incidents of cancer, depression, osteoporosis, obesity, and diabetes, according to a host of studies done for the National Institutes of Health.

Most of us already get chided by our doctors to get more aerobic exercise. This can be everything from brisk walking to running, cycling, fast dancing, riding an elliptical, spin cycling, swimming, cross-country skiing, or anything else that sustains an elevated heart rate for at least 30 minutes. You can even get the benefits of aerobic activity by doing shorter, 10-minute workouts throughout the day. Aerobics use large muscle groups and work the heart, lungs, and core, so it's important to check with your doctor to see if you are okay to start a program. Those who have knee troubles will also do well to get a doctor's approval, as many aerobic activities like running are hard on the knees. Because of the fast pace and many moves that may involve jumping, the knees can take a real beating, as can a heart that has not had much activity for a while, so go slow and increase how much time you work out by five more minutes each week and how intense your workout is, working up to perhaps 80–90 percent heart rate capacity. Don't go all out. The rule of thumb is that you should be able to breathe!

Aerobics can help you keep your blood pressure under control and reduce fatigue by increasing lung capacity and stamina. You can lose weight and activate your immune system and human growth hormone, keeping you healthier and less likely to get sick. It's generally recommended that you do aerobics five days a week, or you can do them three to four times a week with two days in between for weight training and a day off.

Two of the most popular forms of aerobic exercise are walking and running. Walking for 30 minutes a day at a brisk pace, or even 10 minutes three times a day, is all you need, and you can always add five minutes each week to get to an hour. You can walk every day or have a rest day in between where you do some weights. If you are serious about walking, go to the nearest running shoe store and get fitted properly for a good pair of walkers. You will be glad you did.

Running is tougher on the knees and leg joints, but you do burn more calories. People love to run and get that "runner's high" when the endorphins kick in. You can start out with a jog and move up to a run over a period of weeks, always being careful to stretch before and after you run. Before you know it, you may be feeling the competitive bug to train for a 5K, then a half marathon, then a full marathon. Properly fitted running shoes are an absolute must. Don't go buy cheap running shoes thinking you can get away with it; you can't. A trained salesperson can help determine if you have arch issues, if you pronate, or if you need more heel or toe padding or more support on the sides with a wider fit. It's worth the time and the extra money if you desire to make running your exercise of choice. A general rule is to replace your running shoes every 500 miles or at visible signs of wear, whichever comes first.

Running does burn off more calories, almost double that of walking. An example from *Healthline* is that a person who weighs 160 pounds and runs 5 miles per hour burns about 606 calories. The same person walking briskly for the same amount of time at 3.5 miles per hour burns 314 calories. You would have to walk fast to catch up to the runner's calorie burn rate, but running is not appealing for many or may be too harsh on your knees or result in the dreaded shin splints that runners often contend with. Walking will give you a great workout and a boost in energy and is good for your heart and your mood.

Anaerobics

Short, intense bursts of physical activity are considered anaerobic and include exercises fueled by energy sources within contracting muscles and muscle groups. The word means "without oxygen," the opposite of aerobic, and that is because instead of the body receiving energy via oxygenated blood, it gets it when the body breaks down carbohydrates from blood glucose to glucose that is stored in the muscle. It requires much less time than aerobics to get the necessary benefits and calorie burn.

Anaerobics include weight and resistance training, sprinting, and high-intensity interval training.... The main goal is to increase muscle mass and strength....

Anaerobics include weight and resistance training, sprinting, and high–intensity interval training, which we will discuss below. The main goal is to increase muscle mass and strength, which is the result of stretching, contracting, and tearing muscle fibers. It is in the repair of those fibers that muscles become stronger and bigger.

Anaerobics boosts all health markers, including endurance, heart and lung capacity, stamina, and mood and self–esteem, as this type of exercise tones and sculpts muscles for a lean and defined look. If it involves weights, it should not be done on consecutive days to give the fibers time to repair themselves. This type of workout can burn more body fat than aerobics and is highly recommended to increase metabolic rate and help with weight loss, but both are necessary for overall physical health and complement each other. Some people do weight machine circuits at the gym to get both an aerobic and anaerobic workout at once.

Weightlifting Basics

Weight training, or resistance training, is probably the most popular and effective form of anaerobics for its ability to assist weight loss and sculpt the muscles. For older people, who lose more muscle mass as they age, weights can help reverse some of that loss and get them toned and strong again. One big benefit of weight training is that you burn calories even when resting after a workout. Starting a weight training program should require a little research to make sure you know what you are doing. The possibility of injuries is high with lack of proper form or doing too many reps with too high of a weight.

You have many options if you want to do weight training: going to a gym and getting personal training, buying a DVD program, or learning on YouTube are only a few, but your best bet is to start off with lower weights and more reps, working up to higher weights with fewer reps. The only way to truly build muscle is to tax it enough to cause the fiber tears that rebuild it bigger the next time around, and that often requires lifting to exhaustion. The end goal might be lifting so much weight that you can only complete five reps as opposed to using lighter weights and completing 15 reps, but it's that exhaustion point that will bring about the most visible and obvious changes to your body.

Resistance training can involve free weights, resistance bands, kettle bells, medicine balls, giant ropes, and machines; you should always ask the proper way to use these before just jumping on. You can also use your own body weight with planks, push-ups, pull-ups, and burpees. You should always warm up before you do weight work with some light aerobic activity to loosen up those muscles.

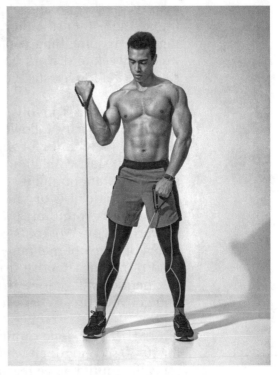

The key to weight training is to work various body groups consistently, starting with lighter weights and more reps, then increasing weight and de-creasing reps. You might start out with three sets of 15 reps per exercise, with a one- to two-minute rest period between sets. A rule of thumb is to inhale before you lift, then exhale as you lift, and never hold your breath. Work out no longer than 45 minutes in order to not overtax your muscles, always end with a good

Resistance training can also be achieved using strong bands.

stretch of the muscles you just worked, and don't work the same body group two days in a row.

Again, it's all about form, so it helps to get a few starter points from a personal trainer if you can. Women should not be afraid of weight work causing giant muscles. It won't happen. What will happen is that you will get the lean, defined look of someone who is athletic, strong, and healthy.

HIIT and SIT

Hundreds of modern scientific studies state that you do not have to exercise for hours at a time to get the benefits you seek: a stronger heart, healthier lungs, a lean body, and more muscle strength. Today, less is more, and people are finding ways to get their exercise needs into a smaller window of time.

Some people do enjoy a one-hour run or spending hours at a time pumping iron at the gym, but if you are not one of them, rest assured that you can get your workouts in within a shorter time frame. High-intensity interval training (HIIT), or sprint interval training (SIT), is something you can do in under 15 minutes three or four times a week and work your body, heart, and lungs even more efficiently than longer, steadier workouts.

HIIT and SIT involve bursts of activity at 80 percent or more of your total capacity, followed by a longer resting period, then you repeat this a few times for the duration of your workout. For example, you might start with 20 or 30 seconds of all-out jumping jacks to get your heart rate pumping, then follow with two minutes of slower activity like sidekicks or knee raises at a much lower rate of intensity, then another round of 20–30 seconds of all-out movement, then the slower activity. Workouts of this nature can be as short as four minutes, but the optimal range appears to be seven to 12 minutes of this kind of repetitive move from high bursts to lower rest periods. The rest periods still require that you move your body, but this is when you get your breath back for the next high-intensity burst.

SIT can be done running or walking, speeding up to full capacity for 20–30 seconds, then walking at a slower rate for a moment or two, repeating until you've reached the end of your desired workout time. Ample scientific evidence exists that these shorter and more intensive types of exercise work better to burn excess body fat while maintaining muscle mass. You can also do them holding hand weights for extra added strength training.

Even in the gym, working with hand weights and machines, it is possible to do HIIT. You do a fast circuit of a group of machines, doing your 20–30 reps at the highest weight possible, then taking a rest period in between of less weight or more simple body movement before getting on the next machine. You can focus on arms one day, then legs the next. Never work the same body group two days in a row to avoid overworking the muscles. They need that critical time to repair the tiny tears that are what make muscles bigger and stronger.

Never work the same body group two days in a row to avoid overworking the muscles. They need that critical time to repair the tiny tears that are what make muscles bigger and stronger.

Spin bikes and even the good old treadmill also work for HIIT workouts. Spin bikes–or any exercise bikes, for that matter–allow you to speed up and slow down and show you your heart rate as you do. Treadmills do this as well, and you can time yourself at a fast burst of walking or running, followed by a longer rest walk or run period.

Tons of HIIT and SIT books, videos, and resources are on the internet and in bookstores, or you can design your own program doing what you like to do (including planks and floor work). Please check first with your doctor to get the clear go–ahead before starting a program, especially if you are older, already obese, or have any current medical issues. Always warm up and cool down, too, and the consensus is to not do HIIT or SIT every day but rather every other day. Rest is just as important for building muscles and keeping the body from exercise overwhelm.

A smart approach would be to ease into a HIIT or SIT with a four– to five–minute, every–other–day workout schedule for a few weeks, then extend the time until you are challenging yourself. Can a shorter workout really improve health markers? Dr. Blake Livingood (yes, that is his name), a well–known chiropractor and champion of integrated well–being who runs his own health clinic, says in his article "6 Natural Ways to Lower Cholesterol" that high–intensity workouts can help lower cholesterol levels and optimize cholesterol ratios, eliminate Type 2 diabetes and regulate blood pressure, improve insulin sensitivity, boost fat metabolism and improve body fat percentage, and boost levels of human growth hormone. He suggests 10–minute workouts, and we can all find 10 minutes in our busy schedules to see those kinds of positive benefits to overall health, can't we? Dr. Livingood states that if we treat sickness and disease, we get sickness and disease. If we build health, we get health. It starts with diet and exercise.

If You Hate Exercising

Join the club. No, really. Join the club. People who hate exercising often just hate doing it alone. Running and walking is so much more pleasurable for some people if they find a buddy or a group to join. That group can be a competitive organization with meeting places and the goal of training for a race or marathon or just a bunch of neighbors or work colleagues who like the idea of walking at lunch-time or after work. Having people to motivate you on when you feel tired or expect you to be at the corner for the nightly run increases the chance that you will get out there and not find excuses if you only had yourself to account for.

Playing team sports or finding sports that must be done in groups is another way to keep yourself accountable to your exercise routine. Whether it be tennis or pickleball, ice skating or touch foot-ball, the social camaraderie is the extra boost needed to keep you coming back for more.

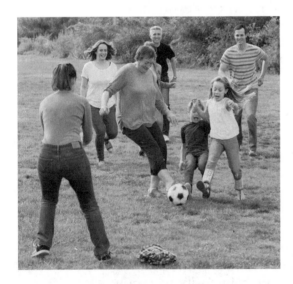
Going to the gym can, indeed, be boring for many people. So, get your exercise by doing something fun you enjoy with others such as playing ball in your backyard or at a local park. Just make sure to do it regularly and not just on holiday picnics!

The best way to exercise has always been the way you will do it, which means finding something you love to do instead of torturing yourself with rote move-ments. If it isn't fun, you won't keep it up. This explains why so many yearly gym memberships end up unused after three months and expensive home equipment gets used enthusiastically for a year, then left in the corner as a place to stack boxes on, hang clothes on, or be sold for one-fifth of the original price at the neighbor-hood garage sale. Sound familiar?

If it is an activity that you really enjoy doing on a long-term basis, you are far more likely to stick to it. You can always add something new later, but at least get started. Do things that you enjoy, and you are bound to keep exercise as a daily part of your life. By the way, do you know where the "10,000 steps a day" goal came from?

The Story behind the Steps

It's propaganda, folks. Sorry, but the origin of the 10,000 steps craze was nothing but a sales ploy. It began back in 1965 when a Japanese company created a device it called *manpo-kei*, which translates into "10,000 steps meter." The device was thought of right before the 1964 Olympic Games in Tokyo; the company wanted to name it something catchy that would sell its product. The name was nothing more than a cool marketing tool, but it took off like crazy and is now an ingrained part of our beliefs about exercising and staying healthy.

Do you really need to walk 10,000 steps a day to get the greatest health benefits? Several studies have tried to find out, including a study by I–Min Lee, a professor of medicine at Harvard Medical School, who looked at more than 16,000 women with a variety of step amounts to see which had more benefits. Each woman wore a measuring device for more accuracy. The women were followed for four years to see how many steps were associated with dying of any cause. By the end of the study, 504 women had died.

One might assume that the more steps these women took, the better, but the truth was a bit different. At the 7,500–steps–a–day mark, the benefits then plateaued and made no difference in life expectancy. Before that mark, the women who only took 2,700 steps a day were far more likely to die than those who took over 4,000 steps a day. Even such a small difference made a big impact on life expectancy.

 Women who did 4,400 steps a day had a 41 percent reduction in all-cause mortality. The range between 4,400–7,500 reaps many benefits, but after that, it's all marketing.

Survivors of the study averaged about 5,000 steps a day and could have gone as high as 7,500 to get the best benefits, but after that, it was not necessary and did nothing to increase the benefits at all. The study also found that the typical sedentary woman averaged only 2,700 steps a day. Women who did 4,400 steps a day had a 41 percent reduction in all–cause mortality. The range between 4,400–7,500 reaps many benefits, but after that, it's all marketing. No matter what, taking as many steps as you can is always going to be better than sitting all day, and wearing a tracking device is a great way to keep yourself on track and motivated.

Some ways to get more steps in:

- Take the stairs whenever you can
- Walk your dog every day
- Park far away from where you need to be, if it's safe
- Walk to the corner store instead of defaulting to driving there
- At home, move from room to room whenever possible and stand at your desk every now and then instead of sitting for hours at a time
- Get a treadmill

Movement Meditations

Movement meditations consist of things like walking and running, paying attention to the present moment and what you are experiencing with the five senses, and practices like tai chi and qigong, two Eastern movement practices, or yoga. Movement meditation gets the body actively engaged while the mind is quiet because all of one's focus is on a mantra being chanted silently or out loud or on the breathing.

Nature offers the best landscape for a walking meditation, with the sights, smells, and sounds being added benefits, but even a busy city street can become a meditative place if you listen to a guided visualization or meditation audio as you walk, keeping in mind to look up every now and then for your safety. The key is to get your mind into a slight trancelike state, a focused wavelength that brings about great calm, even as your body is doing some work. Walking or running meditations are best done alone, as having another person around might be a big distraction, but always do this in areas that are safe, preferably during the day.

First thing in the morning is a wonderful time for a movement meditation. Getting outside as the sun comes up not only keeps your circadian rhythms working properly (more on this in the sleep section), but it also allows you to start your day with a fresh mindset. The exercise you get is the icing on the cake. Some people love to do their yoga or tai chi practices in the light of the morning sun. A back-yard or park would be a great spot, but you can do this inside, too, if needed. Focusing on your breath as you watch the sun come up is a fabulous way to start each day with positivity that you cannot get from turning on the news or checking on stressful emails.

Move first, then do all the things later.

Tai Chi and Qigong

Tai chi is an ancient Chinese martial art made up of a series of gentle, flowing postures and movements done in a graceful and slow manner. Deep breathing during tai chi creates a powerful sense of calmness and inner strength. Originally, it was developed as a method of self-defense but evolved into a form of graceful exercise that anyone of any age can do. Pregnant women and people with back pain, hernias, or fractures should always check with their doctors first.

The "chi" refers to the invisible, subtle energy that is worked with during the movements and postures. Chi is meant to flow through the body with ease, so this practice serves to remove blocks to our access and flow of our own chi. It is sometimes referred to as "qi" and is over 2,500 years old, and the use of "chi" or "qi" helps connect us to the source of universal energy we all have access to and are ourselves made up of. As gentle as tai chi may look, expert masters can throw an attacker to the floor without effort using the movements and their internal energy. This is so subtle; observers cannot even see how they are able to do this.

It is a self-paced system of movements that can be done alone or in groups. As each posture flows right into the next, the body is al-ways in a state of flowing movement and stretching. Tai chi consists of many different styles, but the basic principles are the same. It is al-ways a low-impact form of exercise and stress relief and is not meant to be high intensity.

Tai chi benefits include:

* Lowered blood pressure
* Improved joint pain
* Improved flexibility
* Lowered stress levels

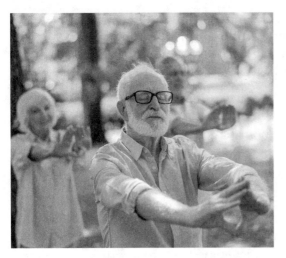

People who are older or who have physical limitations can get the benefits of tai chi through the less disciplined form called qigong, which is more free form and adaptive to people's

- Improved mood and energy
- Improved stamina, muscle strength, and definition
- Enhanced sleep quality
- Enhanced immune system
- Improved congestive heart failure symptoms
- Improved aerobic capacity

It is best to learn the movements from an expert teacher, especially in terms of breath work and balance work, but many instructional videos and programs are out there if you cannot physically attend a class.

Qigong works with the energy of qi or chi that permeates all things. It is also a movement practice that combines meditation with physical exercises and breathing for balance and harmony of the body, mind, and spirit and is a part of traditional Chinese medicine. It is described as a body–mind–spirit practice by the National Qigong Association; the term consists of the words "qi" (vital energy) and "gong" (skill cultivated through steady practice).

Like tai chi, qigong (sometimes spelled qi gong) improves mental and physical health through integrated postures, movement, breathing techniques, self-massage, sound, and focused intent. Many different styles of this practice exist, all of which make up what the NQA calls "an amazing energetic science."

Working with the life force, the energy that is qi has many benefits:

- Tones vital organs and connective tissue
- Improves circulation of blood and body fluids
- Improves blood pressure levels
- Helps alleviate stress
- Heals mental illness and chronic illness
- Deepens our connection with the physical world and universal energy
- Helps us in emotional and spiritual times of crisis
- Helps us cultivate a personal path or journey of self-discovery
- Restores health and well–being

Yoga

Yoga uses controlled breathing methods and specific body postures and poses to build strength, promote flexibility, and relax and focus the mind. Yoga is a spiritual practice that has its roots in ancient India but is hugely popular in the Western world. The first mention of the word yoga comes from the Rig Veda, a collection of ancient spiritual texts. The word comes from the Sanskrit word *yuj*, which means "union" or "to join." Yoga can be traced back over 5,000 years to northern India, but the most prevalent teachings come from a book called *The Yoga Sutras of Patanjali*; Patanjali was considered the father of yogic practice.

Many schools of yoga are found throughout Hinduism, Buddhism, and Jainism, but the more modern version known in the West is hatha yoga, using a form of postures called asanas, breathing techniques called pranayama, and meditation known as dyana. Yoga is

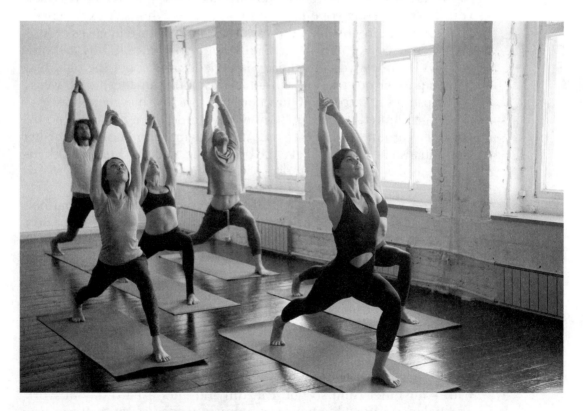

Yoga originated as a kind of meditation practice among Buddhists, Hindus, and Jains. Today, it has largely shed such connections to become a healthy exercise of mind and body in both the East and the West.

Natural Health

considered a form of exercise as well as a spiritual practice, for it works the muscles and builds incredible flexibility and range of motion. In a National Institutes of Health survey taken in 2017, one in seven adults in the United States alone practiced yoga at some time in the last 12 months. Approximately 94 percent do it for the wellness-related benefits, and about 20 percent do it for specific medical reasons. Even children are learning yoga as a way to deal with stress at school and home.

A large body of research points to the health benefits of yoga, and many modern doctors even prescribe it as a healing modality. Yoga helps to lessen pain, improve sleep, increase balance, relieve muscle stiffness, quit smoking, lose weight, release stress, lessen the effects of arthritis and fibromyalgia, and decrease chronic inflammation. It works to restore emotional, mental, and physical health, and for those who practice under an adept teacher or yogi, spiritual health, too.

Finding a yoga instructor and class takes time and research because you don't want someone teaching you asanas who isn't experienced. That can result in possible injuries, so ask around for references or look on review sites like Yelp. It's generally not a good idea to buy at-home yoga DVDs unless you are already knowledgeable about the right way to do a pose or posture. The author of this book can attest to how easy yoga postures may look but how hard they are to achieve and how easy it is to get injured if you don't know how to do them right and no instructor is around to correct you. An instructor who knows his or her stuff can also help you achieve the best results with the breath work involved, as it is an important part of the yoga practice.

However, many yoga websites and educational video channels can help you learn the basics if you cannot attend a class in person. Just use due diligence and do some research, especially reading those product reviews if buying a program, to see how others fared or if many associated injuries occurred. They can help you begin a yoga practice at home, but they do lack the social and spiritual community aspect of a class. It is a lot harder to learn the proper postures from a book or words on a page, so it is always best to have visuals to guide you.

Yoga, done alone or in a class, can become a wonderful practice for toning the body, improving health and well-being, getting in touch with your inner calm so you can unwind after a hard day at work, and balance a busy life with some much needed serenity. It is a way to keep the body and mind happy and the spirit fulfilled without having to adopt any religious beliefs that contradict with your own. Yoga involves physical, mental, and spiritual well-being in an open manner that allows anyone to benefit from it. Some yoga styles are more about burning off fat and high-intensity movements, while others are slow and meditative, so you may want to try a few classes to see what works for you. Many instructors will allow you to sit in and watch one class before committing to more.

Those who practice yoga usually do it for a lifetime because the ancient knowledge behind it works just as well today. The times may change, but finding ways to bring about a harmonic balance between the body, mind, and spirit never do. In the stressful times we live in, it's no wonder that yoga remains one of the most popular and widely practiced forms of movement and exercise.

Types of Yoga

The different types or styles of yoga serve to strengthen and tone the body while calming the mind and nourishing the spirit. They involve a variety of postures, breathing techniques, and meditation.

- Ashtanga: An ancient yoga teaching popularized during the 1970s with poses and asanas that link movement to breath. This is a set sequence of poses always practiced in the same order, focusing on the breath. Decreases stress, tones and strengthens muscles. Can be fast paced and challenging.
- Bikram: A 90-minute technique consisting of 26 poses and two breathing techniques, practiced in a room heated to 105 degrees Fahrenheit. It can be challenging; it detoxes the body by sweating out toxins, which improves overall circulation.
- Hatha: An overall term for yoga practices that use poses, or asanas, and may be a bit more gentle than other styles. While the poses, many of which are done standing, can be physically challenging, the focus is on awareness, calm, and preparing for meditation.
- Iyengar: This practice is all about alignment in poses and uses props such as blocks, pillows, chairs, boosters, blankets, and straps. Postures are done standing and sitting and help with posture, range of motion, and strengthening muscles.
- Jivamukti: A sequence of poses incorporating meditation, compassion, and chanting for a more spiritual yoga experience that involves chanting Sanskrit, body awareness, and deep listening.
- Kripalu: An inward-directed practice to put the student in touch with their bodies with breathing exercises, gentle stretches, and individual poses, ending with relaxation.

- Kundalini: A meditative system for releasing pent-up energy with chanting, asanas, meditation, and a specific goal in mind for the practice of raising the energy at the base of the spine and letting it rise to the crown of the head, where it is released. It often ends with singing. Mantras are used silently or out loud as well as dynamic breathing.

- Restorative: A gentle and restful series of poses that are held for 10 minutes using props such as pillows, blankets, and straps. The four or five poses are meant to bring about a deep, meditative calm.

- Sivananda: This yoga system consists of a five-point philosophy involving breathing, relaxation, diet, exercise, and positive thinking to create an overall lifestyle.

- Vinyasa: A free-form style of Ashtanga, with poses given by the teacher and a focus on light cardio and building muscle tone. This is a more athletic workout style of yoga.

- Viniyoga: The focus is on meditation, breath work, relaxation, body posture, and awareness; it is more of an inner workout. It is great for those who have limited movement or are not up for the more athletic forms of yoga with more challenging poses.

- Yin: The focus here is on holding passive poses for longer periods of time to target deep tissue, joints, fascia, ligaments, and bones.

More modern types include prenatal yoga, which is safe for pregnant mothers who might not be able to do other styles of yoga, and power yoga, which combines its focus on strength and athleticism with Ashtanga yoga postures. Studies going back decades show the benefits of yoga for reducing back pain, improving mood, lessening stress, building muscle tone and strength, expanding lung capacity with breathing exercises, bringing about a sense of calm and inner peace, and increasing immunity and resilience. Yoga and meditation are powerful anti-inflammatory and immune boosters when done alone or together, and a new study in *Frontiers in Human Neuroscience* shows that these practices have a positive effect on the central nervous system and immune system.

Dance Away the Stress

If you hate exercising but love dancing, you are in luck. Dancing, whether alone in your room when no one is watching or with a partner out on the town, is a wonderful way to not only get some aerobic exercise but have fun and relieve stress, too. Dancing also helps to improve your body image and connection to your body by reminding you of the joys of a tango, a cha cha, or the electric slide. Dancing is so popular that Congress officially declared July 31 as National Dance Day.

Dance shows on television pull in millions of viewers, who love to watch celebrities and professional dancers move to the music, some with incredible skill. You don't have to be a pro to learn new dance moves, thanks to YouTube videos, DVDs, and exercise programs that teach the skills to you right in the privacy of your living room.

Dancing for at least 20 minutes is an incredible workout that targets large muscle groups such as the arms, legs, back, and torso. Like any aerobic program, it's about getting a little out of breath, using as many body parts as possible, and even incorporating some power moves such as leaps, jumps, bursts, and squats. No matter what style you choose, dancing benefits in a leaner, tighter, and more toned body, but always keep in mind that you need to do it at least three times a

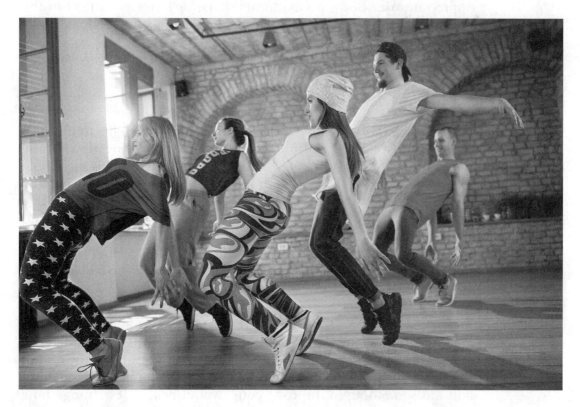

Getting your aerobic workout through dance can make it much more enjoyable and creative for many people who want their exercise routines to be fun.

week for a minimum of 20 minutes. If you have kids, have them join in and get their exercise at the same time.

Even more flowing styles of dance like belly dancing and ballet can be incredibly challenging and work the body, so don't discount them. Belly dancing works the upper body the most and tap dancing the lower body. Jazz dancing is super high impact; ballet is focused on muscles, stretching, and balance. Salsa is about those hips and arms, and good old rock dancing moves just about every part imaginable. Get creative and combine different dance types to come up with your own routine or mix it up to make sure you are covering both upper- and lower-body movements each week. Any type of dance that incorporates rhythmic movements or the use of light hand weights adds even more impact to the workout.

Above all else, have fun. Dancing is a lot more enjoyable as a form of exercise because it doesn't feel like a chore. It truly helps you appreciate your body, no matter its shape or form, as you get in the groove and go with the flow. If you love doing it, you will do it. That's the bottom line.

Just Do It

Any kind of movement or activity can have benefits to physical well-being. Golf, archery, bowling, kayaking, and rowing all work the upper body and expand lung capacity. Horseback riding is incredible for building leg muscle strength and balance. Martial arts work the entire body and provide a sense of self-esteem while teaching an important method of self-defense. Volleyball, tennis, badminton, and racquetball work the entire body aerobically and increase arm muscle strength. Soccer works the legs and lungs. Softball works the upper body and legs and, depending on how often you hit the ball and run, could be considered somewhat aerobic.

The idea is to go do something, whether outdoors or indoors, alone or in a team or group, to move the body. The camaraderie of playing a team sport adds to the physical positives, and at the end of the day, you have the satisfaction of knowing you got off your duff and did something to improve your overall health. It's strange how much we resist exercising only to find ourselves feeling fabulous once we are done with it.

How Many Calories Can You Burn in 30 Minutes of Activity?

Harvard Health Publishing, a division of Harvard Medical School, did a great study of how many calories you can burn in just 30 minutes of exercise. They looked at people in three different weight groups and included numerous types of activity. Here is a sampling of what they found (link to full study is in the bibliography section):

Activity	125 Pounds	155 Pounds	185 Pounds
		Weight of Person	
Weightlifting	90	108	126
Hatha Yoga	120	144	168
Aerobics/Low Impact	165	198	231
Stationary Bike/Moderate	210	252	294
Elliptical Trainer	270	324	378
Aerobics/High Impact	300	360	420
Slow Dancing	90	108	125
Golf, Using Cart	105	126	147
Volleyball	90	108	126
Tai Chi	120	144	168
Kayaking	150	180	210
Swimming	180	216	252
Tennis	210	252	294
Hockey, Field or Ice	240	288	336
Food Shopping with Cart	85	106	126
Cross-country Running	255	316	377
Raking the Lawn	120	144	168
Shoveling Snow by Hand	180	216	252
Playing with Kids/Moderate	114	141	168
Sleeping	19	22	26

You can see from the full chart, which includes dozens of examples such as these, that everything we do burns calories, including sitting and sleeping, and some activities burn more than we probably imagined. It's a fascinating look at how movement is healthy, even when you think it's play.

The body is the vehicle through which we experience life. It be-hooves us to not only feed it right but treat it right, and whether that means taking up a martial arts practice, starting a dog-walking club, or doing jumping jacks and squats after dinner while watching game shows, that treatment must include exercise and movement. It could mean the difference between a beat-up, fume-sputtering old jalopy and a smooth-running, engine-purring sports car. You get to choose which you prefer to drive.

Stress Relief

Life is stressful. It is inevitable that the course of a human life will include both positive and negative stressors, from planning the birth of a child to setting the will of a deceased loved one, from paying bills to looking for and landing a dream job, from getting on a plane to an island vacation spot to walking into the biggest meeting of your life. Stress is a normal reaction to physical, emotional, and mental challenges, even the great ones.

The problems arise when stress becomes our go-to state and we cannot come down from or off the elevated responses we have to a stressful situation. The body is a powerful adjustor, but often, the hormones released under stress, the cortisol and adrenaline that give us the ability to fight or flee, stay high enough to keep us on edge and eventually take a toll on our health. Those stress responses, if they continue beyond the duration of the actual challenge or situation, give us no relief and no relaxation, and the hormones continue to stay in our system, disrupting our sleep, digestion, heart rate, mental clarity, and mood. A 2020 study of 38,000 Finnish adults published in the *British Medical Journal* showed that chronic heavy stress was associated with a decreased life expectancy for both men and women.

Stress comes in two kinds. Acute stress is short term and goes away once the challenge is met or a better response is adopted. It can be positive stress over an exciting new challenge or negative stress over dealing with a flooded basement unexpectedly. We all experience acute stress throughout our lives. Chronic stress is longer lasting and often revolves around marriage and family issues, illnesses, money problems, and ongoing trouble with a work or career. This kind of stress is deadlier because of the possibility that you will adapt to it over time, not realizing that a more peaceful way of living exists. Chronic stress means chronic high levels of the fight–or–flight hormones that make you feel on edge, with tense muscles, a quick pulse, sweating, and anxiety.

Chronic stress is longer lasting and often revolves around marriage and family issues, illnesses, money problems, and ongoing trouble with a work or career.

Too much stress leads to inflammation in the body and a higher risk of heart disease, strokes, cancer, diabetes, skin problems, high blood pressure, insomnia, high blood sugar, heartburn and indigestion, headaches, fatigue, weight gain, and mental issues such as depression and panic attacks. If you already have these conditions, the addition of chronic stress makes them much worse.

Both kinds of stress, when not dealt with properly or gotten under control, can lead to the following symptoms:

- Chest pain and racing heart
- Sweating
- Trouble having sex
- Stomachaches
- Headaches
- Indigestion, diarrhea, and constipation
- Exhaustion
- Insomnia and trouble falling and staying asleep when you do sleep
- Jaw clenching
- Muscle aches and tension
- Panic attacks and mood swings
- Skin rashes, eczema, and psoriasis outbreaks
- High blood pressure
- Menstrual problems
- Easily catching colds and flus

- Stiff neck
- Weight loss or weight gain
- Excessive use of drugs, gambling, shopping, sex, smoking, eating, or alcohol to "wind down"
- Forgetfulness and poor memory recall

So many things in life can stress us out. Weddings, divorces, new jobs, being fired, retiring, deaths, illnesses, moving, having a baby…. If the stress is ongoing and no relief occurs, it is always best to seek the help of a doctor or therapist who can help you work on responses and coping behaviors. This is especially helpful if trauma or violence is involved or if you are not processing grief and moving forward after a long period of time. You will know when stress has gotten the best of you if you stay tuned in to how you feel and what is happening. The signs are all around you, and if you ignore them, it could result in an accident or illness.

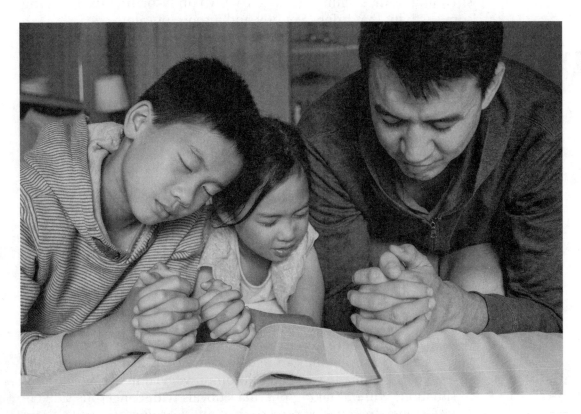

Research shows that, among other approaches, prayer can be a good way to relieve stress in one's life. People who pray regularly and have a strong faith also tend to live longer, and stress relief might be why this is.

You can naturally deal with stress in many ways, as we will explore here in this section. In the herbs and plants list and the natural remedies section are other suggestions for managing stress. You do have control over your body's autonomic nervous system and can manage your heart rate, blood pressure, and mood to become more resilient.

One of the best things to do is try to avoid being overwhelmed before stress occurs. This can be achieved by thinking positive, practicing meditation, praying regularly, talking to friends and loved ones when stressed out, getting out into nature, exercising, eating healthy, and finding some spiritual practice to soothe the soul. Getting into and keeping a routine often helps you regain a sense of control when life seems chaotic. This can be as simple as adopting a morning routine of yoga out on your back patio, structuring your day to include mini-breaks, getting in some exercise early to have more energy later, cutting off all work-related communications before dinner is served, spending your evenings engaged with family or friends, or doing some activity that brings you joy and a sense of calm.

Having more structure can also extend to goals. Stress accompanies feeling overwhelmed, so if you have goals, breaking them down into structured, small bits that can be achieved easily gives you more control and the sense of accomplishment to keep you motivated.

Relaxation techniques such as breathing exercises can be done whenever stress arises, and you can do them at your desk, in your car, or in bed before you get up in the morning. At the end of the day, you can try a cup of herbal tea to soothe the nerves before attempting sleep. Perhaps a phone call or video chat with a good friend and a glass of wine is all you need to wind down. Maybe journaling or taking a long, hot bath is your thing. If you make self-care a regular part of your day, you will find that you handle stress much better when it does show up with a lot less anxiety and lack of control.

Chronic stress leads to physical, mental, and emotional burnout. You feel as if you have hit a wall and it's impossible to get past it; what was a natural response to your environment is now a beast you cannot keep caged. However, one can release all that blocked and stored-up excess energy in many ways and decompress even in the most trying of situations without taking pharmaceuticals with dangerous side effects. Getting stress under your control and learning new ways to be more resilient and adaptive will not only benefit your health but also benefit those who love you and spend the most time with you.

According to Dr. Tony Hampton for his column on the *Diet Doctor* website, you can deal with stress in negative ways by eating too much comfort food, turning to drugs or alcohol, sleeping too much or too little, and not paying attention to your stress responses. You can also deal with it in positive ways, such as eating a healthy diet, getting exercise and movement, breathing deeply, thinking positive, reframing the situation in a more positive way, changing your interpretations about an event, taking supplements like vitamin B and magnesium to help you deal with stress, and being grateful and mindful of the present moment. He suggests you also work to identify your stressors first as a way to face them directly and understand how you can reduce their impact and influence in the future.

Chronic stress leads to physical, mental, and emotional burnout. You feel as if you have hit a wall and it's impossible to get past it....

Dr. Hampton writes, "One of the greatest lessons I've learned to reduce my stress is to take care of my needs first, set boundaries, and say no. When I do, I have much more to give to others. I cannot help others effectively if I cannot help myself first." The idea of caring for ourselves first may feel selfish to some, but it is critical. If we are sick, tired, and irritable, how can we possibly be of benefit to anyone else? Dr. Hampton brings up boundaries and learning to say no. In this hectic, 24/7-connected world where we are always accessible, putting boundaries into place to protect our time and energy is essential. It starts with learning how to say no.

Boundaries

Before you can begin to take better care of yourself, you need to know where you begin and others end. You need to stop living to please others, feeling their feelings, worrying over things you cannot control, and trying to insert yourself into someone else's life or letting someone do the same in yours. You need boundaries. The idea of boundaries often leaves people feeling selfish, as if they are cutting others out and pushing others away. The truth is that boundaries are necessary for well-being to identify where we begin and end when interacting with others. All too often, those lines of demarcation blend and merge, and we find ourselves in a codependent situation where we no longer have a strong sense of identity.

Having boundaries keeps us healthy and mature because it holds us to an authenticity of thoughts, behaviors, and actions that are ours and ours alone, unaffected by the desires of others. Our boundaries let others know what we will accept and not accept, and when someone disrespects us or breaches our personal space, we let them know not to do it again. Establishing strong boundaries is about keeping our life our life and not someone else's but also about respecting that we end somewhere, too, and they begin. It's impossible to ask others to respect our boundaries if we don't reciprocate. Then, when we interact, we do so from a healthy position where we know what we want and are not engaging in people-pleasing, codependent, or enmeshed behaviors.

Once we establish boundaries, and they may be different with everyone we meet or every situation we find ourselves in, then we move on to the next prerequisite for a plan of self-care: learning what to say yes to and what to say no to without guilt or apologizing. Only when we have strong boundaries will we be able to accomplish this and protect our time and energy. We all know the power of saying "yes" to life, to new people and experiences, to going for our dreams, but too often, we find ourselves exhausted and burnt out, pulled in 10 different directions, no longer able to find pleasure in the things we once loved to do. You know the feeling: when life becomes a chore and your calendar is so full, you barely have a moment to even go to the bathroom.

Creating and enforcing your boundaries may be perceived by others as being selfish and spoiled. The truth is the opposite. It's the ultimate form of self-care, being able to spend your time and energy doing the things that are important to you, not to someone else you are trying to please or appease.

Here are some tips to creating and sticking to boundaries:

- Always check in with yourself when asked to do something. Is it aligned with your values and goals? If not, don't do it, and if you feel pressured, ask the person to stop pressuring you.
- Do not let the emotions of others affect your own. Realize where they end and you begin. You can care, but don't absorb. Being enmeshed in the emotions of others is codependency.
- Say what you mean and mean what you say. This creates integrity and lets people know you are true to your word.
- Never try to fix or save another person. You can help and support them through a challenge, but by fixing them, you deprive them

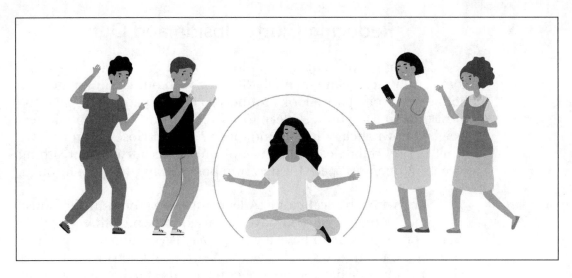

It's okay to set your own boundaries and keep your needs and wants separate from those of peers and family who might try to impose their will on you or drain you of your energy.

of the chance to save themselves and build their own sense of self-worth and resilience.

- Define your own likes, wants, and needs, and don't mix them up with the likes, wants, and needs of others just to be a people pleaser. You give up your soul and spirit when you twist and bend yourself into a pretzel in order to be approved of.

- Seek your own approval and worth. It's great to be liked by others and to have them value us, but if we don't first value ourselves, none of that matters. We will become a bottomless pit that cannot get enough approval from outside.

- Even with children, lovers, and friends, have your own life goals, hobbies, passions, and purpose. You are the only you that you have, and although you will share the path of your life with many others along the way, it is only your path to walk. They have their own.

- Make self-love a priority because when you love yourself, you will not allow others to use you, take advantage of you, walk all over you, or treat you poorly. Boundaries begin with loving your-self enough to realize you are whole and complete just as you are.

Solid boundaries and self-respect lead to being able to say yes to the things you truly want in life with ease and say no without the guilt and shame of hurting someone else. You also serve as a role model for others seeking to enact their own boundaries and start say-ing no to what they don't want to do, even if you are the one asking.

Reducing Clutter Inside and Out

Getting rid of things we no longer need or use can be a game changer physically and mentally. Starting with our environment–our homes and workspaces–look around you at the spaces you spend the most time in. Do you feel clear, focused, free, and light? Do you feel weighed down, heavy, hectic, and messy? Clutter closes in on us if we don't periodically clear it out to not only give ourselves breathing room but open up space for new and better things to come through.

Start with physical clutter. Clear out every room in the house and either donate what you have not used in two or three years to charity or set it aside to have a garage sale. If you donate it, you can write it off on your taxes and have the pleasure of knowing that others will benefit from what you no longer have a use for. If you have a garage or yard sale, you can make some extra money with all the stuff that was weighing you down and cluttering up your space.

Hanging on to items such as clothing comes from a sense of lack and scarcity, that we might not have the money down the road to buy something newer or better. So, we keep things we haven't used in years, clothing that stopped fitting five years ago, and items that until we cleaned out the clutter, we forgot even existed. The key is to let them go and not hang on to them, not suddenly decide we need the pair of black pants we haven't worn in five years, the boots that might come back into style someday, or the puzzles we've done over and over because we feel too guilty to buy new ones. Clearing out clutter in your physical space is freeing and allows you the pleasure of buying new things, knowing that the old are serving someone who needs them.

The clutter in your mind works the same way. What no longer serves you? What thoughts and patterns bog you down, block your happiness, and detour you from success? Too many thoughts can create a sense of disorganization and disorder. Too many doubts and disbeliefs can stop the smallest of goals in their tracks and keep you from ever reaching the bigger ones.

Clutter of the mind can be cleared by prayer, meditation, guided visualization, or just some quiet time in nature, letting thoughts come and go on the breeze through your mind. The art of mindfulness, being in the present moment with no regret of the past or worry of the future, is the most effective way to keep the mind clear, focused, and free of clutter. A good night's sleep works wonders, too.

Clutter is junk. It's stuff we accumulate thinking we cannot get rid of it because someday we might need it, even if that day never comes. Take the declutter challenge and start with one room of your living space at a time, setting everything you haven't touched or used for years into two piles: sell and give away. Then, either sell it or give it away. No second looks back, no hanging on "just in case." If by some chance you do need it later, you can always buy another one new or used.

Then, do the same with your mind, cleaning out the junk that doesn't align with your dreams and goals or make you feel good about your life. Replace old, worn-out patterns and thoughts with new ones that are more positive and empowering. Don't hoard the past or try to collect the future. Stay in the now, and you will always have what you need.

Now that you have the time to say yes to more self-care and well-being, what are some of the ways you can pursue that?

Laughter Is Good Medicine

Imagine a life without humor, without laughter. So much of what bonds us to others is a shared laugh over our life situations and a

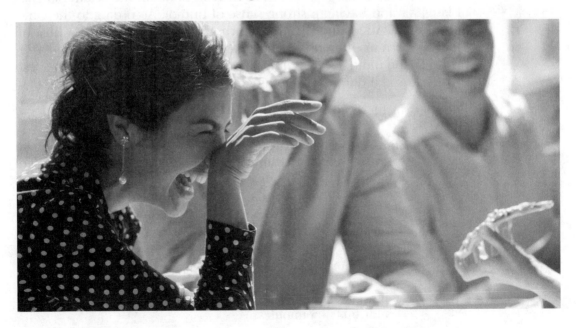

Maybe it is a cliché, but laughter really is a great medicine that can reduce or reverse the negative mental and physical effects of stress.

perspective of being able to find the funny silver linings. Humor and laughter are as old as humanity itself and serve a critical role in our well-being. Having no sense of humor or ability to see humor leads to a depressing, anxiety-ridden existence where release from the challenges and burdens of daily life never occurs.

Like a warm cup of tea before bed or a cool shower in the morning, laughter can calm and soothe or give us the boost of energy and joy needed to keep on keeping on. It's even better when we share laughs with someone else, but even laughing alone to an episode of *The Three Stooges* is enough to improve our physical and mental health in a number of ways.

We naturally gravitate toward people who are always making us laugh or finding the humor in any given situation. We are repulsed by those who are in a perpetual bad, grumpy mood. Our energy seeks out good energy to match to, and when someone is negative and draining, it brings us down with them. Laughter is the best lifter and quicker picker upper around, and those who make us laugh have a way of finding silly, playful joy in the smallest of things. They are more resilient, too, and better equipped to cope with the bigger challenges life throws at them.

Numerous scientific studies have been done on the health benefits of laughter and having a strong sense of humor. According to the University of St. Augustine Health Science, the Mayo Clinic, and a host of other research institutions, laughter has a number of positive benefits for the body and mind and, certainly, the spirit, too. Laughter truly is the best medicine, and it doesn't cost a thing or require any heavy equipment.

Physical benefits of laughter include:

- Stimulates your organs: When you laugh, you take in more oxygen-rich air. This stimulates your lungs, heart, and muscles. Laughter enhances your intake of oxygen-rich air and increases brain endorphins.
- Activates your stress response: Laughter fires up and then cools down the stress response as well as raises and lowers your heart rate and blood pressure for a calm feeling.
- Relaxes your muscles and soothes tension: When you get stressed, your body tenses up and can cause you to feel stuck. A good laugh can relieve physical tension in the body and relax the muscles for up to 45 minutes.
- Improves cardiac health: Laughing increases your heart rate and the amount of oxygen in your blood. This can improve vascular

function and decrease the risk of heart attacks. It also increases circulation.

- Boosts immune system: When you're stressed, negative thoughts can turn into chemical reactions that decrease your immunity to sickness. When you laugh, you adopt a positive mindset that can release infection-fighting antibodies and neuropeptides that help fight stress.
- Lowers blood pressure: Laughter releases endorphins that counteract the negative effects of stress hormones, lowering your blood pressure as a result.
- Helps with weight loss: A common side effect of chronic stress is weight gain. Laughing not only reduces the stress hormones that cause weight gain, but it also burns calories.
- Relieves pain: Laughter allows the body to produce its own natural painkillers.

Mental benefits of laughter include:

- Provides distraction: When you laugh, you aren't thinking about that assignment that is overdue or the big final you have coming up next week. Laughter provides your brain with a break from the worrying thoughts that cause stress.
- Improves your mood and lifts your spirit: Nothing squashes a bad mood quite like a good laugh. Laughing produces a general sense of well-being and can diffuse the anger and depression you were once feeling.
- Reduces stress hormones: Cortisol is the primary stress hormone that circulates throughout our body when we're feeling stressed. Laughter can decrease cortisol levels by increasing your intake of oxygen and stimulating circulation throughout the body.
- Increases endorphins: Endorphins are those "feel-good" chemicals produced by your brain that help boost happiness levels. Laughing increases the number of endorphins released in your body, fighting off stress and promoting a positive mood.
- Strengthens relationships: A shared laugh with friends, family, or a coworker can help you feel more connected to that person and form a strong and lasting bond. Humor is also a powerful way to heal past disagreements or resentments.

Ways to Laugh More

Here are simple ways to increase laughter and humor in your life:

- Follow some funny meme accounts to put a smile on your face every time you hop on social media.

- Create a Pinterest board full of things that make you laugh, like quotes or hilarious pictures.
- Spend time with pets such as dogs and cats. They are a source of laughter and joy for many people. If you don't have a pet, consider asking a friend to pet-sit theirs or volunteer at an animal shelter in your free time.
- On your way to work or school, listen to a funny podcast or audiobook to make the commute go by quicker and get a boost of humor.
- Laughter yoga is a new take on yoga that encourages prolonged voluntary laughter. Try out a class by yourself or take it with a friend next time you're feeling stressed.
- Learning to laugh at yourself is one of the best ways you can add more laughter into your life. Next time you do something that would otherwise upset you, try to find the positive in the situation.
- Your environment can play a huge part in your mood. Reshape your work or study area to include things that make you smile, like a picture with friends from a funny night out or a photo of your dog in a hilarious costume.

Laughter is important, but remember to never, ever laugh at the expense of another person or use humor as a way to shame someone.

- Nothing beats a shared laugh. Invite some friends over for a game night and play party-style games like Charades.
- YouTube is chock full of hilarious videos from jumping cats to funny clips from your favorite show for a fast and easy pick-me-up.
- Watch funny movies and TV shows alone or with someone else.
- Spend time with happy, silly, fun, playful people who love to laugh.
- Jokes are always funny, but dumb ones are great for face-palms and belly laughs.
- Hang out with children. They say and do the silliest things.
- Go to a comedy show with friends.

Laughter is important, but remember to never, ever laugh at the expense of another person or use humor as a way to shame someone. Avoid people who are negative, whiny, and humorless when you can. Moods are contagious, so make an effort to find people who love to laugh and see the humor in life just as much as you do. While not everyone's idea of what is funny is the same, we can all agree that plenty of things are worth a chuckle, snort, or guffaw.

Love Heals All Things

Like humor, love is an all-purpose healing agent with plenty of benefits for health and well-being. It's free and can be easily given away and shared without ever depleting your own source. Love comes in so many forms. Love of self, love of others, love of life, love of nature–all of it is empowering and positive to both the giver and the recipient. Most of the love we experience is expressed through our relationships with family, spouses, friends, colleagues, pets, and community. Expressing love brings the greatest benefits, and it always must start with being loving toward ourselves. We need to give ourselves the same love we so willingly give to others. From that full well, we can then share and spread it out into the world.

Love is not just caring for another, it's about having compassion and empathy and being a support system. It's about finding commonalities even amid differences and having each other's backs in good times and bad. Love is a feeling and an expression, a noun and a verb, and the more we have of it, the happier we are.

We are not talking here about desperate, clingy, romantic attachment sung about in pop songs and written about in romance novels. Love is not all sugary-sweet romance movies with happy endings. Romantic love is often the only love people say they want when it is the least likely to make them happy in a fundamental sense. Harry Reis, Ph.D., coeditor of the *Encyclopedia of Human Relationships*, stated in an article for *WebMD Health News* that "there is no evidence that the intense, passionate stage of new romance is beneficial to health. People who fall in love say it feels wonderful and agonizing at the same time." If we keep in mind the biological reasons for this kind of stressful, intense passion, which is to couple

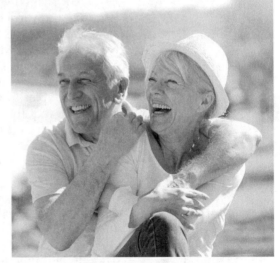

Nothing is better for your health than a long-term, genuinely loving relationship. People enjoying great relationships have less depression and go to the hospital less often than those who don't.

Natural Health

and reproduce, and that it tends to fade over time, we can then define real, healthier love.

Reis goes on to state that evidence shows that people who participate in satisfying, long–term relationships fare better on a whole variety of health measures. This doesn't just mean romantic relationships. Real love is unconditional and expansive and does not attach to outcomes or demand that someone behaves a certain way for us to be happy. Love is, perhaps at its highest level of expression, the ability to be who we are and let others be who they are and care for and support them as they do.

Some of the benefits of love include:

- Fewer visits to the doctor's office: Married people tend to visit the doctor less and spend less time in the hospital, suggesting that good relationships and a sense of connectedness and community keep us healthy. If you are not married, you can get this same effect from having a best friend or a few good friends as your support system. People who have a lot of love in their lives tend to get sick a lot less, too. Researchers at Carnegie Mellon University found that people with a positive mindset get sick after being exposed to colds and flu viruses far less than those who are more hostile.

- Less anxiety and depression: Loving, stable relationships make us less anxious, worried, afraid, depressed, and stressed out. We have someone who cares for us and about us, who supports us through tough times, and who keeps us laughing and happy. Researchers at New York's State University at Stony Brook looked at MRI scans of people in love and compared one group of passionate, newly married couples to those of couples in longer–term relationships and found that the dopamine reward area of the brain was activated in both, but the longer–term loves also had activation in the part of the brain associated with bonding and much less activity in the part of the brain that produces feelings of anxiety.

- Less pain and more healing: Numerous brain studies show that people who are in love and happy experience less pain and have quicker wound healing, which suggests that love and positivity affect the immune system, too. In one study at Ohio State University Medical Center, married couples were given blister wounds, and they healed twice as fast in those couples who had a warm, loving relationship compared to the ones who did not.

Love also makes us live longer and have a higher quality of life. Love gives us meaning and purpose and keeps us bonded to others in our older years, so we feel less alone and afraid of getting sick or dying. In the elderly, fear of isolation is a big factor in unhappiness, especially for those who are in assisted-living situations, so being surrounded by love alleviates the loneliness and increases our ability to handle the challenges of growing older. Having family, friends, or neighbors who you can interact with in your old age is important to keeping your brain active and your heart happy.

A study in the *Journal of Family Psychology* showed that happiness depended more on the quality of family relationships than on level of income. Love is a bigger part of our happiness quotient than our income, although you would never think that from looking at our money-driven media and entertainment industries. Apparently, money doesn't make the world go around; love does.

Love is also not all about experiencing rapturous joy 24/7 and floating on a mountaintop at an ashram. Often, love is more down-to-earth, expressed in the smaller things in life, the little daily joys we experience in between the bigger joys as well as quality time spent with people over quantity. Love is the most important force in the universe, and the more we give, the more we have to give.

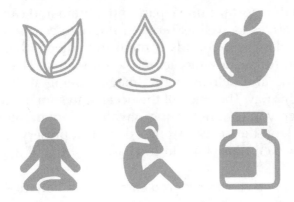

Aromatherapy and Essential Oils

For thousands of years, the use of aromatic oils, essences, and plants has been a source of relaxation and renewal of the body and spirit. Aromatherapy is an ancient practice that uses the power of scent to create calm or to give you more energy, depending on your needs. The scent of smell is the most closely connected to memory, as we can all attest when we get a whiff of homemade cookies and are instantly transported to our grandmother's kitchen, or we smell night–blooming jasmine and remember our first kiss. Smell is often relegated in importance behind sight and hearing but can bring about healing and well–being in ways that sight and hearing cannot.

Aromatherapy focuses mainly on the use of essential oils from flowers and plant parts but can include incense, sage burning, and other methods of delivering potent aromas to the nose and, therefore, to the brain. These aromas can be inhaled, put into a bath, or applied topically on the skin during a massage. The use of this healing modality goes back to ancient times when incense and oils were burned to treat patients physically and psychologically. Our ancestors understood that the power of smell could affect every aspect of health, even more so than anything that stimulated the other four senses.

The science behind it is simple. The olfactory nerves are directly connected to the most primitive part of the brain and can act as stimulants or sedatives as well as serve to improve clarity and memory recall. Many plant compounds contain ingredients that are natural pesticides and fungicides and act in the same manner in the human body: purifying and detoxifying it. Imagine being at the beach on a warm summer's day. The smell of the ocean and suntan oil is palpable, and later when you're at home, just a whiff of suntan lotion can place you right back on the beach. Aromas don't just preserve recent memories; they awaken those long in the past.

Many plant compounds contain ingredients that are natural pesticides and fungicides and act in the same manner in the human body: purifying and detoxifying it.

Essential Oils

The use of essential oils is traced back to a physician and pharmacist named Ibn al–Baitar, who lived in Spain during Muslim rule between 1188–1248 C.E. Oils were used in rituals and ceremonies and in medicinals and focused on the plant life people in the region had access to. The plant parts were used, including the flowers, petals, stems, leaves, bark, roots, and wood. Everything was then distilled in a device that steamed the plant parts over water. The steam vaporized the compounds, which were then returned to their liquid form and collected in a bottle, jar, or vial. The oils that had the most healing properties came to be known as "essential oils."

As a healing modality, using essential oils that target a specific ailment or need can induce the relaxation response or give you an extra energy boost. The smell of fresh lemon or mint has a different effect than the smell of burning wood or hay. Dr. Kurt Schnaubelt, former director of the Pacific Institute of Aromatherapy, stated in *Alternative Medicine: The Definitive Guide* that the chemical makeup of essential oils is what gives them desirable pharmacological properties such as being antimicrobial, antifungal, antibacterial, and antispasmodic. These oils can do everything from promoting the production and excretion of urine to stop a virus or bacterial infection to widening the arteries for improved blood flow and stimulating the thyroid and adrenal glands to work optimally.

Essential oils have been found to stimulate the brain's prefrontal cortex and improve your ability to organize, plan, make decisions, and regulate emotions. They also support increased emotional intelligence and keep the brain processing information at the proper speed while also allowing for greater focus and attention. Rose oil and orange oil seem to do well in stimulating this part of the brain to promote relaxation, and topical essential oils rubbed into the forehead can help increase blood flow in the brain to improve cognition and processing speed.

Essential oils include chemical compounds that aid several ailments and have multiple purposes, including to:

- Ease headaches and migraines
- Stay alert
- Calm the nerves
- Relax tense muscles
- Clear skin issues
- Help hair growth
- Improve sleep
- Curb food cravings
- Purify and detox

They are used not just on the body as oils, salves, and balms or to bring about a state of calm and well-being but in rooms as air purifiers, as cleaners and disinfectants, and to ward off pests. Each essential oil can contain as many as 200 bioconstituents, and some include up to 500. The oils can be ingested, inhaled, or absorbed through the skin, but it behooves you to do your research, as some are okay to be rubbed into the skin but not consumed, especially if you are pregnant or breastfeeding. Ingesting essential oils is usually not recommended unless you are working with a trained and experienced herbalist or aromatherapist. Please use your due diligence. A few drops of one oil may be fine in a cup of tea, but another may be toxic.

Essential oils can be purchased in vials and bottles, or you can try your hand at making them yourself. Distraction can be done in many ways, including steam distillation, cold-pressing, and hydro distillation. Many oils are too potent to put on the skin alone and require carrier oils to be mixed in to make them less volatile. Carrier oils aid absorption but also dilute the concentration of the oil's contact with the skin. Common carrier oils include coconut oil, vegetable oil, olive oil, and jojoba oil.

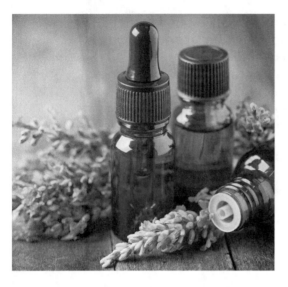

Essential oils come in a number of forms, such as these oils. You can also buy them as balms and salves.

If you choose to buy and blend your own essential oils, it's always helpful to go to an aromatherapy or health food store and try a few out to see if you like the smells. You can dab a tiny bit of the sample oils most stores carry on your wrist, avoiding anything that smells rancid. Only use a tiny bit. If you are concerned about allergies, dab a tiny bit on the inside of your elbow and wait 24 hours before purchasing or using again to see if a rash or reaction appears. If not, don't be afraid to blend two or three oils together.

The dilution guidelines for carrier oils to mix with your essential oils is as follows:

- 2.5 percent dilution: 15 drops of essential oil per 6 teaspoons of carrier oil

- 3 percent dilution: 20 drops of essential oil per 6 teaspoons of carrier oil

- 5 percent dilution: 30 drops of essential oil per 6 teaspoons of carrier oil

- 10 percent dilution: 60 drops of essential oil per 6 teaspoons of carrier oil

For children, never go above 1 percent dilution, which would be 3–6 drops of essential oil to 6 teaspoons of carrier oil, and always do an allergy check on children's sensitive skin.

Inhaling seems to be the easiest method. You can buy a vial and open it, inhaling for a few seconds, or put a few drops into your bath or a bowl of hot steam. Try dropping some oils into a hot bath or shower. You can put a few drops onto a cotton ball to gently sniff. You can also buy beautiful oil diffusers that you fill with water, which turns to steam to dissipate the oil. Try blending two or more oils to create your own favorite scents.

Some of the most popular essential oils are:

- Lavender oil for relief from anxiety and inducing sleep

Tips for Diluting Essential Oils
from Mountain Rose Herbs

Use proper measurement tools and be sure to accurately convert between different types of measurements.

Not all essential oils are equal in potency. For example, cinnamon leaf essential oil is less potent and less aromatic than cinnamon bark essential oil, so it's important to do your research about the nature of the oils you want to use, especially when formulating your own recipes.

Make sure your essential oil(s) are appropriate for the end use of your recipe. For example, a few essential oils react poorly when exposed to sunlight, so these would not be ideal choices to include in a hair serum recipe. Getting to know the basic properties of the essential oils you want to use is highly recommended.

Dilution Chart

Carrier Oil	1% Essential Oil	2% Essential Oil
5 ml	1 drop	2 drops
10 ml	2 drops	4 drops
0.5 oz.	3 drops	8 drops
1 oz.	6 drops	12 drops
2 oz.	12 drops	0.25 tsp.
4 oz.	0.25 tsp.	0.5 tsp.
6 oz.	36 drops	0.75 tsp.
8 oz.	0.5 tsp.	1 tsp.
10 oz.	1 tsp.	2 tsp.

- Jasmine oil for improvement of mood, calming anxiety, and balancing hormones
- Peppermint or spearmint oil for a boost of energy and focus
- Eucalyptus oil for clearing out stuffy noses and soothing sore throats
- Lemon or orange peel added to any oil will give it a citrusy boost for clarity and energy
- Tea tree oil fights off infections and heals skin issues when used topically

Natural Health

- Sandalwood oil is a potent anti-inflammatory that elevates mood
- Frankincense oil calms anxiety, helps ease PTSD symptoms, and elevates mood
- Spruce and blue spruce oil are high in camphene to alleviate respiratory discomfort and acts as an adaptogen, calming or boosting energy when needed
- Roman chamomile oil improves heart health, is a natural antihistamine, calms jangled nerves, and promotes sleep

Several essential oils enhance exercise benefits and improve circulation by relaxing blood vessels, which allows more blood to circulate. Other oils help veins contract to stimulate more blood flow and can improve the function of the lymphatic system by flushing out toxins to reduce inflammation in the blood vessels. Essential oils massaged into the lower back area can support the adrenal glands during stressful times and ease stiff and tense muscles from overexercising or lifting too much weight. Taxed adrenals can mean less support for the muscles supporting the lower back and pelvis.

You can also try some essential oils behind the earlobe on the mastoid bone, which directly affects the vagus nerve to improve circulation and moderate inflammatory response. Stimulating the vagus nerve activates the parasympathetic state and helps to restore balance throughout the body and reduce inflammation in the brain for clearer and more focused thinking.

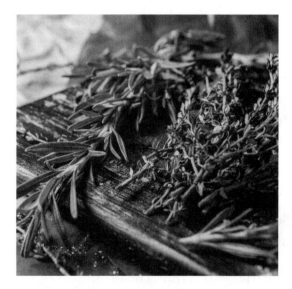

Rosemary and thyme—two herbs easily found at grocery stores or grown at home—are antispasmodics that work to reduce pain.

Antispasmodic herbs such as rosemary and thyme are great for exercise-beneficial essential oil blends as well as herbs that deliver more oxygen to cells such as black pepper and frankincense. Rosemary and thyme also help reduce pain. Clary sage, peppermint, and frankincense are great stress relievers. Dilute them first with a few drops of carrier oil if placing on the skin and rub on your stomach, sides of the neck, lower spine, and the bottom of your feet. You can use these herbs and others in massage oils or dab a few drops on the wrist, sides of the neck, or anywhere you can smell them. Place several drops in a hot bath for a healing, calming experience, or try them in a diffuser.

A 2013 study published in the journal *Evidence-Based Complementary and Alternative Medicine* found that a blend of lavender, Roman chamomile, and neroli oils reduced anxiety and improved the quality of sleep of patients in an intensive care unit.

Essential oils and aromatherapy work, but it may take some practice to find the oils and oil blends that work best for your needs. Don't be afraid to buy oils online or in stores, and always ask if they have samples open for you to smell first. Do the allergy test first before using more liberally if applying topically, and never consume anything without making sure it is not toxic first.

Smell and scent can create a powerful sense of healing and well-being. Scented soaps, candles, sachets, and fragrances all work to evoke memories and feelings and to put us in a slightly altered state of consciousness. Even going outside to smell the flowers or freshly cut grass can transport us to another time and place or soothe and relax the mind, body, and spirit.

 If oils aren't your thing, you can try burning sage or incense to get the same effect, but never do so in a closed space, and be careful of the smoke irritating the throat and lungs when inhaled.

If oils aren't your thing, you can try burning sage or incense to get the same effect, but never do so in a closed space, and be careful of the smoke irritating the throat and lungs when inhaled. People often turn to diffusers of oils to avoid this problem, but incense can be purchased in stick and cone forms and put into decorative burners; this method gives off a lot less smoke than sage bundles.

Peppermint Power: An Oil with Many Benefits

One essential oil that has been used for thousands of years in ancient Greece, Egypt, and Rome is peppermint oil. A well-established body of research has been built up on the beneficial properties of this one oil alone, showing its incredible versatility. Its main component is menthol, which has been used as a medicinal for fighting bacterial infections, inflammation, fatigue, relieving congestions and allergies, fighting headaches, improving energy, battling bad breath, and aiding digestion.

Peppermint oil can be used alone or with other oils in the following ways:

- Boosts energy and mental alertness: Inhale peppermint oil for a quick pick–me–up or add a few drops to a diffuser during the day.

- Relieves muscle and joint pain: The menthol has anti–inflammatory effects that can be rubbed on topically to relieve soreness and pain.

- Fights dandruff: Antifungal and antimicrobial properties in the oil keep dandruff away. Add a few drops to your regular shampoo and massage into scalp.

- Helps hair grow: Adding a few drops to your shampoo doesn't just fight off dandruff, it helps promote new hair growth.

- Repels insects: Volatile compounds like peppermint are great for keeping bugs at bay, especially mosquitoes. Dilute several drops into a carrier oil, such as olive or jojoba oil, and rub on exposed skin.

- Cools rashes and itchy skin: Peppermint oil has a nice cooling effect on skin; a few drops diluted in olive oil can be rubbed directly on affected areas for instant relief.

- Fights acne: The antibacterial and antimicrobial properties reduce skin bacteria and therefore acne. Add a drop or two to some jojoba oil and dab directly on acne.

- Fights toenail fungus: Apply a few drops directly onto the affected nails.

- Fights headaches: Peppermint oil relaxes you and reduces the severity of headaches when inhaled, or mix a few drops with carrier oil and rub directly on temples.

- Reduces nausea and motion sickness: Take one or two peppermint oil capsules before traveling or when symptoms first appear. It also relieves symptoms of IBS, gas, and bloating.

- Freshens breath: You can buy a peppermint oil–based toothpaste, or add a couple of drops of oil diluted with water into a spray bottle and spray in mouth when needed. The menthol has a cooling effect on a sore throat, too.

- Clears up congestion: Diffusing peppermint oil when you have a cold or bug helps relieve a stuffy nose and chest congestion. This works great when kids are sick, as it often helps enough to avoid OTC medications with sugars and additives.

Connecting to Yourself and Others

Mindful Living

Mindfulness requires only one thing: that you stay focused in the present and not in the worries of the past or anxieties of the future. Being mindful is a way of experiencing each moment fully and presently and placing your attention on what is right there in front of you rather than on things that already happened or haven't happened yet. Being mindful allows you to embrace each moment and the opportunities it offers. It is in the present that we notice the beauty of life and the amazing calm and peace that come from nonattachment to things we cannot control.

Talk to anyone on their deathbeds, and they will tell you that the one thing they most regret is wasting precious time worrying about things that never came to fruition. They wish they had been more present to life, to their loved ones, to their surroundings, even to their more difficult emotions because it is in the present moment that we most feel alive and fully engaged with the flow of life. This is one of the reasons why mindfulness during meditation or therapy practices is wonderful for alleviating anxiety and depression: it brings the mind back to something it has complete control over–the moment at hand.

You can practice mindfulness in meditation, yoga, walking, or running, but the great thing is that you can do it right now as you're reading this book. Stop any thoughts or concerns of before or after and just be in the moment. Be fully present to the sights, sounds, smells, and how you feel right now. You will notice how much more you can get into a present–moment state once it becomes a habit and how much better you feel about your life.

Here is a great exercise to practice getting into a state of mindfulness: Stop whatever you are doing. Focus on one thing, such as a chair or tree outside. Say to yourself, "I am sitting here looking at this chair." Now, begin describing the chair in as much detail as you can. What does it look like? How does it feel when you sit in it? Does it have any squeaky joints? Can you adjust the seat height? Closely examine the cloth or leather and the nuts and bolts that connect one part of the chair to another. Remember to breathe deeply the whole time.

You will realize that time passed by more slowly because you were so much more in tune with what you were doing each second as you observed the chair. You can go outside and do this with a flower, bird, pond, or lake. Stay in the present, and if any thoughts to the contrary enter your mind, simply acknowledge them and let them slide on by the movie screen of your mind. Pay them no attention, and they will be gone. By strengthening your ability to stay mindful, you will become more productive with your time and enjoy everything around you that you normally take for granted.

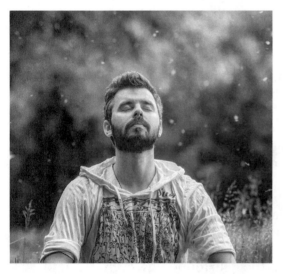

Mindfulness is the practice of just being in the moment, being aware of where you are and who you are.

It is possible to be mindful even during times of conflict by keeping thoughts focused on what is happening in the present rather than allowing thoughts to dwell on the past or future, which brings up resentments and grudges or projects fear and anxiety forward to events that haven't even hap–

pened yet. Mindfulness works wonders in high-stress and anxiety-provoking situations such as meetings with superiors, plane travel, giving a speech to a crowd, or dealing with a panic attack in the middle of the night. Keeping the mind on the present moment is the key to dissipating anxiety, fear, and distress because so much of what leads to those things are regrets over what we cannot change and worry of what has not even happened yet. No matter what is going on, we can deal with it in the moment, then in the next moment, and so on.

Mindfulness at work helps colleagues get along better by keeping the collective focus on the tasks or projects based upon what is needed to accomplish each day. Overwhelm is less likely when goals and deadlines are broken down into what can be done in the present rather than stressing out over what needs to be done over a longer period of time. Mindful living does not say don't make plans; it just says work at those plans one day at a time.

Mindful Eating

Mindful eating can help those who struggle with emotional eating and weight gain by focusing your mind on the moment you have a desire to eat or a craving. If you stop and ask yourself:

- Am I really hungry?
- Am I anxious or bored?
- Am I eating to suppress an emotion?

Then, drink a glass of water. Often, this will be enough to feel a sense of fullness. If not, have a small snack, eating it with mindfulness. Wait 10 minutes and ask the same three questions above. Mindful eating opens your eyes to the ways you might be using food as a soothing or coping tool rather than as something to nourish your body. Numbing out in front of the TV and shoving handfuls of snack food down your throat rarely has anything to do with actual hunger and more to do with feelings and sensations we are trying to "swallow down" with a substance, whether food, alcohol, or buying things on the internet we don't really want or need.

Stress drives us to the fridge or cupboard because we know the comfort of food. When we were little and got a cold or flu, our mothers would give us warm soup or a cup of cocoa to "make us feel better"; perhaps it was the soup or cocoa that did make us feel better, or perhaps it was the love and attention of our parent. As adults, we may not have a parent to comfort us, but we do have access to chicken

One way to tell if you are eating emotionally is to pay attention to how fast you eat and how much food you keep consuming even after you acknowledge to yourself that you are full.

soup and a whole lot of other foods that work to make us feel better, even if only on a surface level.

One way to tell if you are eating emotionally is to pay attention to how fast you eat and how much food you keep consuming even after you acknowledge to yourself that you are full. The stomach fills up faster than the bottomless pit of deep, unprocessed emotions, so you may end up gorging yourself and feeling sick afterward. Staying mindful will cut this off by keeping your attention on how your stomach feels full, at which point you should stop eating. If you still feel anxious and want to reach for more, ask those three questions again and find a healthier way to alleviate your anxieties with a hot bath, a walk around the block, petting your dog, reading a chapter of a novel, or calling a friend or loved one who you can count on for support.

Bringing mindfulness into our eating habits shines a light on why we eat, what we eat, and when we eat. Sure, it's fine to snack at a party while focused on chatting with friends, but emotional eating usually happens when we are alone and vulnerable to engaging in an act that is not about our bodies being hungry but about a deeper hunger that needs to be addressed and worked through.

Teaching Mindfulness to Children

Children live with a lot of anxiety as they go through the stages of physical and emotional growth. Teaching them to stay present and focused on the moment at hand empowers them to face any challenge and better deal with fears and fearful situations, such as a doctor visit, a big test at school, or making new friends. Mindfulness gives children a powerful tool to assist them in their self-development and allows them to feel more in control. It also improves their ability to focus, pay attention, follow instructions, calm and soothe themselves, regulate their emotions, and respond better to events and situations.

First and foremost, kids have to see their parents practicing mindful living or they won't bother. Parents are role models who lead by example, and kids tend to mimic their parents' behaviors and actions when young. So, establish your own mindfulness practice and share openly with your children what you are doing and why.

Look for easy mindfulness exercises and play you can do with your children. If these are too complex and complicated, they won't understand them and therefore won't adopt them as new behavior. You want to keep it simple, make it fun, and let them know the many benefits they will get from mindfulness practices, whether meditation, yoga, deep-breathing techniques when they feel scared, or staying present and attentive to their environment when crossing a busy street.

Help your kids develop their own ideas on how they can be mindful in their everyday lives and allow them to have some control over what that looks like. This is about building their skills and not

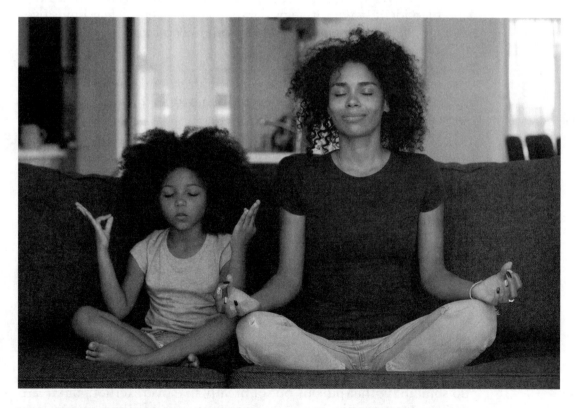

You can teach mindfulness to your children, but you should make sure to keep it simple and fun so they will be more likely to continue to practice this skill later in life.

expecting them to fully embrace mindfulness in every aspect of life. If they are being bullied at school or just found out they are having surgery, mindfulness may go right out the window and require a lot more patience and time, so remember that this is a progressive practice and don't expect perfection after only one week.

Let them try some of the things you might in your own practice, such as mindful walks in the park or on the beach, making gratitude lists before bed, praying before bed, doing breathing exercises together while watching a movie, practicing mindful eating, taking notice of how they feel at any given moment, or just stopping and saying five things about their immediate environment.

Noticing and naming is a fun game kids can play on long drives, sort of like "I Spy," and keeps them focused on the present moment rather than whining about the long trip. Noticing and naming their feelings is a critical step in learning how to identify and regulate their own emotions. If they can say "I am feeling really scared right now" and then identify why, it helps dissipate the power the fear holds over them, especially when followed by some deep belly breaths to calm them down.

Always remember that they are children, and it may take longer for them to develop new habits and behaviors. Practice mindfulness with them and strive to make it fun.

Breath Work

You breathe without thinking, without effort, every moment of your life. On average, we take about 16 breaths per minute, 960 per hour, 23,040 per day, and 8,409,600 per year. That is a lot of breathing and lung activity, yet how often do we really focus on our breath or recognize how shallowly we are breathing, which means we are not getting enough oxygen to our vital organs, including the brain?

Because breathing is automatic, or "involuntary respiration," we assume it is going to continue to happen and that we never need to pay it any attention. The only time we do think about it is when we do something that puts us out of breath, like overexertion, or we are gasping for air in the ocean as we swim for shore. Then, we get how critical breathing is.

Shallow breathing is common and related to stress. It's fast, lung–based breathing that does not take in adequate amounts of oxygen or hold it in the lungs to make us feel our best. When we check in with our breath and change it, breathing in more deeply into the abdomen, holding it for a few seconds, and fully exhaling, it is as if the light switch was turned on. We have more energy and vigor, our thinking is clearer, and we feel better in general and much less stressed.

Breath work refers to breathing exercises and techniques that help us improve our mental, physical, and spiritual well–being. We take voluntary control of our breath and purposefully breathe in ways that are more conducive to well–being. It is conscious, systematic, con–trolled breathing and can be done anywhere at any time.

We take voluntary control of our breath and purposefully breathe in ways that are more conducive to well-being.

Breath work activates the body's parasympathetic nervous sys–tem, slows down your heart rate, and lowers your blood pressure for an overall feeling of calm. Breath work can help the body's immune system work better, lower stress, assist in better sleep patterns, enrich creative thinking, release negativity, process pain and trauma, and connect us with a higher power or level of conscious awareness. It is an integral part of meditation and is used in shamanic traditions, and in yoga it is called pranayama, the practice of directing the breath, but is also taught and practiced on its own. Some of the most popular techniques are:

- Belly breaths or diaphragmatic breathing: Sit up tall and breathe in deeply through the nose, if possible, with one palm placed over your lower abdominal area. Feel the breath going into this area, lifting your hand. Do not breathe into the lungs. You want to breathe into the diaphragm while relaxing the neck and chest areas. Hold the breath there for four seconds to allow higher ox–ygen intake, which will then nourish your body's cells and organs, then fully exhale from the mouth with your lips puckered, as if pulling the abdominal area in with an invisible string. Do this 10 times and see how different you feel. Even a handful of belly breaths can sharpen your mind and energize your body.

- Sigh power: Inhale deeply, filling your lungs and abdomen with as much air as you can take in. When you feel that's all you can inhale, take a quick extra breath. Exhale while sighing out loud, letting all the air escape your lungs and abdomen. Do this for one or two minutes when you feel extra anxious or stressed.

- Circular breathing: Breathe in and out continuously with no breaks or pauses. Inhale, then exhale, and do not retain the breath.

- Box breathing: Inhale deeply for four seconds. Hold your breath for four seconds. Exhale for four seconds. Hold for four seconds before taking the next breath. Do several rounds to increase alertness and mindfulness.

- Empty the tank breathing: Inhale for a count of three, then slowly exhale to the count of six. Keep your focus on the breath as it leaves the body. Release as much as you can. Then, repeat several times until you feel calmer. This breath activates the parasympathetic nervous system and calms the sympathetic nervous system.

- Spirit breathing: Breathe in through the nose into the belly and imagine your breath is "prana," the life force entering your body and filling you with energy connected to your higher self. Hold the breath for four or five seconds and imagine the prana moving through your body, strengthening and nourishing every cell and muscle, bone and organ, tissue and fiber. Then, slowly release with an "ahhhhhhhh" until your belly is empty of air. Repeat as often as you wish.

- Holotropic breathing: Inhale and exhale for the same amount of time, accompanied by music or an instructor's guidance. You can vary the speed of the inhales and exhales, but they must be the same. The purpose is to produce a similar high to using drugs without the drugs by altering your state of consciousness with your breath and the accompanying external sounds.

- Rebirthing breathing: Best accompanied by a seasoned instructor or program, this kind of visually guided circular breath work focuses on releasing pent-up trauma and clearing out blocked-up stress from the traumatic experience of your birth. As you breathe, your birth is reimagined in a way that releases emotional trauma and baggage that you have carried with you since birth. It is advised to do rebirthing with someone who knows the process and can supervise your progress.

If you need a little extra guidance, many YouTube instructional videos can walk you through the steps as well as a host of guided breath work programs for purchase. Breath work has few risks, but never hold or retain your breath too long, and stop if you feel faint or dizzy and return to normal breathing patterns. The best thing you can do for your health, whether body, mind, or spirit, is to breathe more deeply into the belly and become fully aware of the power of the breath as it moves through you, something you can retrain yourself to do through practice and habit.

No matter which technique you use, it is about increasing awareness and mindfulness. As you breathe, you can be aware of thoughts in your mind, but do not attach to them. Allow them to drift by as if clouds in the sky. Feel any emotions that arise and breathe into them. If using intuition work, pay attention to that still, small voice within and take notice of any words, images, or phrases that pop into your mind. You can also do breath work with a guided visualization to set intentions or goals such as losing weight, quitting smoking, or overcoming shyness.

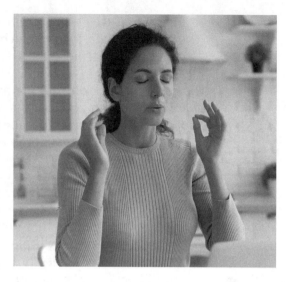

Conscious breathing exercises help to calm the mood, lower blood pressure, and boost your immune system.

We can survive without food for weeks and water for days but only three minutes at most without air. Breathing is life, and when we choose to find ways to make the best of our breath, we experience well–being and a stronger connection to the life force all around us.

Letting Go

Living mindfully also allows us the gift of letting go. A famous saying goes, "What we resist, persists." Much of our stress and worry can be alleviated if we let go of our need to redo the past or control the future as well as our desire to control other people. Trying to get others to behave and act as we want them to is a futile exercise because people are all not cookie–cutter products we can move about on the countertop at will. Even our children, to some extent, are not ours to control, especially when they get older. We must learn to let go and to do it gracefully.

It is never easy to stop clutching and grasping at what we want to keep forever, but that isn't how it stays anyway. Think of a cupped hand with water. You can hold some of it without spilling it. Now, clench that hand into a fist. The water squirts out of every possible opening, and you are left with a wet hand. Life is the same. What we grasp and hold too tightly, we can choke out of existence. It is an illusion that we can control others or control what happens outside of our immediate locus, which is only how we think, behave, and respond to life around us. That's it. To think otherwise is to suffer.

You can look back on your life and see numerous examples of how something you panicked over never happened or it happened completely different from what you feared, and you realize how much time and energy you wasted.

Staying mindful of the moment at hand helps keep us from dwelling too much in the past, where grief and regret can set up house and lock us in so that we can never move forward, or fretting anxiously over a future that will no doubt be much different from what we are afraid of or will play out in such a way that we will handle it just as we have everything else in our lives. You can look back on your life and see numerous examples of how something you panicked over never happened or it happened completely different from what you feared, and you realize how much time and energy you wasted. You can also see how the past had its powerful lessons; life should not contain regrets, as long as you strive on a daily basis to be the best you can be in the now. The now, the present, is where life meets us at and where we have control.

The Serenity Prayer, written by American theologian Reinhold Niebuhr, sums it all up nicely: "God, grant me the serenity to accept the things I cannot change, courage to change the things I can, and wisdom to know the difference." Accepting what is, recognizing what is within our ability to change, should we wish to, then having the courage to make those changes is critical to a life well lived and a state of well-being. Letting go of all else is pure wisdom.

The Art of Detachment

Detachment and nonattachment are two names for a similar concept of not attaching too much to any goal, outcome, or expectation. In many spiritual traditions such as Buddhism and yogic practices, detachment is a way to end all suffering because while we can still pursue goals, dreams, and hopes, we do not get so attached to them that it could destroy us if they happened differently. It is a way of being in the world that allows you to live without being bogged down by the fears, desires, doubts, and obstructions that come with wanting things to be an exact certain way before we can feel good. It is not a running from but a running toward a more open perspective of what the world has to offer if we get out of our own limited tunnel vision of what we think it should look like.

Some falsely believe that detachment means you are aloof and not invested in your intentions or your relationships with others. The truth is that you are invested in everything, but you leave the "how it all unfolds" up to a higher source: God, the universe, or a spirit. Nonattachment to outcome does not mean you are not concerned or invested in the process. It is letting go of the thoughts and emotions that say things MUST be a certain way for you to be happy and not allowing life to unfold as it will.

It [detachment] is letting go of the thoughts and emotions that say things MUST be a certain way for you to be happy and not allowing life to unfold as it will.

Approaching the world and your life with a sense of nonattachment means you act on the things that matter but don't become depressed or distraught if they unfold another way. An example might be setting the intention to meet the love of your life and being detached enough from the outcome that you allow that person to come into your life naturally rather than force the outcome on someone that may not be right for you at all. Another example might be wanting to achieve a certain career goal and not allowing yourself to be open to other career opportunities that might be even more exciting and promising.

This approach is especially powerful in relationships, where we so easily become codependent on others for our happiness and fulfillment or seek to force our spouses and children to behave a certain way so we can feel better. Loving from a place of detachment means you love someone unconditionally and allow their own lives to unfold as they should without you micromanaging everything, which only serves to make you miserable when they don't act and behave according to your schedule or rules.

We can experience greater inner peace and overall well-being when we stop attaching our joy, happiness, and fulfillment to specifics that may or may not fill those needs. When we detach from outcome and focus on the process, doing our part and releasing the result to the universe at large to fulfill, we find that sometimes people, circumstances, and things come into our lives that we never imagined could.

Try journaling, setting intentions, praying, and working with goals in all areas of life with a sense of detachment to specific out-comes. Focus instead on the essence of what it is you want from those experiences you seek, such as finding love instead of hooking up with Jane or George (who might be incredibly toxic in the long-term) or experiencing an increase in overall prosperity instead of making more money on a job you hate, and let the universe decide how to best bring them to you and in what form.

Create Your Way to Better Health

Humans were born to create things. When we are children, we create freely, whether it be doing macaroni art, coloring in our coloring books, writing stories, playing musical instruments, or telling ghost tales by the campfire. As adults, we consider creativity a nonessential act compared to working and earning money, and creative play is either relegated to an occasional hour on the weekend or completely ignored.

Engaging in creative activities isn't just for fun; it improves brain function and mental health. Cognitive theory suggests that being cre-ative is the basis for all human life and is therefore not something to push off until next week. Having fun comes with incredible benefits like getting totally lost in a project or en-deavor and exploring the imagination's ability to go beyond the five senses.

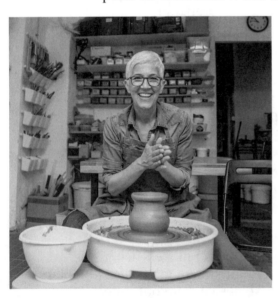

Creativity creates flow, that sense of losing track of time because you are so into what you are doing in the present moment. Writers and artists know this state of flow well, but it is accessible to anyone. Creativity reduces anxiety and calms the chatter of the monkey mind and doing something creative such as art or crafting has a meditative effect on the mind and body. Creative acts can include gardening, painting the house, sewing or knitting, and even cooking, all of which focus the mind.

Doing anything creative can be immensely satisfying and therapeutic, nourishing both body and spirit.

Other types of creativity such as journaling can help alleviate anxiety, depression, and PTSD by expressing difficult feelings and emotions on paper to process them. Writing daily about life improves the functioning of the immune system and increases well-being. Listening to music, or playing it yourself, engages focus and improves communication between the brain's two hemispheres. Creativity improves memory and resilience in older adults and can help those suffering from dementia find a way to connect with their surroundings and experience an increase in cognitive functioning while having a little fun.

The Centers for Disease Control and Prevention (CDC) has conducted surveys that show that anxiety and stress during the 2020–2021 COVID-19 lockdowns skyrocketed, and many people turned to creativity to help destress. Art and play therapies have been used for decades by therapists and psychologists to treat anxiety and PTSD in adults and children.

Some people have hobbies or jobs involving creative pursuits, but even if you don't perceive yourself as creative, you can experience the benefits of being in a flow state from doing things such as reading and doodling while chatting on the phone, making up crazy dances while doing housework, or writing funny limericks to post on social media. No rules exist as to how you can be creative and find ways to express yourself, which is what creativity is all about.

Social Connection

In a study done at Brigham Young University, head author Julianne Holt-Lunstad showed "substantial evidence now indicates that individuals lacking social connections … are at risk for premature mortality." The rate is even higher than for those who suffer from obesity. Loneliness, then, contributes to higher rates of death. It's hard to believe in our socially connected world with cell phones, computers, apps, and social media keeping us plugged in 24/7 that we are actually lonelier than ever. Lunstad predicts that loneliness will reach epidemic proportions by the year 2030 if no actions are taken.

With Facebook, Instagram, Twitter, Snapchat, Facetime, chat rooms, messenger apps, and numerous ways to keep in touch with others, are we missing the crucial element of person-to-person contact and bonds and friendships that are based on spending time together, not over screens? Human beings thrive on social connection, and when that connection becomes detached and artificial, we all suffer.

Clearly, this suffering is reaching epidemic levels that threaten our physical and mental health and well-being. Sure, it's great to have friends and followers on social media from all over the world, but the connection is a tenuous and artificial one that lacks the depth of being with someone face-to-face, experiencing life together, laughing and crying with one another.

Elderly and poor people who often do not have computers or cell phones suffer the most, but everyone appears to be lacking as far as the old-fashioned, personal contact that once kept communities and neighborhoods strong and family units and friendships lasting more than just a few years, if that long.

Well-being is impossible if you are lonely and lack contact with others that is meaningful. Social isolation is as much a killer as any virus. Lunstad notes that "although living alone can offer conveniences and advantages for an individual, this meta-analysis indicates that physical health is not among them." She cites another study that "has demonstrated higher survival rates for those who are more socially connected." A 75-year Harvard University study with men found that it is universally clear that without loving and supportive relationships, the men were not happy. This no doubt applies to women, too, who tend to be more social to begin with.

We need connection to survive and thrive. We need
alone time, too, but balance and the opportunity to be
with other human beings is essential, not just over a screen
or via a voice chat.

We need connection to survive and thrive. We need alone time, too, but balance and the opportunity to be with other human beings is essential, not just over a screen or via a voice chat. To stop the loneliness epidemic in its tracks, we need to reach out to those who are unable to connect to the outside world and make sure we are not getting too used to being stuck inside in our comfort bubbles.

We may be able to live without other people in a physical sense, but mentally, emotionally, and spiritually, we would suffer tremendously. We were meant for relationships with ourselves, others, and the planet. This includes exposure to pets, too, as they can provide connection and love we might not always have access to otherwise. Pets love us unconditionally and are the best snugglers and listeners around. People who lose a pet are found to grieve as deeply as those who lose a human loved one; that is how strong our bond is. In this technology-heavy age, we find more and more reasons to hide out in our homes, rooms, dorms, and spaces and only go "out there" when necessary. This mindset is killing us, as the above studies show, and certainly does not make for a well-lived life.

For those seeking more connection who may not have family and friends nearby, some ideas include resources such as Meetup, social media site groups that get together locally, neighborhood email newsletters and websites that feature activities of every possible sort, and local organizations for volunteering or spending time with like-minded souls. If you are not on a computer, you can call your city and ask them to send you a catalog of classes or events the city puts on. Check the phone book for community groups and civic centers, which can provide you with ideas on activities and groups in your area. Reach out to neighbors and get to know them. Ask your city government about volunteer opportunities, as that is not only a great way to spend time with others but for a good cause such as a neighborhood cleanup. If one doesn't exist in your area, start your own.

Perhaps the days of front-yard coffee klatches and block parties are gone for many people, but one can reach out and connect in new ways. One way technology can be used for good is to find groups and hobbyists and ask who is in your area. Start a get-together group that meets regularly, or look for classes through your city that you can take to meet others who like the same things you do. Opportunities to meet new people and make new friends are everywhere.

The age of technology is not going away, but we don't have to lose our humanity because of it.

News and Media Fasts

Our nonstop access to screens and media in all its formats has created a new level of stress requiring an occasional detox or fast. We take in too much negative and bad news, and it plays havoc on our well-being to the point where we become fearful, anxious, and unable to relax. The worries of the world and the weight of the world threaten to smother us, resulting in bad moods, depression, irritability, anxiety, and lack of quality sleep. Often, we replace news and social media with bingeing fictional shows without realizing that they, too, affect our moods and peace of mind. Watching violent or scary shows or dramas that expose other people's problems isn't always conducive to your own well-being and, if indulged in too much, detach you from your own life, the good and the bad.

In general, our triggered behaviors don't serve anyone or anything, yet we expose ourselves to them daily.

Between the news, the binge shows, and social media, we can get triggered by something in so many ways and experience a past trauma or hurt or react negatively and regret it later. In general, our triggered behaviors don't serve anyone or anything, yet we expose ourselves to them daily. If we survived abuse, seeing a barrage of news reports or Facebook posts about abuse can set us back and lead to physiological symptoms such as speeding heart rate, shortness of breath, fatigue, changes in eating and sleeping patterns, inability to do our work or care for ourselves and our families, and overall malaise. Sometimes, we just must disconnect.

Just as a detox or fast can help to purify the body and rejuvenate our immune systems, a news fast does the same for our emotional health. Too much negative news, whether from family and friends posting on social media or nightly news striking terror into our hearts over the latest shooting or natural disaster, takes its toll on our nervous system and robs us from our peace of mind. Watching the news before bedtime also robs us from our ability to fall asleep.

Don't worry about falling behind if you take a fast from news and media and something happens. You will find out somehow, and by fasting, you filter out all the unnecessary minutia that is not necessary for your survival. A news fast can be a week or even just one day if you cannot imagine going more than 24 hours not checking Facebook or turning on CNN. A regularly scheduled news fast will do you wonders and, over time, you might just find yourself extending the amount of time you are off the grid and unplugged from the onslaught of stressful stories and communications. You will feel more balanced and calm, and you sleep much better without constant exposure to wars, shootings, crime, corruption, and economic woe, not to mention the bombardment of ads for pharmaceuticals and products you don't want or need.

That doesn't even cover all the energy suckers and time wasters of social media. It's no wonder that most people never reach their goals in life. They're too busy glued to one screen or another as if their lives depended on them. Yes, this kind of obsession has all the hallmarks of an addiction, one that is incredibly diffi-cult to break free from. One day at a time, one news fast at a time. People who fol-low you on social media can be alerted that you will be offline ahead of time, so they don't worry. Others don't need to know every bit of your business. The whole idea of unplugging is to remove distractions long enough to catch your breath, regroup, and renew your spirit before diving back into the nonstop bar-rage of news and nonsense.

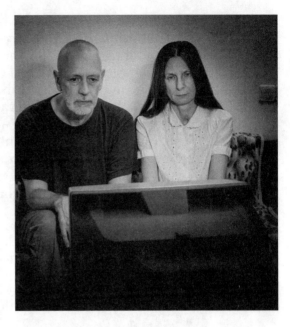

Try fasting from news and social media for one day, then see for how long you can increase the time. Work up to a week. Check in and see how you feel, why you are anxious when you are not plugged in, and what changes for the better when you consistently tune out screens in order to tune in to the world around you in person, with mindfulness and awareness. If you are unable to tune

The news media know that bad news gains audiences, and so much of what you see on TV can be upsetting. Try turning off the TV for a period of time and see how that affects your mood.

out even for a day, you could be addicted to your phone or to being constantly connected. It is a real addiction, one that is affecting not only adults but also our teens and children.

Once you decide you are ready to tune back in, try to limit your consumption of news and social media and focus on positive stories and people to follow. Sure, you need to know what is happening out there, and you can easily get caught up with a quick view of your local news, but to focus on the negative so much takes its toll men-tally, physically, and emotionally, requiring even more work to replace unhealthy coping skills and distractions with those that can nourish your spirit and calm your soul.

Therapy Is Not a Bad Word

So much negativity is still attached to seeking therapy when we are experiencing challenges in life, whether physical, emotional, or mental. Therapy comes in a variety of forms, all of which allow us to express what we are feeling with a third party who is not a family member or friend and who is trained to listen and respond with solid, workable methods for processing our pain and suffering and moving beyond it toward healing and well–being.

The most popular form of therapy is psychotherapy, or talk therapy, and often, just getting the pent–up emotions out of our head help us see more clearly. Having a trained professional to assist us as we do this can bring us a different perspective or walk with us through a grieving process that we could not do alone. The following therapy types open the door to a deeper healing through a variety of methods– one that might appeal to you over others.

- Cognitive behavioral therapy (CBT): The power of CBT comes from uncovering and acknowledging our unhealthy and self–destructive thoughts, feelings, and behavioral patterns. When we understand when these patterns originated, usually in childhood, and what they are, we can then make small, doable steps toward reprogramming our thoughts and emotions and, therefore, our be-

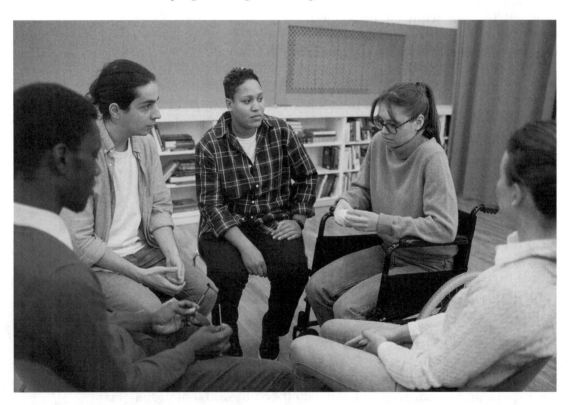

Everyone needs a little help sometimes, especially when trying to go through a life crisis. Do not be embarrassed if you need the help of trained counselors or therapists.

haviors to see different results in our lives. CBT does not involve taking medications and is a great way to move past the many ways we self-sabotage and embrace new "programming" that is much healthier and constructive and includes positive thinking and challenging old paradigms. According to the National Alliance on Mental Health, CBT is effective for treating anxiety and depression, bipolar disorder, eating disorders, and dealing with past trauma. A similar form of CBT called dialectical behavior therapy focuses on regulating emotions by being mindful and learning new ways to cope with situations and challenges. DBT is used in treating addictions, substance abuse, and mood disorders, including suicidal tendencies and PTSD. Phobia exposure therapy is also a type of CBT where the therapist works with the patient to overcome a fear or phobia by exposing him/her to the object of fear as a method of desensitization.

- Eye movement desensitization and reprocessing (EMDR): EMDR is a form of therapy often used to treat PTSD. The patient recalls traumatic situations from the past while performing specific eye movements that serve to disrupt the emotional response to the past trauma. The author of this book's own son used EMDR to successfully overcome childhood trauma from surgeries and the subsequent PTSD he developed.

- Family and marriage therapy: Relationship issues are the focus of family or marriage therapy, where the patient may see the therapist alone at times and with members of the family or their spouse at other times. This is used to understand and interact more positively with loved ones and to find constructive and productive ways to overcome challenges and difficulties in the relationship. It is also called interpersonal therapy and can be used to treat depression and social anxiety.

- Psychodynamics: Psychodynamics involves the therapist asking questions of the patient to learn their patterns of thought and feelings, then creating ways to change those negative patterns to more positive and productive behaviors. This can also focus on emotions that are triggered by past events, often unconsciously, and learning how to identify triggers and choose new, more constructive responses.

- Art and play therapy: Art therapy and play therapy involve using art and playing games to help the patient express their fears and challenges and process them through a medium of their choice, such as drawing, painting, or playing with building blocks. This is a wonderful form of therapy for children who may not be able to verbalize what they are thinking and feeling.

- Animal-assisted therapy: Trained therapy pets often make the best therapists, especially for children and nonverbal adults, and are used in hospitals, nursing homes, and medical facilities to provide comfort and support for patients who are undergoing chemotherapy or surgery. It is a wonderful way to help those with PTSD and anxiety disorders.

- Group therapy: Group therapy involves a trained therapist leading a group discussion with individuals sharing their stories and comments in a supportive environment. Group therapy works well for addiction and substance abuse and for showing anyone in treatment for any disorder that they are not alone. It helps the patient see new perspectives and glean new ideas on how to cope and process their own experiences more positively.

These different types of therapy offer help from someone who understands how to process and work through challenges of every possible kind. If you think therapy is right for you, contact your healthcare provider, as many do cover psychotherapy and may even have on-site therapists at affordable rates or on a sliding scale.

Nature Power

The average adult in the United States over their lifetime spends the equivalent of 44 years looking at a screen, according to a recent study. The statistic looked at the breakdown of the average day of 4.5 hours watching TV, around five hours on computers, and over three hours on gaming devices. Our ancestors spent almost all their time outdoors among the elements, but in our technological age, we are doing the exact opposite, and it's taking a toll on our physical, mental, and emotional well–being. We don't have to become outdoor nomads again to benefit. Even taking a walk outside every day or spending an hour in nature improves many health markers, and we just plain feel better. We can also bring nature indoors with little gardens, fresh flowers, and growing our own herbs on the kitchen counter.

Scientific studies on the benefits of nature abound. One study recorded in the *Proceedings of the National Academy of Sciences (PNAS)* showed the benefits of time in nature. The study, titled "Nature Experience Reduces Rumination and Subgenual Prefrontal Cortex Activation," was published in July 2015; the abstract is below:

> Urbanization has many benefits, but it also is associated with increased levels of mental illness, including depression. It has been suggested that decreased nature experience may help to

explain the link between urbanization and mental illness. This suggestion is supported by a growing body of correlational and experimental evidence, which raises a further question: what mechanism(s) link decreased nature experience to the development of mental illness? One such mechanism might be the impact of nature exposure on rumination, a maladaptive pattern of self-referential thought that is associated with heightened risk for depression and other mental illnesses. We show in healthy participants that a brief nature experience, a 90–min walk in a natural setting, decreases both self-reported rumination and neural activity in the subgenual prefrontal cortex (sgPFC), whereas a 90–min walk in an urban setting has no such effects on self-reported rumination or neural activity. In other studies, the sgPFC has been associated with a self-focused behavioral withdrawal linked to rumination in both depressed and healthy individuals. This study reveals a pathway by which nature experience may improve mental well-being and suggests that accessible natural areas within urban contexts may be a critical resource for mental health in our rapidly urbanizing world.

Stepping away from the screens and getting outside should be our first nature, but we are so trained to do more work and hole up indoors on our gadgets.

Stepping away from the screens and getting outside should be our first nature, but we are so trained to do more work and hole up indoors on our gadgets. We choose to get together now over Zoom and FaceTime and lose the experiences of having lunch at an outside café or breathing in fresh air with a walk on the beach with a friend. We are overexposed to indoor air pollution and toxins and underexposed to sunshine, vitamin D, and the feel of breezes on our skin. Many ways to get back to nature don't require expensive travel, equipment, or learning new skills. That's the great thing about nature. Accessing its many gifts is as easy as going outside and kicking off your shoes.

Animal Healing

You don't necessarily have to travel to a park to connect to nature. Even just bringing a domestic pet into your life can have many benefits. Numerous scientific studies show that owning a pet can do wonders for lowering stress and experiencing greater well-being. Pets provide us with something to snuggle with, companionship, hilarious antics, and warmth when they cuddle up to us on cold nights. Pets provide affection that is unconditional and give us a reason to get outside and walk or move around more.

According to CNN's February 2020 article by Sandee LaMotte, "The Benefits of Owning a Pet–and the Surprising Science Behind It," having a fur baby in the home brings joy and positive feelings along with higher survival rates, fewer heart attacks, less loneliness and depression, lower blood pressure, higher self–esteem, better sleep, and more physical activity. This is according to Professor Harold Herzog of Western Carolina University, who has studied the positive effects of pet ownership for years.

An analysis of over 4 million pet owners in America, New Zealand, the United Kingdom, Canada, and Scandinavia found that dog ownership was associated with a 24 percent reduction in all causes of death, and if the person had suffered a heart attack or stroke, having a dog made them 31 percent less likely to die of cardiovascular disease. Dr. Glenn Levine, the chair of the writing group of the American Heart Association's scientific statement on pet ownership, said that while nonrandomized studies could not prove that owning a dog directly leads to reduced mortality rates, "these robust findings are certainly at least suggestive of this."

A 2013 official statement from the American Heart Association stated that dog owners were 54 percent more likely to stay active and get the recommended amount of exercise, suggesting that having a pet in the house is good for the body as well as the mind and spirit.

While some studies show conflicting results about the benefits of owning a pet and point to negatives like house training, barking and behavioral issues, and having another mouth to feed and body to take care of, in general, most pet owners believe they get more positives than negatives and point to better mood and fewer feelings of loneliness and isolation.

Though getting a pet from puppyhood can be stressful and costly, children love to grow up with a dog or cat they can call their own. Older animals make wonderful companions and are more likely to be homebodies for those who cannot get out of the house much. Energetic pets are great for athletic, outdoorsy types. Pets don't have to be the usual dogs and cats. They can be anything from guinea pigs

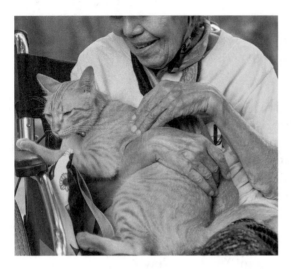

The positive effects of pets such as cats and dogs has been known for some time. Animals are often used as emotional and mental therapy for the elderly, ill, and disabled.

to ducks to lizards. The type of pet you choose may be based on the level of commitment and time you are able to give, and if you travel a lot, it might not be a good idea until you are more settled, as pets don't like to be left alone. Their feelings and needs must be taken into consideration, too.

Stroking a cat's soft fur or petting a dog can no doubt relax your nerves after a stressful day. A snuggly pet won't make the demands of children go away, yet you get the companionship and free face licks. For emotional support, nothing beats a wonderful pet to be there for you when no one else is around. Pets listen without talking back and don't ask for money or the car keys. They can't wait to see us when we get home from work and don't care how bad we look or whether or not we've had a shower. They require care and love, but the care and love a pet can bring are so much that they become as much a part of the family as the kids.

The animal you connect with does not have to be a dog or cat, of course. It can be a bird, or a horse, or even farm animals. Many people have found it therapeutic to go swimming with dolphins, playing with ferrets, having a pet rat, creating a coy pond, or bonding with ducks or geese, just to name a few possibilities.

Earthing and Forest Bathing

Maybe our ancestors were a lot smarter than we give them credit for. They lived close to the earth and her cycles and rhythms and understood that nature provided more than just food to eat and water to drink. The hippies of the 1960s spoke of "flower power" and "getting back to the garden," but our hunger for faster, cheaper, and easier ignored their pleas to connect with Mother Earth and instead pursue technology that has us now slaves to the indoors. To experience real well-being, maybe it's time we got back to the garden, the beach, the woods, or a waterfall.

Earthing

When we were children, we loved to go barefoot outside. As adults, we rarely remove our shoes and socks long enough to benefit from "earthing," a grounding technique that connects you directly to the energies of the planet beneath your feet, complete with a growing body of scientific research behind it.

Living things are electrical beings. Beneath the surface of Earth is energy that we cannot observe unless we are experiencing static from our laundry or we get a shock from touching metal on a super-hot and dry day. Earth's own surface conducts energy, which seeks the path of least resistance, so when you stand barefoot on the grass, dirt, or sandy beach, you are absorbing that energy.

The human body holds positive–charged electrical energy. When you are barefoot, the transfer of electrons from the earth into your body happens because nothing impedes it, such as cement, shoes, socks, or pavement. Your skin acts as a conductor to receive Earth's natural electrical and limitless supply of free or mobile electrons. These negative charges create a stable internal bioelectrical environment for normal functioning of bodily systems, including regulating circadian rhythms and balancing cortisol levels.

When you are barefoot, the transfer of electrons from the earth into your body happens because nothing impedes it, such as cement, shoes, socks, or pavement.

The human brain, heart, and neurotransmitters rely on electrical activity and signals to operate, so earthing improves overall health, and its anti–inflammatory properties fight the proliferation of free radicals and reduce inflammation that leads to disease. Our ancestors walked barefoot or wearing the skins of wild animals they had caught. The direct contact they had through the perspiration–moistened animal skins, according to the 2012 issue of the *Journal of Environmental Public Health*, allowed free electrons from the earth to enter the body and equilibrate with the electrical potential of the earth. This served to stabilize the electrical environment of the organs, tissues, and cells in the body.

Sleeping directly on the ground improves sleep cycles and normalizes cortisol rhythm, but you must be directly on the grass or dirt to get the best results or have as little as possible between your skin and the ground. This might help explain why so many people have insomnia and other sleeping disorders because in the modern world, we now sleep on beds and platforms well above ground level unless we are camping.

The neutralization of free radicals reduces acute and chronic inflammation and slows the aging process by improving the circulation of blood and oxygen throughout the body, better distributing nutrients to where they are needed, and flushing out waste and toxins. Earthing is well studied for reducing stress and normalizing cortisol levels.

To benefit from earthing, go outside and walk or stand on grass, dirt, or sand without shoes or socks on. You can stroll along the beach or through the park or do some gardening while standing on the soil. Spend at least 10 minutes barefoot, and the more often, the better. Connecting our bodies directly to the energy of Earth is as old as human beings are, yet we spend so much of our time today sitting at desks in offices or cubicles or at home walking on flooring or carpet that we have lost the amazing energetic charges of the planet we live on.

Negative Ions

Spend some time near the ocean or other moving bodies of water to benefit from the presence of negative ions. A large body of scientific research documents the positive effects of negative ions and how they benefit our health and well-being. Waterfalls give off an energizing burst of energy as they release ions, charged air particles, molecules, or atoms with a negative charge to them. These air molecules are exposed to things like moving water, sunlight, and radiation, and break apart. Negative ions, which contain an extra negatively charged electron, are found in nature, such as forests, mountains, and bodies of water like lakes and the ocean, but they are also found during thunderstorms, which is why the air after a storm often feels so crisp and clear. Negative ions rid the air of dust mites, pollens, allergens, bacteria, and viruses and attach themselves to positive ions to neutralize them.

The human body is made up of positive and negative ions, but modern life exposes us to way too many positive ions, thanks to our technology negatively influencing our body's magnetic field. When we spend all our time in front of or near electronic devices, we become tired and lethargic from all the positive ions and lose our energy and vitality. We also experience weakened immune systems. All of this can be rectified by getting outside in nature more often, preferably barefoot. Negative ions produce biochemical reactions such as the increased production of serotonin, which improves mood and makes us more resistant to diseases.

You can have some of the benefits of negative ions by purchasing a negative-ion room purifier or putting a water feature or two in your home or backyard, but nothing beats getting outdoors. Have you ever had a "forest bath"?

Forest Bathing

The Japanese have a mindfulness practice called "forest bathing." No, you don't take a bath in the woods, although that can be quite relaxing. Forest bathing involves engaging all your senses in the beauty of the woods. Called *shinrin-yoku*, which means "taking in the forest atmosphere," this experience involves all five senses as you

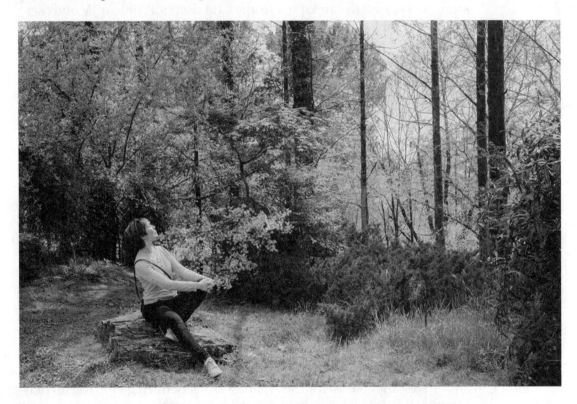

Shinrin-yoku is the practice of "forest bathing." To do this, simply visit a wooded area (preferably with no signs of humans) and allow yourself to take in the beauty and sensations of the woods.

smell the scent of the plants and trees, touch the soft moss or rough bark, taste the clean air, hear the sounds of woodland creatures, and see the beauty and lushness of the natural environment free from the marks of human existence.

The concept was first introduced in 1982 by the Forest Agency of Japan as a way to encourage people to get outside and spend time in nature to decrease levels of stress. In Japan, forest bathing is a popular practice, and people can even receive free medical checkups in the forest. Forest bathing benefits the body, mind, and spirit. Camping and spending time in nature hiking or fishing is a form of forest bathing when the senses are all engaged, but it is important to leave cell phones and gadgets at home.

The pioneer of research into forest bathing is Dr. Qing Li, the president of the Japanese Society of Forest Medicine, who has done many studies into the effects of this practice on mood, stress, and the immune system. In one of his studies, he used a Profile of Moods scientific questionnaire with 65 "feeling" words and asked participants to describe how weak or strong they experienced each word during the week. Those participants who had at some point during the week engaged in forest bathing showed a decrease in words indicating anxiety, anger, and depression and an increase in words describing vigor, health, and positive moods. Li also found in another study that habitual forest bathing increased the body's natural killer (NK) cells, which fight cancer.

The takeaway here is that spending any time in nature is so beneficial, whether barefoot or not, near bodies of moving water or not, deep in the forest or not.

The takeaway here is that spending any time in nature is so beneficial, whether barefoot or not, near bodies of moving water or not, deep in the forest or not. A quick walk in the park helps, as does a monthly trip to the seashore. Obviously, the more you can get outside and make a habit of it, the more benefits you receive. Nature heals, and earthing, negative ions, and forest bathing are three ways that science is catching up to this fact.

In another study for the Japanese Society of Hygiene, researchers conducted field experiments with study participants across Japan and underwent evaluations of their pulse, heart rate, blood pressure, and other markers in different environments. Measurements were recorded at the same time each day for consistency, and the results showed that compared to a city, many more profound benefits occurred when the participants engaged in forest bathing. The researchers stated in their findings that "the results of field experiments also provide a platform for interested enterprises, Universities, and local governments to promote the effective use of forest resources in stress management, health promotion, rehabilitation, and the prevention of disease."

Maybe one day, your doctor will say, "Take two hours in the forest, and call me in the morning."

Benefits of Sunlight

We are trapped in our homes and office spaces, rarely going outside except to head to lunch or the local coffee shop. Our health is suffering because of it. Getting adequate natural sunlight has huge health and well-being benefits. About 10–20 minutes of exposure with major body parts such as arms and legs bare and without sunscreen offers the most benefit without concern for sunburn or skin damage. If you have fair or freckled skin, you may need to spend less time in the sun. Sunlight provides the following benefits:

- Helps the skin produce vitamin D
- Improves sleep quality
- Improves eye health
- Anchors the body's internal clock and circadian rhythm
- Reduces anxiety and stress
- Boosts mood and libido
- Regulates appetite and metabolism
- Helps strengthen the brain, bones, and immune system

Early morning exposure to the sun for even five minutes does wonders to keep your circadian rhythm and internal sleep clock working well. You want to tell your brain it's daytime as soon as you get up in order to get that boost of wakefulness and energy. You can walk or run in the morning sun, go on an afternoon hike, swim in a pool or lake, or just lie on a lounge chair and relax with a cool drink, but the bottom line is, don't shun the sun. Your body needs it, and limited daily exposure is good for the mind and the spirit, too.

Sunlight affects us in other ways: it can soothe the spirit. A Japanese word, *komorebi*, refers to the ephemeral experience of sunlight

as it is filtered through a canopy of tree leaves. This same mystical experience might happen watching the way sunlight reflects in dappled
light off the tops of tall palm trees.

You can get creative and take photos of each morning's sunrise to
post on social media. Start an Instagram or Facebook page devoted to
your sunrise snapshots. Share the joy of each morning. It's a great way
to start your day and give others a nice visual to start theirs with a smile.

Sleep Your Way to Better Health

A long with diet and exercise, sleep is the third leg of the triangle of health. Sleep is so important to physical, mental, and emotional health that it is often recommended to get more sleep even if it means getting less exercise. A current pandemic of epic proportions involves insomnia, poor sleep quality, and sleep deprivation, which is taking a huge toll on human health and on our healthcare system.

We are told we need approximately seven to eight hours of un-interrupted sleep per night, but who really gets this on a regular basis? We fall asleep later, get up during the night more often, and wake up groggy and tired, then we either drink too much coffee or caffeinated beverages to stay awake during the day or we nap, which makes it harder to fall asleep at bedtime. It's a vicious circle, one made even worse with all the cell phones and gadgets that we use at night, dis-rupting our natural sleep cycles.

Some basic statistics about sleep from the Sleep Foundation and the CDC are most telling:

- Adults between the ages of 18–54 need between seven and nine hours of sleep a night. Over the age of 65, seven to eight hours.

Over 35 percent of adults report sleeping fewer than seven hours per night.

- Half of all Americans report feeling sleepy during the day most days of the week.
- REM sleep makes up between 20–25 percent of sleep in healthy adults. We average about two REM cycles each night dreaming.
- During sleep, the body's temperature drops by one to two degrees Fahrenheit, and metabolism drops by about 15 percent.
- 32 percent of working adults report sleeping fewer than six hours of sleep per night.
- Over 42 percent of single parents sleep fewer than seven hours per night compared to 32 percent of adults in two-parent households and 31 percent of parents without children.
- Active-duty military members are 34 percent more likely to report insufficient sleep.
- Between 10–30 percent of adults report chronic insomnia.
- Between 30–48 percent of older adults suffer from insomnia.
- Women are twice as likely to suffer from insomnia.
- Between 135,000–200,000 people suffer from narcolepsy.
- Approximately 9 percent of adults suffer from some type of sleep apnea.
- About 69 percent of adult men over 40 get up to go to the bathroom at least once per night. That number rises to 76 percent of women who do the same.
- Approximately 57 percent of men snore, and about 40 percent of women do.
- Premenstrual women, pregnant women, and menopausal women lose more sleep and report night sweats that make sleep quality even worse.
- Babies need between 12–17 hours of sleep each day. Toddlers need 11–14 hours.
- Preschool-aged children are recommended to get between 10–13 hours of sleep a day, and school-aged children between nine and 11 hours.
- Between the ages of 10–12, average total sleep per night drops by 40–50 minutes.
- Approximately 27 percent of children snore.
- Over half of all middle schoolers and about two-thirds of high schoolers get less than the recommended amount of sleep for their age group.
- Driving drowsy causes over 6,000 car crashes every year.

- Nurses who work 12.5-hour shifts are reported to commit more than three times as many medical errors than those who work 8.5-hour shifts.
- 75 percent of adults with insomnia also suffer from depression.
- 40 percent of people with insomnia are believed to also suffer from mental disorders, and 90 percent of people with PTSD have insomnia.
- More than two servings of alcohol per day for both genders decreases sleep quality by 39.2 percent.
- About 8.3 percent of adults take medication to help them sleep at least four times per week.
- 20 percent of adults tried a natural remedy for sleep problems in the past year.
- Sales of melatonin supplements in the United States alone rose from $62 million in 2003 to $378 million in 2014.
- 28 percent of U.S. adults have used a smartphone app to help them sleep in the past year.

These statistics represent a small sampling of Americans, but the message is clear: people are losing sleep and suffering for it. Exhaustion during the day, less productivity at work, more difficulties dealing with daily tasks, disease, bad moods, mental disorders, weight gain, less desire to exercise, too much caffeine or stimulant use, and higher levels of inflammation due to the body's lack of downtime all are symptoms of poor sleep quality and quantity.

Causes of Poor Sleep

So many factors play a role in poor sleep: age, stress, illness, worries about money or relationships, what's going on in the world, and job issues are common. Having a poor sleep schedule or no sleep routine prevents quality sleep, as does a lousy diet and blood sugar imbalances. People who exercise sleep far better than those who are sedentary, and chronic pain sufferers get far less sleep than those without pain keeping them awake. Other causes are thyroid problems, hormonal

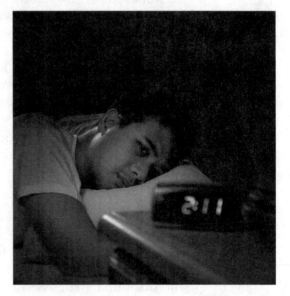

Experts say you need seven to eight hours of sleep per night, yet most Americans do not get this or do not get restful sleep.

imbalances, LED light exposure, sleep apnea, obesity, gut and digestive issues, heart palpitations, restless leg syndrome, nutrient deficiencies, and too much caffeine or drug stimulant.

Of the actual sleep disorders, the most common are:

- Insomnia
- Sleep apnea
- Restless leg syndrome
- Narcolepsy
- Sleepwalking

Lack of sleep is linked to many chronic illnesses including heart disease and stroke, diabetes, obesity, anxiety and depression, and autoimmune disorders. The body and brain cannot function at optimal levels with so little restful and rejuvenating sleep, and mental and cognitive functions begin to suffer after only a few days of less than stellar sleep. Brain fog, memory loss, lack of coordination, falling asleep during the day, dizziness, blurred vision, irritability, and bad moods are the results of sleep loss or of waking up too many times during the night to ever get the deep sleep that is needed.

"Coronasomnia" affected millions who were already dealing with job losses, lockdowns, sick loved ones, and fearmongering in the media.

Too little sleep makes it harder to learn, fight off colds and bugs, lose weight and maintain weight loss, keep a positive mood, and find the drive to have sex. You may also notice how blurred and unfocused your vision is when you had a bad night's sleep or experience double vision. Going without sleep for several days can lead to hallucinations. The author of this book experienced hallucinations after being sleep deprived from childbirth for several days before receiving treatment.

For many of the issues we grapple with, we end up taking a pharmaceutical pill to treat the symptoms and then deal with side effects that make it even harder to sleep. This is true of chronic pain and insomnia. Drugs we are prescribed for a variety of issues, including high blood pressure, depression, anxiety, and cancer treatment, often contribute to our inability to sleep. Some drugs, such as diuretics for blood pressure, cause you to urinate more, which means more trips to the bathroom in the middle of the night. Before taking any drug, it's always a good idea to ask about side effects, especially if you are already having trouble falling and staying asleep.

During the COVID-19 pandemic of 2020–2022, more people reported sleep issues and insomnia because of stress and anxiety, and sleep prescriptions increased over 20 percent from previous years. "Coronasomnia" affected millions who were already dealing with job losses, lockdowns, sick loved ones, and fearmongering in the media. This chronic, unrelenting stress had a hugely negative impact on getting a good night's sleep because stress activates the autonomic nervous system, which causes the release of hormones like cortisol and adrenaline, the "fight-or-flight" hormones that keep us on edge. It then becomes impossible to relax enough to get some shut-eye.

Lifestyle changes during the pandemic contributed to bad sleep overall, as people who were working from home and kids who had to do their schooling online now were staying up later and sleeping in later, and their sleep clocks were disrupted for months. With little time for everyone to relax and being locked inside without access to the sun and light, our bodies couldn't figure out when it was time to wake up and when it was time to wind down. Routines and structured habits, especially for children, who need more sleep than adults, were disrupted and, combined with less time outdoors where our internal body clocks could get their share of light, it created a scenario where more people stayed up longer, then fell into fitful sleep for shorter periods of time, if they slept at all.

Before the pandemic, almost one-third of Americans were sleep deprived. Sadly, more kids and teens are being added to the mix because of online gaming and bingeing shows on their phones. Adults are guilty, too, of staying up for hours watching 10 episodes back-to-back of a new series, but younger people are more susceptible to the sleep deprivation of electronic gadgets and the excessive blue light they produce, which tells our brains to stop making melatonin, which helps us get sleepy. It's a vicious circle that the lockdowns made worse but will no doubt continue once all is back to normal.

Since more people are up later, they tend to raid the kitchen later, meaning their bodies now must digest meals when they should be in rejuvenating sleep mode. We are told to stop eating at least three hours before bedtime to get the best sleep possible, but that rule is broken every time we sneak a late-night snack because we are awake and hungry. Sleep deprivation leads to an increase in the hunger hormone, ghrelin, and a decrease in leptin, which fights cravings and hunger. The foods you crave most when exhausted are comfort foods, which are high in calories and sugar or carbs.

Because poor sleep raises stress hormones and increases glucose production as a result, you end up with higher blood sugar levels....

This adds to the growing obesity epidemic since the body never gets a break from the feeding phase so it can go into the fasting phase of utilizing excess fat for fuel. Those excess calories get stored as fat because you are not moving enough to burn them off. Because poor sleep raises stress hormones and increases glucose production as a result, you end up with higher blood sugar levels, making the extra pounds you pack on all but impossible to get rid of.

Insulin resistance, a huge factor in obesity and weight gain, increases after just one night of partial sleep deprivation and, over time, leads to weight gain even if you are eating right and exercising. Symptoms of prediabetes can begin to show up with only five days of sleep disturbances, and blood pressure rises, too. Imagine weeks, even months, of poor-quality sleep, and you can see how we have so much chronic disease and illness.

It's easy now to see how lack of sleep can hurt us physically, mentally, and emotionally, yet we don't seem to care enough to make the necessary changes to get better sleep.

Healthy Sleep Habits

When is the last time you went to bed, fell asleep right away, and woke up the next morning feeling refreshed and ready to take on the day ahead? It's probably been a while if you are like most Americans. People who get adequate, quality sleep wake up at the same time each morning, often without the aid of an alarm clock. They feel rested and have the energy to get moving without an entire pot of coffee as a crutch. They do not experience as many hunger cravings during the day; have better concentration, focus, and memory; and are in a much better mood.

Getting healthy sleep changes everything. You have better clarity and cognitive functioning. You remember more. You have more energy. You feel more positive and happier. You are rested and experience less anxiety and irritability. Life is just so much better. If you cannot recall those happier days of getting decent sleep, bringing those days back and establishing a sleep routine that works for you can be done in many ways.

Going to bed and waking up at the same time every day reestablishes your circadian rhythm. Having a set routine before bedtime can help you wind down from the day and prepare yourself and your bedroom for a good night's sleep. A warm bath, listening to calming music, doing a guided meditation, deep breathing, dimming down the lights, writing in your gratitude journal, praying, or light reading are all ideas that can be incorporated into a bedtime routine.

Other ideas include:

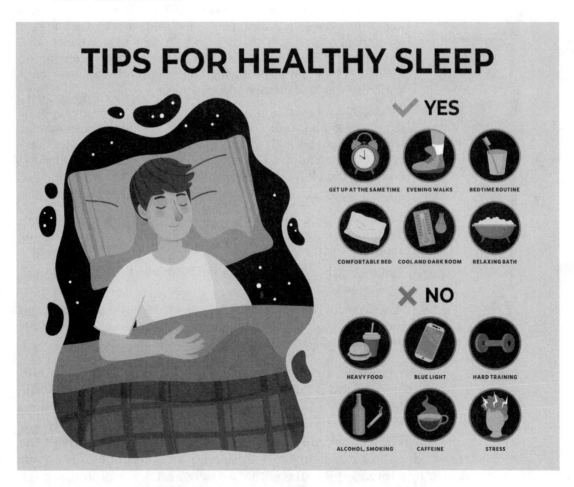

There are a number of simple things you can do to promote better sleeping habits.

- No food or alcohol for at least three hours before bedtime.

- No phone or gadget use for an hour before bedtime, and keep them shut off during the night to avoid EMF effects.

- Make the bedroom a cool, dark place for best sleep, and use blackout curtains or an eye mask if needed.

- Avoid drinking water later in the evening, or you'll be making a few trips to the bathroom during the night.

- Use earplugs if a lot of external noise is an issue.

- No vigorous exercise for at least four hours before bedtime. It's best to work out in the morning or during the day.

- Get daily sunlight exposure, especially first thing in the morning, to help reset your circadian rhythms that tell your body and brain when it's time to wake up and when it's time to sleep. Light is the most important regulator for good sleep because it triggers biological processes that cause you to feel wide awake. Darkness, in turn, triggers processes that tell you it's time to sleep, including the release of melatonin to assist you in doing so. Screwing up the body clock and not allowing your natural rhythm to work is a surefire way toward sleep deprivation.

- Although it is best not to have your phone on, some great phone apps for iOS and Android such as Calm, Headspace, and Breethe will help you relax with soothing sounds, music, and stories. However, turn the phone off at least one hour prior to going to sleep, and keep the phone away from your head while you sleep.

- Journal away stresses of the day before bedtime.

- If you are tossing and turning, it is better to get up and do something to get yourself tired again instead of lying in bed stressing about how you cannot sleep.

- Gentle stretches and light yoga can help calm the body and spirit for a good night's sleep.

- Have a cup of chamomile and lavender tea to calm the nerves and soothe the spirit without the grogginess that comes from pharmaceutical and over-the-counter sleeping aids.

Sleep hygiene, or the things you do to get good sleep and enough of it, is a must if you ever want to experience health and well-being. It doesn't matter how clean and healthy you eat or how often you work out if your body and brain never get the time they need to slow down to a crawl and rebuild and refresh. If you try many of the above ideas and still struggle with sleep, it may be time to see your doctor or a therapist if you feel that anxiety and depression may be a large factor. A comprehensive blood panel and other tests may indicate that nutrient deficiencies or other problems must be treated to help you get back to sleep.

Managing stress is critical, so any ways that work to alleviate the buildup of stress from the day's activities and release them before bedtime work except for turning to substances like food, drugs, and alcohol. Find healthy ways to let go of the day and relax, and incorporate routine and structure so that bedtime isn't a guessing game. The easier you can make it to get into bed and be ready for some shut-eye, the better. Teach your children these same skills, too, while they are young, so they don't fall prey to bad sleep habits that will plague them for life.

Getting good sleep has both short-term and long-term benefits, and the biggest one is being able to live longer. Nobody wants to live longer if they are sick, tired, and miserable all the time, and good sleep improves mental and emotional well-being as much as it does physical health. The hours spent sleeping may seem unproductive to our driven, overambitious culture, but sleep helps generate more ideas, greater creativity, and higher productivity during the day.

Brain-detoxing Effects of Good Sleep

Sleep allows your brain to detox in several beneficial ways. Getting adequate sleep helps brain cells perform autophagy, which is the system's method of getting rid of dead and damaged bits of protein and metabolic waste. Sleep also contributes to ridding the brain of toxins by improving the ability of the lymphatic vessels that surround the brain to deliver waste to the lymphatic system.

Getting the brain detoxed of waste and old, dead cells and nourishing the growth of new cells and stronger neural connections is directly related to the amount of quality sleep we get.

When we sleep well, our special nervous system cells, the "glial" cells, rush in to scavenge waste bits in and around the brain. Finally, sleep assists cells to detoxify metabolic waste, eliminate dysfunctional neuronal cells, rebuild new neuronal connections, and improve neurotransmitter sensitivity. Getting the brain detoxed of waste and old, dead cells and nourishing the growth of new cells and stronger neural connections is directly related to the amount of quality sleep we get.

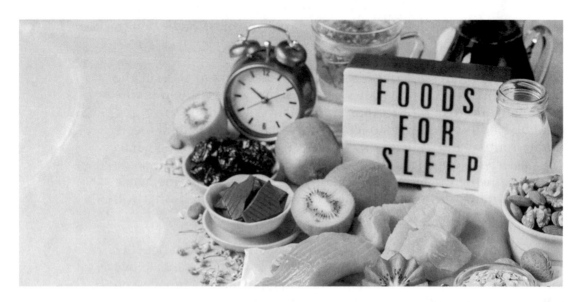

Foods that are high in tryptophan, magnesium, calcium, and vitamin B6 are condusive to better sleep.

The brain works overtime to keep us functioning. Sleep provides it with the downtime it needs to renew and do some hohousecleaning.

Sleep loss and deprivation is one epidemic you have a lot of control over, so why would you not take that control and eliminate the bad habits and mindless actions that keep you from getting better sleep?

Foods for Sleep

Several foods assist in falling and staying asleep. They contain four main vitamins and minerals known for promoting sleep: tryptophan, magnesium, calcium, and B6. Some even help the body produce melatonin, the hormone that governs the circadian rhythm/sleep–wake cycle.

Tryptophan is an essential amino acid that the body cannot produce, so it must be obtained from animal- and plant-based protein sources in the diet. Of all the body's amino acids, it is found in the lowest concentration but is vital for metabolic processes and has a positive impact on mood, memory, premenstrual issues, learning, cognition, and treating sleep disorders. It can even help alleviate anxiety, which adds to insomnia.

No scientific proof exists that eating turkey at Thanksgiving causes tryptophan-induced drowsiness, which may better be ascribed to taxing the body with overeating. Many foods contain far more tryp-tophan than turkey, and they do not have the attached reputation of making you fall asleep in front of the television after consuming them.

Taking tryptophan as a supplement is not recommended since it interacts with other medications and supplements that influence the production of serotonin. Instead, try eating these foods for dinner or closer to bedtime:

Magnesium

- Soybeans
- Bananas
- Yogurt
- Avocadoes
- Kiwifruit
- Nuts and seeds such as almonds, sunflower seeds, pine nuts, cashews, Brazil nuts, flaxseed, and pecans
- Wheat germ
- Salmon, tuna, mackerel, and halibut

Calcium

- Dairy such as milk and cheeses
- Yogurt
- Sardines
- Soybeans
- Fortified cereals and breads
- Okra
- Broccoli
- Green snap peas
- Fortified orange juice

Vitamin B6

- Flaxseed
- Pistachio nuts
- Bananas
- Avocadoes
- Spinach

- Lean meats and poultry
- Dried prunes
- Tuna, salmon, and halibut

You won't achieve quality sleep by eating the above foods if you also indulge in those that destroy a good night's sleep such as processed and high-sugar foods, spicy foods, and heavy meals high in fat too close to bedtime. The body must work harder to process toxins and sugars and digest a huge meal, which cuts into sleep time. Foods with high water content should be consumed with dinner to avoid late-night pee breaks that interrupt sleep, but you can also try teas such as valerian, chamomile, tart cherry, passion fruit, and peppermint to soothe and calm you before bedtime. One cup should be enough. More than that, and you'll be visiting the toilet more than the pillow.

Supplements for Better Sleep

A few well-known and tested herbs and supplements can provide relief for insomnia and sleep troubles. Because the body relies on chemical signals to regulate its many systems, it suffers when deficiencies prevent the body from making the necessary hormones, neurotransmitters, and proteins. The presence of toxins such as aluminum found in vaccines and arsenic and other heavy metals in waters, pesticides, and molds, many of which find our way into our diets or environments, wreak havoc on the body's ability to absorb the nutrients needed to ensure a healthy brain and functioning system, including sleep.

The body must work harder to process toxins and sugars and digest a huge meal, which cuts into sleep time.

Melatonin is the hormone most associated with sleep. Most of your melatonin is made in your gut and not the pineal gland, which means your gut health is directly related to sleep quality. Melatonin is naturally produced in the body according to the circadian rhythm that detects light/day and dark/night, but thanks to people being indoors too long and using brightly lit gadgets at night, our natural cycle has been disrupted. Melatonin normally is released during the night, but because of our lifestyles, the body doesn't know when to release it or doesn't release enough. Supplementing with melatonin can help reset the body's clock but should be used as a method of helping the body once again learn to do it on its own and not as a long-term treatment or an excuse to ignore good sleeping habits. You can find a little melatonin in foods such as grains (rolled oats, barley, rice), nuts (walnuts, peanuts), and seeds (flaxseed, mustard seeds, sunflower seeds).

We discussed the importance of magnesium in the supplements section, but it is a rock star for promoting a calm brain and sleep. It works by regulating melatonin and GABA levels in the brain, which induce relaxation and promote sleep. The brain must have adequate magnesium to signal the body that it is time for sleep. You can combine it with calcium and zinc as a Cal-Mag-Zinc supplement taken before bedtime. Even though plenty of foods are high in magnesium, the modern diet just doesn't get enough for most people, so taking a supplement makes sense. Magnesium and vitamin D are believed to be the top two deficiencies experienced by large numbers of people in modern times.

GABA is an inhibitory neurotransmitter that signals the brain to relax. GABA works best if levels of zinc, B6, magnesium, glutamine, and taurine in the system are adequate.

GABA, L-theanine, and 5-HTP are amino acids that promote sleep. They can all be taken in supplement form. GABA is an inhibitory neurotransmitter that signals the brain to relax. GABA works best if levels of zinc, B6, magnesium, glutamine, and taurine in the system are adequate. GABA and L-theanine also enhance immunity, and all three, along with tryptophan, lessen anxiety and induce relaxation.

5-HTP assists the production of serotonin, the chemical messenger that sends signals between nerve cells. Low serotonin leads to depression, sleep disorders, weight gain, and anxiety, so getting enough 5-HTP is critical. These supplements have become very popular as a sleep aid but also because they help with weight-loss efforts by counteracting the production of hunger-inducing hormones. This amino acid also increases your melatonin production to better regulate sleep. 5-HTP and GABA taken together create a synergy that has been found in studies to significantly reduce the amount of time it takes to fall asleep and increase the duration and quality of sleep.

Amino acids are multipurpose and because they have such a positive effect on so many of the body's systems, they no doubt improve sleep quality. However, as with anything you put in your body, check with your doctor first if you are taking other vitamins, supplements, or medications and if you are pregnant or lactating.

In the herb section are many contenders for "award for best sleep aid," but valerian is the most widely used as a supplement. It relaxes and promotes sleep without leaving you feeling groggy the next morning. Valerian contains sedative compounds such as valeric acid, valepotriates, acevaltrate, isovaltrate, and valtrate. It promotes deep sleep without brain fog the next morning, and it is a lot cheaper than most pharmaceutical sleep aids. The *American Journal of Medicine* published a large-scale review of all clinical trials done on valerian and sleep and reported, "The available evidence suggests that valerian might improve sleep quality without producing side effects."

Valerian doesn't just help you sleep. It also relaxes the muscles and relieves muscle tension, which can keep you from relaxing enough to doze off, and it prevents restless leg syndrome, which can interfere with sleep, by improving blood circulation. When taken in supplement form, valerian increases deep REM sleep, but taking more than the recommended dosage on the bottle will not make you get more sleep. It will make you oversedated and groggy, so follow the dosing and take about an hour before bedtime for optimal results. If you don't want as much of a sedative punch, try it in tea form and see how you tolerate it and if it works for you.

Other herbs include chamomile, lavender, rose hips, peppermint, and lemon balm. Adaptogen herbs such as Ashwagandha also promote sleep and relaxation. Other adaptogens to try are magnolia bark, rhodiola, cordyceps, and reishi mushrooms. Valerian can be taken as a tea or supplement, while the others here may only be available in natural form or as a tea. Ashwagandha is a powerful and popular supplement that is selling well in gummy form as well as in pill and tea forms.

Always check with your doctor if you take pharmaceuticals or over-the-counter medications to see if they counteract with any herbs or supplements or if you are pregnant or breastfeeding. Never give any supplements to children without discussing it with their pediatrician for proper dosage and side effects. When buying supplements, never take more than the daily dose on the bottle. The most widely reported side effects of any of the above are drowsiness, brain fog in the morning, stomach cramping or pain, allergic reactions, and anxiety/jitters. Just because these are natural or found in the human body doesn't mean that taking them in pill form won't cause a reaction.

Sleep Aids and Therapies

White-noise devices, whether via a phone app or a small table-top model, can help soothe the mind and mask distracting external sounds enough to bring about sleep. White noise consists of low-, medium-, and high-frequency sounds that can create consistent tonal blankets of sound in equal amplitude across all frequencies that prevent you from waking up from an external sound like a door slamming. These devices are great for people who cannot relax in complete silence or who live in noisy cities or out in the country, where the sound of night critters can drive you mad in the pursuit of calm.

White or ambient noise is often used in hospitals to help patients relax and fall asleep and has been shown to reduce the amount of time it takes to fall asleep by approximately 40 percent. It works on adults, children, and babies. You don't need to buy a device, though, because the gentle hum of an air conditioner or whir of a ceiling fan provide the same benefits.

Pink noise is sometimes preferred. Pink noise decreases in amplitude by half the amount every time the frequency doubles for a resulting blend of intense low-frequency tones and softer tones at a higher frequency.

If this kind of "noise" isn't your cup of soothing tea, so to speak, you can also try sound devices that allow you to choose from a variety of soothing sounds such as rain, thunder, croaking frogs, chirping crickets, waves lapping the shore, a trickling stream, the hoot of an owl, or wind blowing through the tree-tops. These natural noise devices, often combined with a night-light, can be changed at will to personal preference and block out sound while engaging the brain in a gently hypnotic, soothing manner. However, any noise machine might block out sounds you may want to hear, such as a baby crying or child's call for help in the next room or the sound of breaking glass downstairs. You can test the volume so that it is at a level

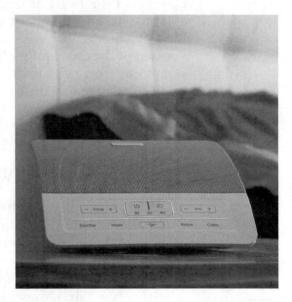

Noise machines like this one can produce sounds to aid in sleep, including white noise or the sounds of ocean waves, rain, thunder, babbling brooks, or gentle breezes.

where you can hear something you need to while not hearing all the distractions you don't, and set a timer so that once you do fall asleep, the machine isn't running all night.

Other than devices, apps, and supplements, cognitive behavioral therapy (CBT) can also help with insomnia and sleep disorders. A study called "Insomnia Treatment: Cognitive Behavioral Therapy Instead of Sleeping Pills" for the Mayo Clinic found that CBT is an effective and safe way to get to sleep because it helps find the underlying causes of insomnia and works on processing them through talk therapy and behavior modifications. CBT teaches you to recognize why you cannot sleep and to change thoughts, beliefs, and behaviors that are stopping you from relaxing, such as negative and fearful thoughts, overthinking, worry, and ruminating.

CBT teaches you to recognize why you cannot sleep and to change thoughts, beliefs, and behaviors that are stopping you from relaxing....

CBT is preferable for long–term treatment or if other forms of treatment don't seem to work well. Addressing underlying behavioral issues is at the heart of mental health disorders such as depression and anxiety, and the more you come to understand why you think the way you do, the easier it is to change the way you think and rid yourself of the cause rather than popping pills to alleviate short–term symptoms. You can also try biofeedback to control your thoughts using a machine that measures biological signs such as heart rate and muscle tension. You can even find a home biofeedback machine to use to identify and change thoughts and patterns affecting sleep.

Can Plants Help You Sleep?

The answer is yes if they are plants that clean the air and detox your bedroom from harmful chemicals and toxins. Try keeping one or more of these plants near your bed:

- Aloe vera: Cleanses the air overall
- Peace lily: Cleanses and purifies air
- Weeping fig: Purifies air and removes formaldehyde and benzene
- English ivy: Cleanses air of allergens and pollutants
- Jasmine: The scent is known to reduce anxiety

- Lavender: The scent calms the nerves
- Snake plant: Removes carbon dioxide during the day and releases more oxygen at night for better sleep
- Boston fern: Purifies air by filtering out xylene, formaldehyde, and toluene toxins
- Areca palm: Detoxes and purifies air of major toxins

How about Your Bed?

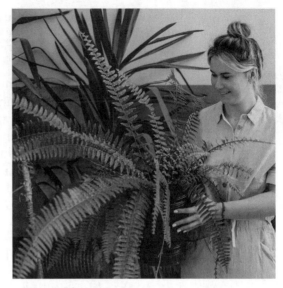

Boston ferns are a popular decorative plant in many homes, but they also serve as air purifiers.

Finally, are you sleeping on pillows that are too soft or too hard? Is your mattress old and nonsupportive or too firm and uncomfortable? Are you using pillowcases and mattress covers that are anti-allergic and keep dust mites away? Is your bedspread too heavy or not heavy enough?

You spend half your life in bed, so it behooves you to make it one that invites sleep and relaxation. Buy a new set of pillows if you are sleeping on one that is solid as a rock or so poofy that your face gets buried in it. Go to a bedding store and lay your head against foam, feather, down, and other synthetic pillows to see which one feels like it will give you the support your head and neck need. Some people prefer firm pillows, and others prefer soft. Pillows come in dozens of types and styles, including body pillows for side sleepers.

Speaking of sides, are you sleeping on your back? Your stomach? Your side? Do you toss and turn, change sides throughout the night, or wake up with an aching lower back every morning? Sleep positions tend to be an individual preference, but if you aren't getting quality sleep, it might be time to turn a new leaf, or position.

Is it time for a new mattress? If money is tight, you can buy a mattress topper. They come in 2-inch, 3-inch, and 4-inch sizes and sit right on top of your existing mattress to provide the feel of a new mattress at a fraction of the cost. Opt for one that is gel based and cooling. If your box spring squeaks every time you turn over in bed, you can forget about sleeping through the night. Beds on frames too high off the ground may be an issue if you roll over a lot while sleeping. If you snore, you may do better with an adjustable bed rather than a flat mattress.

If only we put the same amount of time and effort into the bed we sleep on as we do the cars we drive. Tonight, when you go to sleep, take an inventory of your bedding and see if any areas can be improved on. Even a new, fluffy pillow or a different material comforter can make a difference. Spending money on your bed is one of the most beneficial things you can do for your health and well-being. Where you sleep and what you sleep on makes all the difference in HOW you sleep.

Is Your Bedding Toxic?

It's hard to imagine your pillow and mattress having the power to make you sick, but bedding is a big problem when it comes to toxins in the home that prevent optimal health. You spend long stretches of time in bed, and you shouldn't have to worry about chemicals and contaminants getting into your lungs and on your skin. When it comes to toxic chemicals, look at your mattress, pillows, and sheets/blankets. Many of the chemicals used in these products contain carcinogens that cause cancer, especially memory-foam mattresses and synthetic pillows. The industry doesn't do much regulation, so it is up to you to do your homework and make sure your sleep environment benefits your health.

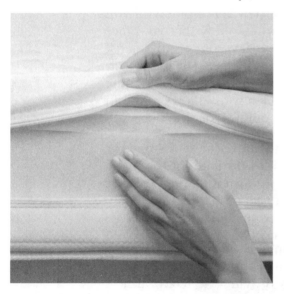

Foam mattresses, including popular memory foam ones, contain toxic VOCs that release gases you can breathe into your lungs.

The biggest offenders are called volatile organic compounds (VOCs) and often have a strong telltale odor like the smell of a new car or a newly painted room. That strong smell is an indicator of the presence of VOC gases being emitted from the products, and since these items are used indoors, the gases become concentrated up to five to 10 times higher than they would outdoors. VOCs can cause headaches, eye infections, throat irritation, respiratory issues, damage to the liver and kidneys, and cancer. Here are some of the places these nasty VOCs might be found in your home.

Polyurethane Foam Mattresses

Mattresses made from foam, especially memory foam, are filled with polyfoam or polyurethane foam, which is a huge source of VOCs that you are exposed to all day and night. This release of VOCs into the air of your home or office is called off-gassing, and you breathe the vapors in. Polyurethane also releases polybrominated diphentyl ethers (PBDEs), which break down and enter the body through off-gassing and are highly toxic. Many states have banned materials with PBDEs, usually anything flame retardant, but mattresses are still permitted to contain them. Some of this comes from the past push to make bedding materials flame retardant, but in the added security of fire-retardant bedding, we are now breathing in higher levels of chemicals.

Mattresses may also contain chemical pest repellents to ward off bedbugs and dust mites. Boric acid is one such pesticide that is often not revealed by your mattress salesperson. Synthetic latex is used to make the mattress mold to the fit of your body, but it is not natural and contains petroleum-based styrene and butadiene, both of which are carcinogens and harmful to the skin, eyes, and respiratory system.

Pillows, Too

Your pillows also include flame retardants and polyurethane, which can disrupt the function of your thyroid and cause cancer, ADHD, and neurodevelopmental issues. Because your eyes, nose, and mouth come in greater contact with your pillow during sleep than with your mattress, the inhaling of VOCs and PBDEs is especially dangerous. Memory-foam pillows contain formaldehyde, a known skin irritant and carcinogen that also causes respiratory difficulties. Your mattress contains formaldehyde as well. Chemicals added to your bedding as deodorizers and fragrances should also be avoided. You also need to watch out for mold, fungi, and bedbugs, too. Fungi, up to 16 different types, is often found in feather and synthetic pillows and can cause lung infections.

Sheets and Bedding

Some types of sheets are chemically treated with formaldehyde to be wrinkle-free and static-free and should be avoided. Also, avoid sheets and bedding that are labeled "blended fibers," as they contain a mix of natural and synthetic fibers. Your best bet for bedding is natural cotton or flax products but be aware that these may also be treated with pesticides and other chemicals. It behooves you to do some research and look for all-natural, VOC- and pesticide-free products that contain cotton and flax that are not grown as GMO crops. Cotton, linen, and bamboo sheets are great options, as they are made of 100 percent natural fibers and contain no synthetics or treatments.

Pillows should be made of natural filling and casing and check to see if they've been chemically treated. Organic cotton and wool are good options, as is kapok, a fluffy material that comes from *Ceiba pentandra* trees and is hypoallergenic. You can also look for millet- or buckwheat-filled pillows. It's always good to encase them in an anti-allergy casing but be sure to check that you are buying one free from chemical treatments.

When you buy a new mattress or bedding of any kind, be sure to keep bedroom windows open for several hours to air out some of the VOCs. Bedding should be washed before use. Natural VOC- and pesticide-free bedding may be a bit harder to find and more expensive, but it is well worth it knowing you are getting a healthier night's sleep.

Though sleep problems can have mental, emotional, and physical causes, they can be treated and alleviated without resorting to dangerous chemicals with a long list of equally dangerous side effects. Improving diet and exercise help improve sleep, as does relieving stress and finding positive coping skills. It's just another reminder that the body, mind, and spirit need a more holistic form of healing that roots out the cause and doesn't just put a band-aid on symptoms. Treat one, and the rest benefit; ignore one, and they all fall down.

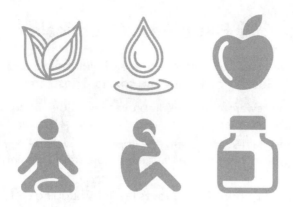

Brainpower

The brain is the most important organ in your body. Just as any other part of the body, it must be exercised and strengthened. In addition to diet and working on lessening stress, you can do other things to sharpen your brain and make it work better even as you age. Keeping the brain active is key to warding off diseases like dementia, memory loss, and Alzheimer's.

Diet and exercise both directly affect the workings of the brain. As we have already seen, a healthy diet feeds it what it needs, and exercise increases the levels of two common neurotransmitters: glutamate and gamma–aminobutyric acid (GABA), both of which are responsible for chemical messaging within the brain. Deficiencies in our neurotransmitters lead to depression and depressive disorders, and when glutamate and GABA are restored to optimal levels, our brain health is restored. Exercise also increases the amount of mood-related serotonin and norepinephrine, which make us feel better mentally and emotionally.

Even if your cognitive functions are rock solid, you can try to improve your brainpower and induce different brainwave states for their benefits in a number of ways. Entraining the brain is one method of optimizing the way the brain responds to stimuli, processes infor-

Hacking Your Happiness Chemicals

The chemicals in the brain work to create a sense of well-being and happiness when they are not blocked by illness and toxins. These are:

- Dopamine—the reward chemical: Improves levels by eating healthy, achieving goals, completing a task, and exercising self-care.
- Endorphin—the pain-killing chemical: Improves levels by exercising, watching an entertaining movie, laughing more, and listening to uplifting music.
- Oxytocin—the love hormone: Improves levels by hugging and physical touch, petting an animal, socializing with others, and helping others or engaging in charitable acts.
- Serotonin—the mood-stabilizing chemical: Improves levels by getting sun exposure, meditation and mindfulness, being out in nature, and being with people you love.

mation, recalls memory, and allows you to learn new things and build new neural pathways.

Brainwave Entrainment and Binaural Beats

In physics, entrainment is the tendency for two oscillating objects to lock into phase, or synchronization, so that they have similar vibrational frequencies. They are said to oscillate in harmony, pulsing in synchrony. This principle can also be seen in the fields of chemistry, astronomy, biology, and even psychology.

Ancient civilizations in Greece, Egypt, pagan countries, and Native American traditions all used the power of rhythmic sounds such as beating drums, shaking rattles, and humming and chanting tones and words at just the right frequency during rituals to alter the consciousness of those in attendance. Binaural beats were discovered around 1839 and another method called isochronic tones was discovered in 1999, but they have their roots in the past, including research done in the 1960s into the use of brainwave entrainment to alleviate pain.

Binaural beats are auditory illusions perceived when two different pure-tone sine waves with frequencies lower than 1,500 hertz, with less than a 40–hertz difference between them, are listened to dichoti-cally (a tone through each ear). The listener perceives an auditory il-lusion of a third tone, the binaural beat. All of this originates in the inferior colliculus part of the midbrain and the superior olivary com-plex located in the brain stem, where auditory signals from our ears are integrated to precipitate electrical impulses along the neural path-ways of the brain. It's a bit complex, but the result is a tone that alters brainwaves and creates a receptive state.

Isochronic tones are often said to be superior to binaural be-cause they use the brain's natural processes to alter your own brain-waves without a lot of effort or expensive devices. These are regular beats of a single tone that is turned on and off rapidly, resulting in sharp sound pulses that can be used with binaural beats to create deeper brainwave entrainment. Altering brainwaves leads to better sleep, deeper meditation, more productive focus throughout the day, relaxation when needed to reduce stress, clear thinking during chal-lenging tests or on the job, improved ability to handle stressors, re-lease of endorphins and feel–good chemicals, optimal healing, improved short- and long–term memory, mastery over emotions, and so much more and remind us that our brains are the most powerful tool we have for physical as well as mental and emotional change.

The human brain can experience entrainment, too. This can bring about increased memory recall, deep relaxation, and positive well–being. Brainwave synchronization is the entrainment of the brain's wave frequency with an outside stimulus, resulting in a dif-ferent brainwave state. We see this with the use of binaural beats when two audio signals to the brain cause a response directly related to the frequency of the introduced signal. Two tones that are close in frequency then generate a beat frequency at the difference of the frequencies, generally in the subsonic range. For example, a 500–hertz tone and 510–hertz tone will pro-duce a subsonic 10–hertz tone in the middle of the alpha range.

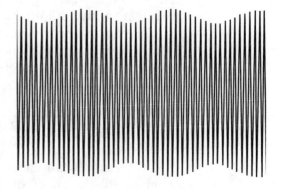

This brain basically hears two tones, then combines the two tones into one. Each ear hears only one steady tone. These entrainment frequencies can bring about many changes in the person,

A diagram of the sine waves comprising binaural beats.

physically or mentally, comparable to meditation practice or biofeedback. Just listening to approximately 15 minutes of binaural beats or brain–entrainment recordings can alter the state of your brain to increase clarity, focus, and problem–solving abilities.

Target frequencies that affect the brain:

- Delta (0.1–3 Hz): deep sleep, lucid dreaming, increased immune functions, hypnosis
- Theta (3–8 Hz): deep relaxation, meditation, increased memory, focus, creativity, lucid dreaming, hypnagogic state
- Alpha (8–12 Hz): light relaxation, "super–learning," positive thinking
- Low beta (12–15 Hz): relaxed focus, improved attentive abilities
- Midrange beta (15–18 Hz): increased mental ability, focus, alertness, IQ
- High beta (above 18 Hz): fully awake, normal state of alertness, stress, and anxiety
- Gamma (40 Hz): information–rich task processing and information processing (some paranormal investigators claim that gamma is active during paranormal experiences!)

In the scientific sense, binaural beats are auditory brain stem responses originating in the superior olivary nucleus of each hemisphere of the brain. These beats are not heard in the ordinary sense of the word (the human range of hearing is between 20–20,000 hertz) but are perceived by the brain at low frequencies (less than 30 hertz) on the EEG spectrum. People who regularly use binaural beats have reported achieving altered states of consciousness due to the changes in brainwave activity from the combined tones. Some people say this can be deeply relaxing, and others may be given a boost of energy and creative inspiration; this is not a one–size–fits–all experience. Since no side effects occur, it might be worth trying in order to increase brainpower, improve mood, and even assist in better, deeper sleep. Many binaural beats videos and programs are on the internet that you can try, and devices can be purchased to assist you.

The Power of Puzzles for Brain Health

It seems almost counterintuitive that after a hard day's work or dealing with the kids, you would want to sit down and do a jigsaw puzzle, yet numerous scientific studies show that doing puzzles, whether crossword, jigsaw, or word search, provide similar benefits to meditation and some forms of yoga and sharpen memory. They even help stave off brain disorders such as dementia and Alzheimer's.

The concentration and focus required to do a puzzle and the joy of watching a "bigger picture" come together create the perfect balance between the rational, logical left brain and the intuitive, visual right brain. The result is a mindfulness state that alleviates anxiety and stress while sharpening the brain's ability to locate shapes, colors, sizes, words, and phrases. The brain's reward system releases dopamine when the puzzle is complete, and the whole process is planted in present–moment activity that takes all distractions out of the picture, pun intended.

Doing puzzles, whether you are a senior, child, or anything in between, moves the brain out of the wakeful beta brainwave state and into alpha, the state associated with focus and meditation. This creates therapeutic effects on the brain and the body, lowering heart rate and blood pressure and, for someone with dementia, offering a state of calm restfulness while also stimulating the brain and memory recall. The July 15, 2019, issue of *Live Smart*'s article "Can a Puzzle a Day Keep Dementia at Bay?" by Betsy Mills, Ph.D.; studies in the 2019 *International Journal of Geriatric Studies*; the AC-TIVE study on cognitive protection; and the PROTECT study on brain aging involving observational studies and a battery of tests all show increased cognitive function in seniors who do puzzles involving words and numbers, even if they only do them once a month. Word puzzles increased grammatical reasoning in the test subjects, and number puzzles increased executive functions such as organizing and planning.

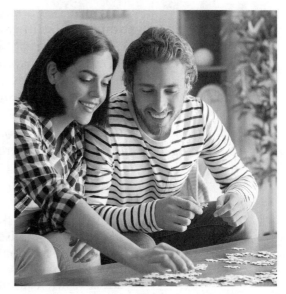

Jigsaw puzzles, which offer the visual completion shot of dopamine release, which is the feel–good hormone, have been shown in many studies to increase memory recall, increase problem-solving ability, and decrease generalized anxiety. The sorting, organizing, and selecting of puzzle pieces allow the mind to switch off from other worries and con-

Solving puzzles, like word puzzles, crosswords, or jigsaw puzzles, stimulates the brain and can keep your mind healthy. Just like exercising your muscles, your brain needs to be worked so it doesn't get flabby.

cerns and focus single-mindedly on the one task at hand, giving the person doing the puzzle a sense of control and calmness. Even children benefit from holding the pieces, looking at and feeling the shapes, and putting them in the right places, which improves their visual-spatial reasoning. They learn the organizing process and how to focus their usually chaotic attention while having fun seeing the result.

These benefits have been reported in both online puzzling and good old-fashioned tabletop puzzles and crossword and word-search books, but the old-fashioned way has the benefit of allowing the brain some time away from computer screens and exposure to EMF, which is especially important for children, but any puzzling will help. During the COVID-19 lockdowns, puzzle companies couldn't keep up with the demand as more people discovered the fun and relaxation of putting together a puzzle, giving new life to an old industry, and families realized they could sit down together and have a blast doing a puzzle, never knowing that they were sharpening their brains and lowering their stress at the same time; it's a win-win situation.

Exercises for the Brain and Memory

A number of brain exercises help improve cognitive function, memory, clarity, and creativity, and none of them require expensive equipment or an extra trip to the gym. Because the brain is the most complex organ in the body, regulating body functions, processing incoming sensory information, and being in charge of what we think, believe, remember, and do, it makes sense to keep it in prime shape, just as you would your muscles. Exercises for the brain also protect against age-related degeneration and the diseases associated with it.

Here are some ways to work that brain:

- Meditate: Training the brain to focus attention is not only calming to the body but also to the brain itself. It slows the aging of the brain by increasing its ability to process information and gain clarity. Meditation also fine-tunes the memory and alleviates stress, which leads to inflammation, which leads to overall fatigue and illness. Give your brain a break every now and then.

- Games and puzzles: As discussed earlier, jigsaw puzzles, crossword and word-find puzzles, memory games, board and card games, and any game that involves the brain all boost cognitive ability and delay the onset of memory decline. Games that engage the memory strengthen the brain's ability to recognize patterns and recall short- and long-term memory, and guessing games such as charades and trivia increase the ability to make connections and process information. Whether it's bridge, Cards against Humanity, chess, checkers, Sudoku, Trivial Pursuit, Monopoly, or backgammon, any game that is both engaging and fun and requires some brainpower is a positive step toward better brain health—and yes, that includes video games.

- Music: Whether listening to it or playing it, music has the power to increase calm, energy, and creativity. Obviously, the best music for brain boosting is something upbeat that makes you feel good. This can be pop tunes for some, classical music for others. A 2018 study published in *Brain Science* journal showed that when a person listens to music they enjoy, it engages and connects various parts of the brain, which leads to better cognition and a sense of well-being. Crank up the tunes and dance around; put on a quiet, melodic instrumental; or pick up an instrument and play it yourself.

- Learning new skills: Learning how to play a musical instrument, garden, speak a new language, paint the house, or design a website all improve the brain by creating new neural networks required to tackle a new task. Older adults who take up a new hobby or learn to speak a language have been shown in numerous studies to have better memory function. This can be anything from scrapbooking to nature photography or enhancing personal vocabulary. The enhanced connectivity the brain learns when taking up a new interest or hobby, especially one that requires dexterity and hand–eye coordination such as drawing, archery, painting, target shooting, or embroidery, delays the onset of Alzheimer's and dementia and slows the aging of the brain.

- Take a new route: Something as easy as driving to the grocery store a different way or walking a different neighborhood block encourages the brain to find new ways to do the same things. It also teaches resourceful thinking and resilience.

- Social interaction: As we get older, we tend to spend more time alone. This is especially true of seniors confined to assisted living. Daily social interaction is good not only for the brain but also the spirit. When we are talking with others, our brains stay engaged and sharp, and studies have shown that social activities lessen the effects of cognitive decline and dementia. The brain needs stimulation and interaction, and if we look at how fast elderly people decline when left alone, it's obvious that being around people is one of the best ways to get that stimulation.

- Movement: Whether the gentle flow of tai chi or an hour of pumping iron, moving the body in any form increases the flow of oxygen to the brain and strengthens focus, attention, and cognitive skills. Even a walk through the woods requires the brain to up its processing ability as information is taken in by the senses. Sports and exercise also require planning and organization skills, and changing up the movement routine improves adaptability skills. Move the body to strengthen the brain.

- Eating right: It goes without saying that eating a healthy diet improves the health of the entire body. Foods that cause inflammation are particularly damaging to the brain, so cut out the sugars and processed junk. It will not only make your body feel better, but it will also make your brain sharper and more clear.

- Sleep: As we saw in the sleep section, along with diet and movement, sleep is the most important thing for health and well-being, yet so few people get a good night's sleep on a regular basis. Without quality sleep, we lose memory recall and cognitive function. Just look at yourself the morning after a night of bad sleep, and you can see the effects: grogginess, brain fog, walking into walls, needing coffee to "wake up." Lack of quality sleep also negatively impacts memory recall and consolidation, the process in which our short-term memories are transformed into long-term memories.

Visualization pushes the brain to create and imagine images while listening to music or a narrator's voice.

- Take an omega-3 supplement: Fish oil, krill oil, or just increasing foods like sardines and salmon benefit the brain by slowing the mental decline that comes from too much inflammation. The omega-3 fatty acids eicosapentaenoic acid (EPA) and docosahexaenoic acid (DHA) found in these supplements and food sources prevent inflammation, relieve stress and anxiety, and improve memory recall.

- Try a brain trainer: You can access numerous apps and online brain-training programs for free or a small fee. These apps and programs boost memory, build cognitive skills, improve focus and concentration, build problem-solving skills, and reduce the risk of dementia in older adults.

Other ways of taking good care of your brain include getting your vitamin D levels checked. Many studies exist showing low vitamin D levels lead to a reduction in cognitive functioning and a greater risk of developing dementia. You can also cut back on alcohol consumption to help your brain, thanks to a lower level of inflammation and sugars your body must process, which is usually at night when it needs to wind down for sleep.

Practicing visualization and mind-fulness also strengthen the brain. Visual-ization pushes the brain to create and imagine images while listening to music or a narrator's voice. Like meditation, which it can be combined with, the brain learns to focus and achieve clarity. It is also helpful for increasing organizational and planning skills as we usually visual-ize things we hope to manifest in our physical environment, whether weight loss, a new job, or a bigger house. Visu-alization also prepares the brain for po-tential challenges that might arise. For example, if you must give a speech or fly to a new city, visualizing a successful speech or a smooth flight helps you cope better, adapt to the situation when it happens, and make better decisions along the way.

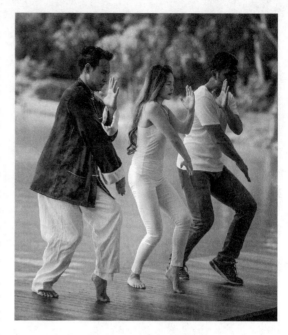

Movement exercises such as tai chi or qigong work the muscles, increase oxygen flow, and improve focus.

Mindfulness also keeps the brain focused on the present moment and re-duces stress and the monkey-mind chatter that causes it. Staying in the present moment improves recognition–memory performance and concentration skills and removes thoughts of worry and regret for the past and future, both of which are out of your control.

A healthy body without a healthy brain is only half healthy. We live so much of our lives inside our heads: in our thoughts, emotions, and perceptions. It behooves us to take good care of the brain just as we would our figure or physique. We live longer, and we age better. This takes us to....

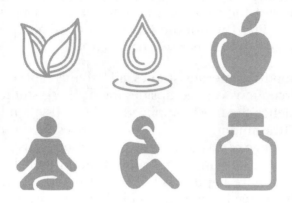

Positively Healthy Aging

Age is inevitable. The truth is that growing older is a luxury not given to all, yet we fear and dread getting older so much that we exhaust ourselves trying to find ways to look and feel younger. We get surgery and buy expensive creams. We work out to exhaustion and buy clothes that are clearly meant for teenagers. We go through midlife crises and become more depressed with each birthday, then go to extremes to create the perception of youth. In a weird way, we kill ourselves to live.

It doesn't help that Americans live in a society that looks down upon its elder citizens as if they no longer have a purpose. Seniors are considered throwaways if they can't breed or work anymore. We fear aging and death, so we shun those going through those things, not realizing that we are on the same path and will one day be on the receiving end of the negative treatment we impart on older people when we are young. It's a cycle no one escapes from unless they die young.

Is it possible to instead embrace age and enter that part of our existence with a sense of adventure, anticipation, and gratitude that we even get to grow old in the first place? To be grateful for each year, even the ones where we lose our youthful beauty and attractiveness, while being totally ignorant of the new beauty of wisdom and experience? So many die young, even children, that we forget that each year we blow out the candles is another year that we were graced with the gift of life. The question is, how do we age positively and perhaps even add to the years we have left?

According to numerous studies, a U-shaped curve of happiness turns our perceptions on age upside down. These studies show that people experience the most happiness in their 30s, then it dips in the 40s and 50s (the midlife crisis years) and rises in the 60s and 70s. People after the age of 60 consistently show more satisfaction, happiness, and well-being than at any other time in their lives. Seventy-year-olds show more happiness than 30-year-olds, which is in stark contrast to the image of aging and elderly people we get.

One of the reasons we may have a skewed perception of aging is our expectation that we will be miserable when we get older. No matter the age group, if a built-in expectancy of fear and anxiety over getting older is present–having to go into a nursing home, coming down with dementia or Alzheimer's, being alone and sick, and all the other negatives we think about when we investigate our future–that is why so many people believe they won't be happy past the age of 30.... Yet, we are.

 Older people remember more positive images than younger people and have a stronger sense of emotional well-being and purpose than younger generations....

Susan Charles, who has a Ph.D. in psychology and is the chair of psychological science at the University of California at Irvine, did a landmark longitudinal study across adult life spans with USC Dornsife professor of psychology Margaret Gatz that showed that the negative emotions of anger, fear, anxiety, frustration, and stress don't increase with age, they diminish. Positive emotions like pride, calm, elation, and excitement remain stable across the life span, with a slight decline in people who are in the very oldest age group. This expectation that happiness will decline with age presents itself even when experience proves it to be a falsehood. By focusing only on the negatives, as society and media tend to do with the subject of age, we see only pain, suffering, loneliness, and illness to look forward to. The truth is that this reasoning is faulty and does not cover the bigger picture that embraces the positives of aging.

Another study by Charles with additional colleagues showed that as we age, our brains become more focused on the positive and are wired to concentrate on positive stimuli. Older people remember more positive images than younger people and have a stronger sense of emotional well–being and purpose than younger generations, who may still be trying to find their way through the maze of life. Older adults are better at regulating their emotions and minimizing their exposure to upsetting things, which makes life more manageable and a lot happier. They also are more mindful and live in the moment, making the most of the time they have left and learning to see and find the best in every experience.

In "Is Aging the Secret to Happiness," Mark Stibich wrote for the *Verywell Mind* website that older people tend to be happier in part because they have not always had happiness all their lives. Starting around age 50, they report that happiness comes to them along with wisdom and an adjustment of expectations that often leave their younger counterparts filled with worry, anxiety, and fear. They become the "eternal optimists" in the fourth quarter of life at a time when society tells them they should be filled with fear and worry.

One of the reasons we look so negatively upon age is our inherent fear of death and change. It is also directly tied to society's obsession with ageism, which distorts views on getting older and focuses only on the gifts of youth. A survey taken by the World Health Organization found that over 60 percent of people say that older people don't get any respect, with the lowest levels of respect found in the higher–income countries. Seniors see and hear the constant barrage of messages telling them they are no longer useful and a waste of space compared to young folks, and it's no wonder they fear aging and meet it with depression and anxiety.

Today, we are seeing a resurgence of positive aging as we realize that health is not just "not being sick" but also adopting a healthy lifestyle and view of aging that empowers us. We are also being encouraged to look at age as just a natural phase along the path of life and to embrace its gifts and insights. Youth may have the energy, but age tells you where to direct it. Youth may have their dreams, but age figures out a plan to make them a reality. Youth may have the beauty, but age has the grace and serenity that make exterior beauty less important than the beauty within.

All ages have their challenges and their gifts. To shun those who are over 60 not only adds to the already hard–to–overcome negative perceptions of older people but also keeps the cycle going for when we get old. Here are some ways to keep more of that youthful energy and vitality and to age positively and powerfully:

- Stay active with movement and exercise, at least 30 minutes every day, and include weights to build muscle and strengthen bones. You can move in so many ways, from tai chi to running, but find what you will do consistently and make it a habit.

- Keep the brain toned and sharp with games and puzzles and keep learning new things to build new neural networks. Look for ways to challenge your brain and change up routines to build resiliency.

- Eat healthy foods, get enough sleep, and get out in nature more often. A healthy diet and plenty of rest work wonders to keep you energetic and vibrant, and spending time in the sun boosts your vitamin D levels to protect bones and the heart.

- Lose excess weight to avoid diabetes and other diseases associated with obesity.

- Cut back on alcohol and stop smoking to cut down on the risk of many diseases, make your skin look younger and healthier, and give your lungs and liver a break so they can heal.

 Dating sites and apps are around for seniors who wish to meet a companion or the love of their later life.

- Stay close to friends and family and build new connections for social interaction. Spend time with children and pets for the love only they can give.

- Play more.

- Meditate and find ways to experience calm and serenity daily.

- Stop sweating the small stuff and be mindful, accepting what is and not trying to fix or change everything and everyone. Get rid of stress anywhere you can. Declutter your mind and your life.

- Set new goals and challenges physically and mentally to give yourself a sense of purpose.

- Find positive ways of coping with stress and anxiety such as breath work, biofeedback, and meditation.

- Be good to your skin and avoid harsh treatments, creams, and plastic surgeries that make you look garish and fake. Age gracefully and age well.

- Stop dyeing hair with harsh chemicals and consider going naturally gray or using temporary dyes with fewer toxins.

- Engage in a gratitude practice such as daily journaling to remind you of all the blessings you've incurred over your life span.
- Find ways to volunteer your time, energy, or wisdom and insight. Mentor younger people. Share your success tips and how you reached a goal or dream on social media or a blog.
- Get adequate sleep and find ways to improve sleep quality if you are struggling with insomnia.
- Stop putting off the things you want to do and do them now because tomorrow is not guaranteed; haven't you waited long enough to go for your dreams?
- Accept your age and don't rail against it. Find the gifts and treasures in being your age. Age mindfully, with no regrets of the past or fears of the future.

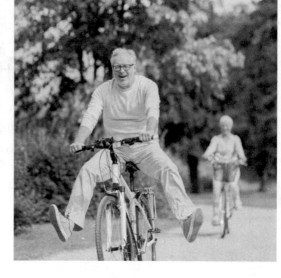

Staying physically active and involved in life as we age is a key part of enjoying your later years.

Thanks to social media, many support groups and pages have formed for people of all age groups to share their thoughts and interests. Dating sites and apps are around for seniors who wish to meet a companion or the love of their later life. It is easier than ever to reach out to others when we feel isolated or alone and set up in-person meetups with like-minded souls.

If you think older people can't chase a new dream or start a new venture, remember this:

- Samuel Jackson didn't get his break in Hollywood until he was 43.
- Stan Lee, when he passed at 95, was still actively involved in the Marvel Comic Universe he created in his late 30s, when he created his first comic.
- Julia Child didn't release her first cookbook until the age of 50 and got her own cooking show much later.
- Ray Kroc started the McDonald's franchise when he was 52.
- Colonel Sanders franchised his little fried chicken venture into Kentucky Fried Chicken at the age of 62.
- Arianna Huffington started her namesake publication at the age of 55.

- Laura Ingalls Wilder wrote the first *Little House* book and published it at the age of 65.
- Grandma Moses, whose real name was Anna Mary Robertson Moses, began her painting career at the age of 78, and in 2006 one of her paintings sold for $1.2 million.
- Harry Bernstein achieved writing fame at the age of 96 for his memoir *The Invisible Wall: A Love Story That Broke Barriers.*
- Martha Stewart didn't publish her first book until she was 41.
- Duncan Hines didn't achieve the fame of having his own line of cake mixes until he licensed the rights to use his name at the age of 73.
- Charles Darwin was 50 when his classic *On the Origin of Species* was published.

No rules exist as to when the clock on success stops. Success later in life may not mean fame and fortune to you, but it could mean discovering your purpose, starting a new business, traveling the world, or any other new and exciting endeavor you can imagine.

Setting Life Goals

Having goals gives you something to work toward, look forward to, and pursue with passion. Goals can be anything from meeting the right person to getting a great job, from finding the perfect shelter dog to adopt to writing your first novel or selling your first house as a realtor. Goals are linked to our passions and desires and to the things we hope to acquire and achieve, whether physical objects or experiences. Well-being is itself a goal to work toward by taking small baby steps and keeping track of our progress.

Setting goals requires self-knowledge of what is important to you and what you hope to achieve in the short and long term in different areas of your life such as career, finances, love and relationships, health, spirituality, and personal growth. Self-help books abound with ways to set goals in small, bite-sized pieces and how to take action on them. Here are some tried and true methods for getting goals down on paper and then doing what needs to be done to manifest them in your life:

- Write them down: Start by writing down the goal. Many people use journals to divide into the different life areas listed above, then they list 10 or so goals they wish to achieve under each area. Ten is a good number for overall goals, but for short-term goals and when you are building your goal-setting muscles, you can start with two per section.

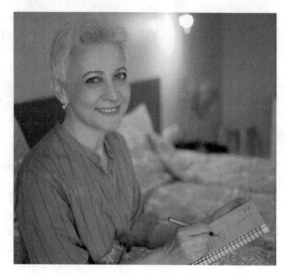

- Don't just write down the goal it-self but how it will make you feel once you've achieved it: Often, it is this feeling and essence of the goal that is more likely to keep you driven and motivated when you lose focus.

- Make sure they are your goals: This is not about anyone but you and the things you want to achieve, do, be, and have. When we set goals that are more about pleasing or impressing others, we won't have the resilience and strength to keep working on them for the long haul. Goals that are more about others are not going to instill in you the excitement and enthusiasm of your own. Listen to your heart and go for what you want.

Write down your goals and keep track of the steps you are making toward each goal. Don't forget to reward yourself for your progress!

- List under each goal baby steps: It can be incredibly intimidating when you set a big goal unless you break it up into small actions that don't scare the crap out of you. A goal too overwhelming is a goal that will never be met, so make a list of the many small actions you can take, even just one or two a day, to get you closer to the big end result.

- Set deadlines: Baby steps won't matter if they don't come with fixed deadlines. If you think you can achieve goals by winging it, you will be disappointed. Giving yourself hard and fixed dead-lines will give you more motivation and impetus to reach those deadlines. Once you do, revel in the feeling of accomplishment.

- Reward yourself: Each time you complete 10 baby steps or so, give yourself a reward. It can be a cup of your favorite latte or a new pair of shoes. Celebrate the baby steps and be proud of how far you are moving toward your goal. The journey and the process are just as important as the destination.

- Share carefully: Some people love the pressure of posting on so-cial media about the goals they have set for themselves. They need the accountability of going public. Others find that talking about or sharing their unfulfilled goals takes some of their power away and the often negative responses they get from others can threaten to derail their confidence. If you want to tell someone about your goals, make sure it is someone you trust who is supportive. You can also find an accountability partner and keep each other on track. Unless you are a great self–support system–and, ultimately, the achievement of your goals does fall on your shoulders–having some cheerleaders who believe in you can go a long way toward keeping you upbeat and inspired.

- Align goals to your higher vision: Goals can be small, like getting a new car, or they can be big and grand, like starting a nonprofit to feed the poor. They should always be in alignment with the highest and best vision of your life. Having a goal requires a lot of blood, sweat, and tears, so it behooves you to make it something that will add value and meaning to your life and not just add more stuff. Each goal should move your life forward, and never should a goal cause anyone else harm if it comes to pass.

- Keep it where you can see it: Once you have your main goals and baby steps, write down the main goals on index cards or small cards you can keep in your wallet, purse, or desk drawer, and look at them often throughout the week. This will keep you excited and on track. You can also make adjustments to goals as you go by revisiting them often. Some goals may fall by the wayside, and others may demand priority attention. Don't be afraid to redo your goal list as you grow and change.

- Stay open to the hows: Having goals means getting specific about what you want, but achieving them asks that you keep an open mind about how that happens. You may think that achieving the goal of speaking French by the summer when you go to Paris will happen by ordering an online language program, but be open to possibly meeting a French person in a coffee shop who would love to tutor you in the language in exchange for piano lessons or showing them how to cook. Life has a way of providing the hows to your whats when you keep your eyes and heart open. The goal is the goal, not the way you got there.

- Set smart goals: Setting S.M.A.R.T. goals means:

S: Specific or significant

M: Measurable and meaningful

A: Attainable

R: Rewarding and relevant to you

T: Time–bound and trackable

Using this S.M.A.R.T. chart is a great way to assure that you are setting goals that matter and are realistic (becoming a leopard or stopping time are not attainable goals, for example). If you are going to go through the time and effort of pursuing goals, they should be all these things or chances are that you will abandon them or waste time going after less important pursuits, only to later regret that you weren't smarter about pursuing your goals.

Additional tips for goal setting include the following, courtesy of the *Mind Tools* website:

- Keep operational goals small: Keep the low-level goals that you're working toward small and achievable. If a goal is too large, it may feel as though you are not making progress toward it, and you may give up on it.

- Set performance goals, not outcome goals: Goals should be something you have control over, or you will be disappointed if you cannot achieve them. Outcome goals may not be within your control and more about external factors, so focus on your own performance for your goals.

- Set realistic goals: Set goals that you can achieve.

- Put a time stamp on goals: Perhaps one-year goals, five-year goals, and 10-year goals. Also, make sure to have shorter-term goals, so you feel like you are making progress and get that sense of achievement.

Goals don't have to be big and groundbreaking to have meaning for you. This is not a competition. They are as individual as you are. One man's goal to bike across Europe may not appeal to the woman who has a goal of learning how to speak two languages by next June. A goal of running for political office is right for one person, while a goal of cleaning the entire house before company arrives is just as important of a goal to another. A goal can be as simple as getting through another day with a chronic illness or finishing a jigsaw puzzle before bedtime. No one is judging or comparing your goals to anyone else's.

The great thing about goals is that once you have achieved a few, the feeling of accomplishment and pride will carry through to encourage and inspire you to pursue more goals. Take the time to celebrate and acknowledge each goal you meet and learn from the goals that didn't manifest. Sometimes, you will find that it was something you can correct; other times, it was just out of your hands and not worth the regret. Learning to fail spectacularly is important to goal setting. Failure is how we adjust our sails on the oceans of life, and that applies to the things we want and the goals we set. It's nothing to be ashamed of or to avoid. Ask any inventor. Had they given up on their goals, we might not have light bulbs and radios.

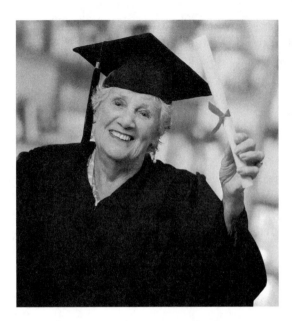

You can achieve your goals at any age, and the feeling of accomplishment you'll experience will be its own reward.

Goals are important because they give life depth and richness and bring out our own individual expression as we move toward what we want to experience in the life we have been given. They are the reasons we jump out of bed in the morning eager to take on the day. They bring us happiness and inspire others to pursue their own goals, especially our children.

A goal achieved is a gift received.

Mindful Aging

The older people get, the more they tend to live in the moment because of the stark realization of how much time they may have left on the planet. It's too bad that younger people cannot have this same realization because the truth is that death can come for us at any age, but after being alive for decades, a greater appreciation occurs for the finer points of each moment we may have ignored before, always seeking the big moments as a way to gauge how successful and happy we were.

Mindful aging keeps the brain and body healthier, too. Because the focus on positivity, gratitude, and well-being is not based on chasing other people and their approval, older people often go against the stereotype of bitter, angry curmudgeons, and science explains why. In a recent study by Natalie J. Shook and her colleagues at West Virginia University, 123 adults between the ages of 25 and 35 and 117 adults between the ages of 60 and 91 were studied. They all lived in the same general area, and most were female. The participants were questioned about mood, mindfulness, their perspectives of the future, and how often they felt positive and negative emotions.

They were also asked how often they stayed mindful to their awareness of the moment and how often they lived in the past or future with regret and worry. The results showed that the oldest participants were more aware of the fact that they had fewer remaining years, yet they had more positive emotions because their focus was on the present, which translated to a greater sense of well-being. Shook wrote that this "cultivation of mindfulness may be an adaptive means of maintaining emotional well-being when faced with life's challenges." Instead of being crippled by a fear of pending death, it made these people more aware of time and how important each moment is.

Several intriguing studies have looked into the genetic aspect of aging well. In 2009, Elizabeth H. Blackburn and her colleagues from the University of California at San Francisco won a Nobel Prize for their discovery of telomerase, the protective enzyme in cells that replenish and lengthen telomeres, the protective tips at the end of chromosomes. Telomeres help cells divide in a healthy manner, becoming shorter as the cell divides. Eventually, they shorten enough so that the cell dies.

 Our mental states have a powerful influence on the length of our telomeres.

Telomerase not only replenishes but relengthens them, and the result is a healthy cell. Because stress, depression, and anxiety are associated with shorter telomeres as well as cancer, heart disease, diabetes, and other major illnesses, finding ways to lengthen them can improve our quality of life. Our mental states have a powerful influence on the length of our telomeres. In additional studies done at the University of California at Davis, meditation was found to improve the length of telomeres, and another study showed that a wandering mind leads to shorter telomeres.

This means that we have more control over how we age than we think and that control comes from positive mental states. Aging with fear and dread is not a positive mental state. This might explain why two people of the same age with similar circumstances can look so different and experience such different perspectives of what the rest of their lives have in store for them. Though much of the genetic "damage" may have been done in the past, shifting attitudes and putting mental health front and center can lead to the lengthening of telomeres, meaning that the past does not always equal the future and that it is always beneficial to start now, today, to improve health and well-being for the time we do have left.

Coming to a place where you can not only accept your age but celebrate it with gratitude opens the door to a life that is just as exciting and filled with possibilities as the days of youth, but now you have the wisdom, insight, and experience to know how to better navigate any challenges to come. If you struggle with fear and depression over aging, see a therapist or doctor who may help you get to the root of your fears and assist you in working through those fears, reframing your attitudes about growing older, and looking forward to whatever life has in store for you in the years to come.

Look at each birthday as another reason to feel grateful and excited. Look for people your age and older who can be positive role models of how to age well. Avoid negative stereotypes and perceptions of age found all over the news and social media. Seek out stories of people doing amazing things in their "old age" or even those who are quietly happy and calm. Big goals don't have to be a part of your plan. Maybe you just want to feel great about the life you lived and the life still ahead of you. Leave the comparisons and approval seeking to the insecure youth.

When it comes to aging, you are what you think, and if you think aging is a curse, it will be. If you think it's a gift, you are far more likely to experience overall satisfaction when those negative expectations are removed. Perspective and mindset are important for physical and emotional resilience and well-being. Understanding that each life phase is a blessing and something to be embraced because again, what is the alternative, helps foster more self-love and appreciation at a time when society might be the least appreciative. Besides, do you really want to spend your days chasing your youth and trying to make yourself look younger when you could be doing things that bring out your passion and zest for life and renew your adventurous spirit? Do you feel better being terrified that you won't wake up tomorrow, or would you rather focus on what you might do tomorrow to bring yourself more joy?

Surrounding yourself with friends, family, and a support system that respects and celebrates age creates a community that helps you live a longer, happier life, but even if you live alone, you can find ways to meet aging with grace and cultivate a stronger sense of well-being. You got this far. You're still alive. It is your right, and an incredible privilege, to grow old happily.

Nurturing the Spirit

"We are spiritual beings having a human experience." You have no doubt heard that saying at some point in your life. What does it mean that we are spiritual beings if so much of our lives are spent focused on human things like going to school or work, raising a family, making money, and paying taxes? Everything we do is on the human plane, including the ways we experience health: eating right, exercising, and alleviating stress. Does a spiritual part of us really exist, and if so, how do we access it if we don't currently feel any kind of connection to it?

What is Spirituality, Anyway?

Spirituality is having a sense of something beyond the physical existence and the five senses, something that suggests that more exists to life than meets the eye. It can be a belief in a higher power, a deity, the universe, or the force, but it is based on a deeper connection between all things and all people. Spirituality is a source of relief, comfort, joy, creativity, and conscious awareness and may be different for everyone because it is not about rules, doctrines, or rituals, although religious beliefs are a spiritual system that you may choose to follow. It may come from a specific religion or from a general approach to the world that speaks to a deeper connectivity.

This is about cultivating a sense of connectedness to the self, to others, and to the world around us in a way that signifies that something greater and grander than we are may exist. This may be a god or goddess, higher power, higher self, deity, or simply a state of conscious awareness beyond that of everyday existence. Spirituality can be the recognition of things that are unseen but give life more meaning and purpose and show us that we are more than just flesh, bones, and blood.

Spirituality is as much a part of a healthy, balanced, and harmonious life as physical health and mental wellness because it speaks to the deeper aspects of who we are, why we are here, and how we express ourselves in the world. It speaks to all the ways we experience the unseen; the inner knowings, intuitions, and synchronicities that have no external causation; the awe and grandeur of nature; the oneness we feel holding our baby for the first time; the expansiveness of possibility; and the ego breakdown and bliss of falling in love. Tending to our spirit is tending to the intangibles that shape the tangibles and the whisperings of the heart and soul that beg to be heard on equal ground with the body and the mind.

Tending to our spirit is tending to the intangibles that shape the tangibles and the whisperings of the heart and soul that beg to be heard on equal ground with the body and the mind.

Attending to the spiritual side can mean seeking out a specific path or belief system, or it can mean going it solo and becoming your authentic self. It can mean traveling to the far corners of Earth to study under gurus and spend hours in silent meditation, or it can mean going inward during meditation to speak to your inner self and asking its guidance. As many ways to explore individual spirituality exist as the number of individuals, with ample opportunities to discover and learn.

It begins with going within and sitting in silence long enough to hear the voice that emerges. That voice, your voice, will tell you exactly what it seeks and how to find it. That voice whispers the great mysteries of life and urges you to look for answers to deep questions about life after death, meaning and purpose, the nature of the universe, and other truths that can only be found beyond the realm of the logical and rational. The world of spirit is often associated with awe, nature, happiness, wonder, joy, full expression, authenticity, interconnectedness, compassion and empathy, internal guidance, and the desire to make the world a better place.

Whether you choose a path that is traditional, modern, or something in between, spirituality nourishes what the physical and mental cannot, yet they all work toward a harmonic convergence of holistic well-being. You can do your own spiritual thing alone or join a community of like-minded individuals and find a deeper level of existence beyond the day-to-day concerns. You cannot take a spiritual path belonging to another. It must be your path, and you can make of it what you wish. Before you can even choose a path, you need to tune out the external world and tune in to the divinity within, which is almost impossible in this day and age of gadgets and technology that give others 24/7 access to us.

Only by taking the journey within can we hope to find the way outside of ourselves. Self-awareness is at the heart of spirituality because without first becoming aware of our true self, we can never become aware of its connection to every other self and the greater forces that make up the laws of nature. If we are disconnected from our interior world, we won't see the connections to others in our exterior world and will always see ourselves as alone and separate.

Spiritual growth allows us to see how our lives are more than just a series of days and moments and that what we believe, say, and do is significant. It may be a grand quest for enlightenment or ascension or a journey inward when so much of our lives are spent focusing outward. When we embrace the spiritual aspects of ourselves, we begin to see and experience time in a different way because we become more focused on the present moment. We understand more about how our own thoughts and beliefs create the physical reality we experience and how we have cocreative power to change that with a force greater than we are. We come to know that physical matter is not the entirety of reality or of who we are and that forces, energies, and frequencies are at play all the time in the field of potentiality that we can tap into.

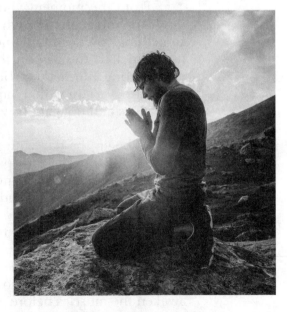

Having a spiritual awakening can be a big, bold event that totally shifts your paradigms and perspectives, or it

The quest for the spiritual is the act of finding more in one's life than just surviving from day to day.

can be a quiet dawning of realization that takes you out of your ego and opens your eyes to the majesty of life beyond the five senses. It can be a gaining of wisdom through experience and contemplation and the opening of the mind and heart to the fact that we may be human, but we are human "beings," and the being part is just as important as our need for survival and the basics in life.

Where do you begin to find your spirit? The most important thing is to tune in to your inner voice of intuition, to the still, small voice within that may indeed be a higher force guiding you, and to slow down long enough to hear the calling to a greater adventure. If you are too outer-focused and distracted by the events and circumstances of the material world or always have your attention on your cell phone and social media, you may miss those inner callings and prompts and either delay or detour spiritual growth if you don't shut it down altogether. Spirit tends to whisper, not yell, so you must listen.

Tapping into the world of spirit beyond our five senses can be done in many ways. Let's start with how we start our day.

A Positive Start to Each Day

From the moment you awaken, are you dreading the coming day? Are you regretting what happened yesterday or stressing over something you need to do next week? Each morning is a new opportunity to start the day on the right foot with positive thoughts and empowering affirmations. How you begin your day sets the tone and mood for everything that happens afterward as you face your worldly challenges and obligations with work, family, and goals.

To begin the day with focus, clarity, and calm intention, before you get up to exercise or put on the coffee pot, take 10 minutes to meditate. Calm the mind and quiet the spirit enough to get centered and reflect on the day ahead from this grounded place. Listen for the voice of intuition with any guidance, direction, wisdom, or insight, and shut out all externals to connect with the internal knowing: your inner GPS.

After a quick meditation, try a gentle morning stretch routine to awaken the muscles before going to the gym or getting on the workout equipment. Don't skimp on stretching, for it does more than wake up the muscles; it gets more oxygen flowing to the organs and the brain. Maybe you prefer to do morning yoga or tai chi or go for a run as the sun comes up. How you begin the morning to clear out the mind and energize the body can make all the difference between having a productive day or one that is chaotic and cluttered.

 How you begin the morning to clear out the mind and energize the body can make all the difference between having a productive day or one that is chaotic and cluttered.

Turn your morning shower into a way to increase blood circulation, invigorate the body and mind, increase energy and alertness, and make your hair and skin dewy and shiny. How? Turn the water from hot to cold for about two minutes at the end of each shower.

Choose a word or phrase of the day to repeat throughout your day to bring you back to your center and keep you focused on your intentions. This can be anything from "joy" to "so blessed" to "I got this!" Let it be your mantra to guide and direct your energy and focus. Repeating your mantra also brings you back into the mindful state of the present moment where you can make better decisions and keep your day on track.

In the morning, do some deep breathing to get the oxygen moving through your bloodstream and into your brain. Then, when the challenges of the day arise, and they will, stop and do some breath work to reinvigorate the body and brain.

How you begin the day is how the day will unfold. Begin it with stress and a cluttered mind, and the day will be stressful and crazy. Begin with a serene and centered body, mind, and spirit, and you will have a much better, happier, and more productive day ahead.

Gratitude

Be grateful. Literally. Daily if you can. People who are grateful are happier, healthier, and just all-around nicer. Focusing on what blessings you have and slowing down long enough to see what is working in your life removes your focus off of what you don't have. You begin to realize just how much abundance already exists right here, right now, including loved ones, material goods, and your own gifts and talents. It's all a matter of maximizing what is and minimizing what isn't.

The power of gratitude is not ignoring bad things or denying challenges, including scarcity and lack, illness and disease. Rather, it is a way to bring the mind back to thoughts that empower it, not drain it, adding to the current stresses and challenges. It is all about shifting focus and perception to what serves and not what drains.

You might ask what you can be grateful for in a world full of war, poverty, violence, and despair. Begin with small things right in your own environment, like your family and the fact that you have a roof over your head and enough money to pay today's bills. Even if you don't have that, you woke up breathing, and you can be thankful for so many things, such as the air you inhale, the nature that exists around you, and your own resilience. Though it may be a cliché, counting your blessings makes you feel a lot better than counting your curses, doesn't it?

Starting a powerful gratitude practice is as easy as keeping a nightly gratitude list. Start by simply writing down five things each night before you go to bed that you are grateful for that day. These can be anything that comes to mind–events that occurred that day, people you met, ideas you came up with, something that made you laugh out loud–or you can just look around the room and write down five things you are glad you have: your bed, your TV, your spouse, your kids, your full refrigerator, chocolate pudding…. The magic of the gratitude list is that you simply cannot keep it to five things once you get started. Five becomes 10, which becomes 20, then 30, and before you know it, you've listed 50 or more things you are so happy to have in your life and you go to sleep feeling quite prosperous indeed, thank you very much!

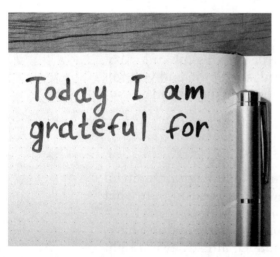

Take a little time to write down the things you are grateful for each night. This will remind you of all the things in your life that are going right.

We are so intent on getting more that we often forget we already have enough. We are so driven to want what we don't have that we often ignore the great things that are right in front of us. We are so determined to become more that we often are blind to the fact that we are there already! When we take the time to see how blessed we are, it opens up our hearts and spirits as wide as can be, ready to accept even more. It inspires us to share some of it, too. Gratitude combined with charity makes for a very potent form of joy that, as you will find, comes back around with more blessings to share.

Try the gratitude list for one week and see if you don't feel a lot happier and more in tune with the present moment of your life. Buy a fun journal to keep your list in. You can even look at it the next morning or write a morning list and then review it at night. Some people write down things they are grateful for that have not yet happened to train their brains to notice things that will help lead them toward a specific goal.

See if your perception window opens a bit wider and you start to notice more things to be grateful for. Watch for synchronicities and serendipities that come with a new and more positive mindset, one that seeks out abundance and prosperity in all its forms. You may find that you just can't keep your list down to five items, no matter how hard you try. Furthermore, once you begin to see how many small and simple miracles occur in your life each day, you will adopt a permanent gratitude attitude that will change your perception and change your life.

Our brains seek to create patterns and order out of chaos. Gratitude is a way to direct the brain to seek out more things to notice that we can be grateful for, including things that were right in front of our faces that we just never perceived as such, as we were too caught up in worry and concern. Marcus Tullius Cicero once said, "Gratitude is not only the greatest of virtues, but the parent of all others."

Journaling

A recent analysis of books that sell the best on Amazon revealed that journals, lined and blank, are a huge market. People love to journal, and journals exist for capturing creative ideas and thoughts on paper, for recording nightly dreams to look for patterns, for keeping track of weight loss and exercise gains, for logging food eaten each day, for recording the path to recovery from an illness or addiction, for writing down intentions and goals, and for everything else under the sun. The act of writing something down not only gives it more power, as in goals and intentions, but brings more clarity when struggling to decide or overcome a problem. Seeing something in writing helps the brain formulate new ideas and sparks new angles of looking at a situation that may reveal a solution you hadn't thought of.

Journaling also helps to disempower negative and traumatic feelings and experiences. When something bad happens, we keep it locked in our heads where the rumination only makes the pain worse. Taking the painful thoughts and emotions out of our heads and putting them onto paper not only clears clutter from the mind but allows you to look at the problem with enough detachment to begin the healing process. It also helps you come to terms with and process events and reframe them to put them in the past where they belong. Journals are like diaries for adults. The diaries we kept as kids were the private repositories of our innermost feelings and thoughts, the ones we felt we couldn't share with anyone else in the world.

Journaling is a way of releasing and letting go, as it gets things out of the dark and murky corners of the mind and into the light of day where they can be examined and processed with clarity.

Difficult feelings and emotions suddenly seem simpler and more manageable when they are written down. Dumping and releasing our deepest anger, resentments, and fears onto paper helps them to dissipate their hold on us, and seeing an obstacle we believe to be insurmountable in writing triggers sudden epiphanies about how to get around or over it. Journaling is a way of releasing and letting go, as it gets things out of the dark and murky corners of the mind and into the light of day where they can be examined and processed with clarity.

Daily journaling relieves the mind of worry and concern. Combined with a gratitude list, it can be a powerful way to put to bed the problems and challenges of the day so that we can start fresh and new tomorrow. It can also get our dreams and goals down on paper, which makes them feel more tangible, so we can then get to work on the steps and timelines it will take to achieve them.

Journaling is meditative writing and reflecting on paper. It is also a great way to ask a question and write out the various possible answers in order to gain enough clarity for the brain to find the best solution. Keeping all your thoughts inside your head builds steam to the point where you feel like you can't think clearly or straight. Letting them have their run on the page allows them all to be heard and acknowledged so that you can pinpoint new ways to meet with old problems or solve a challenge that has eluded you because the solution was stuck in the quagmire of unexpressed thoughts.

Journaling can be a way to get down intuitions and insights after a meditation session when you might ask a question of your higher mind. Writing down the thoughts and images that come to mind will reveal the answers to those questions if you take the time to pay attention.

The author of this book has a line of fun and funky "journals with attitude" for every occasion called *Attitudenals* that are available on her website.

Giving Is Good Medicine

One surefire way to experience more mental, emotional, and spiritual well-being is to become more of a giver. A 2008 study by Harvard Business School professor Michael Norton and his colleagues found that giving money to someone else lifted the happiness of the participants far more than spending it on themselves. Sonja Lyubo-

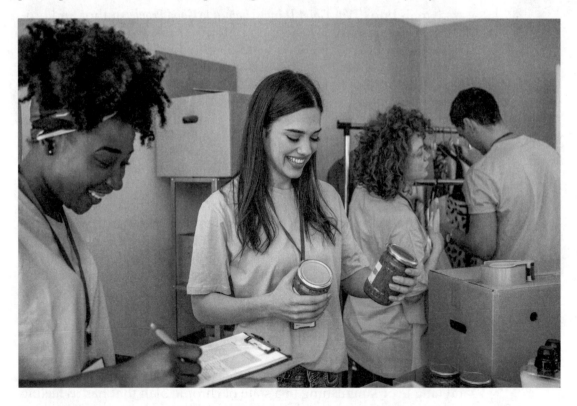

If you aren't able to give money or goods to a cause, volunteering your time is just as valuable—possibly even more valuable than just money.

mirsky, professor of psychology at the University of California at Riverside, asked people to perform five acts of kindness each week for six weeks and found a significant increase in the happiness levels of the participants. According to a 2006 study at the National Institutes of Health, when we give to charities, it activates regions of the brain associated with pleasure, social connection, and trust and increases those feel-good endorphins, producing what has become known as the "helper's high."

Giving to others also helps us see how blessed we are and increases our levels of gratitude. Sharing our blessings makes us feel a sense of purpose and that we influence those around us positively. Giving doesn't have to only mean offering physical objects like food or money to someone but also giving our time to charities as volunteers, visiting people in hospitals and nursing homes and sharing our stories with them, spending time with shelter animals that have yet to be adopted, and so much more.

In his book *Why Good Things Happen to Good People*, author and professor of preventative medicine at Stony Brook University Stephen Post writes about the increase in health benefits in people with chronic illness when they give of themselves. Being able to help others decreases our depression and makes us feel useful, and it takes some of the attention off our own problems by focusing on the needs of others. Seeing how we can assist others in meeting those needs is an empowering and enjoyable experience that helps lower our own stress levels and, according to one 2006 study at Johns Hopkins University, lower our blood pressure at the same time.

Giving reminds us of our connectivity to others, and for those who might be living alone, it is a wonderful way to create social connection and share in the lives of others. Even if all we can do is send $10 to a favorite charity, we feel as though we have done something of value and given some part of ourselves, which makes us feel a lot less alone in the world.

Slowing the Speed of Life

The constant speed of life can easily lead to a state of burnout and fatigue or languishing in a state of chronic blah that has us feeling as though we are going through the motions, aimless and without purpose, joy, or enthusiasm. When we go, go, go all the time and never slow down to catch our breath, we pay the price. Foggy think-ing, lack of energy, too much or too little sleep, zero joy in doing the things we once loved, short tempers, breathlessness, depression, anx-iety, and a sense of being stuck and going nowhere: these are all symptoms of running a sprint at full speed that has no finish line in sight.

Add to that malaise the constant ability of people to contact us via our social media and cell phones at all hours of the day and night, and little is left in our wells. We suffer from extreme adrenal fatigue and utter mental and emotional burnout. Then, when we are bom-barded nonstop with negative images on the news, the complaints of friends and family, and the pressures of daily life in general, we feel as though we are shutting down and disconnecting.

Nothing is wrong with slowing the speed of your life to improve your ability to cope and achieve more well-being. Nothing is standing between you and more peace of mind except your beliefs that you must plow ahead like a monster truck at a rally but at full speed. We all need a reset every now and then, or we may never get back our vitality, energy, and zest for life. Stopping the world for a day or two and getting off the hamster wheel can do wonders for your overall health, but making time each day to slow down and sit with yourself is even better. Doing something every day has so much more power and impact than doing it twice a month.

We all need a reset every now and then, or we may never get back our vitality, energy, and zest for life.

Many people have a fear that if they slow down, life will speed by so fast that they will never catch up again, but think about times when you have been down with the flu or a loved one was in the hospital and you stayed with them for a few days. Did you catch back up to your life again? Yes, because your life is always right where you are. The only thing speeding by is the illusion that you might be mis-sing out on something if you step away or that you might lose a race that offers no reward but exhaustion.

Consider taking time off and going on a vacation, but also be sure to infuse each day with a little self-care and a time to slow down the pace and enjoy what is right in front of you. Symptoms of mental, emotional, and physical distress are telling you that to function at full capacity, you need to get out of the rat race and walk at your own pace, even crawl if that's all you can muster. Otherwise, those symptoms can turn into a full-fledged illness or medical disaster.

Slow down. If you don't feel inspired or productive right now, take a break. If you can't focus on your project, step away for a bit. Nobody is keeping score. It's not a race, and you're not wearing a marathon bib with a tracker built into it. Be less hard on yourself for taking some downtime and realize it is just as much a part of success and well-being as action and movement is. You can't keep driving a car on an empty tank, no matter how big the tank is. If it's empty, it's empty, and you need to refill the tank. How do you do that? By stopping at the nearest station, not speeding by but stopping.

Life was meant to be lived at different speeds for different situations and times. Every now and then, get off the freeway and take a gentle side road to look at the scenery you miss when you're driving at breakneck speed to get to a destination that once you're there, you will be too tired and burnt out to enjoy.

Prayer

Nothing is mysterious about prayer. It is simply the opposite of meditation. Think about it. When we pray, we talk to God, the universe, our higher power, or even our innermost self. When we meditate, we listen for the response. However, many people equate prayer with rules and regulations, believing that to "please" God, prayer must be done perfectly or in a state of total submission and surrender, or they look at prayer as begging and pleading for something from an external source. In Larry Dossey's landmark book *Prayer Is Good Medicine*, he discussed how prayer for oneself and for other people can have a powerful healing effect on illness and trauma and that it can be measured scientifically.

Studies on brain activity during prayer and meditative prayer show that people who pray often have a change to their frontal lobes, the area of the brain that controls concentration and focus. In deep prayer, a shift in consciousness occurs and the parietal lobe kicks in, resulting in a feeling of spiritual transcendence or a sense of oneness with all. Prayer done on a repeated basis with a clear intention leads to a thicker frontal lobe and improved memory, problem solving, motor skills, language skills, impulse control, rationality, and social and sexual behavior. Over time, prayer can shift the way you positively perceive the world and your place in it.

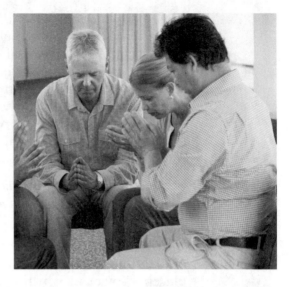

Prayer has the ability to calm and destress, and it may even improve your intellect. Collective prayer may boost this effect as everyone shares in the experience.

Like meditation, prayer calms the spirit and the mind, which leads to less stress and anxiety, lowered blood pressure and heart rate, and increased well-being. It deepens the connection with the life force that you are praying to, no matter your beliefs, and strengthens your intentions toward your goals and dreams. The act of asking, backed by belief, influences the way you act, think, and behave and makes you more open to new ideas and opportunities. Prayer is a form of intention setting, whether you are setting the intention of getting through a traumatic situation or praying for a great new job that won't make you sick every morning. It's a discussion between you and your innermost self, which is connected to the greater source of all knowledge and insight.

Prayer can be thought of as plugging in to the quantum field of all possibility, where you imprint upon that field the desire or goal you have in mind; an intimate chat between you and the god of your choice; or an acknowledgment of blessings received and a nice, big "thank you" to the universe. The ego is removed, and you become more self-aware and aware of a higher level of connectivity to everything around you.

Collective prayer, like collective meditation, operates from the belief that many minds working together for a shared intention can impact the physical realm. Groups of people praying for a particular outcome often cite the power of the many for the result. If individual consciousness is connected to every other individual consciousness, then collective prayer operates in this web and spreads the intention to everyone involved.

Dozens of studies into the collective power of prayer and meditation have been conducted. One standout study occurred in 2001, published in the prestigious *British Medical Journal*. The study divided

3,393 people admitted to a medical center in two groups. The first group was prayed over; the second was not. They were prayed over, however, four to 10 years after admission to the center, and the study concluded that those prayed over had significantly shorter hospital stays. The study conclusion stated, "Remote, retroactive intercessory prayer is associated with shorter stay in the hospital and shorter duration of fever in patients with a bloodstream infection and should be considered for use in clinical practice."

Prayer doesn't hurt, and it certainly seems to help those who engage in it.

While other studies showed prayer had no effect, the jury is still out, although many scientists point to the power of suggestion and placebo power in which a patient is given a placebo and gets well simply because they believed they had received a life-saving drug. The mind is a powerful machine that is capable of beliefs so strong they can help heal us. Prayer doesn't hurt, and it certainly seems to help those who engage in it. It's not harmful to try it, and it's likely that it will bring you a deeper sense of calm and serenity, especially when the spiritual or religious element of something greater than oneself that you are communing with is present.

But not all prayers are answered: a mother praying for a dying child, a homeless man praying for a job, a child with cancer praying for another year to live. Not all prayers come true, although some may argue that we do not know the bigger picture involved in the destinies or paths of those involved. Other times, something you pray for may not come true, only to find out later that you dodged a bullet and your life would have been far worse had it come true. "Prayer hasn't stopped wars and violence," people will say.

Yet, if prayer done regularly makes you happier and more connected, perhaps that is how the world gets changed over time. If you feel better, you act better, and you have a more positive influence on every person you come in contact with. Instead of spreading more hate, anger, and violence, you become a conduit of love, joy, and well-being and, like a virus, the feeling becomes contagious and spreads, infecting a larger and larger group of people. It grows exponentially if only enough people take the time to make praying a habit.

Cultivating Intuition

What exactly is intuition? It is an inner knowing about something that cannot be readily explained in terms of external circumstances or evidence. In the old days, women's intuition often led to being called a witch in a negative sense, yet that very same intuition was used in discerning the right healing herbal remedies or answers to someone's pressing questions that witches became known for. Such a catch-22 to have an ability to help others yet be called evil for it because it seemed foreign to those who never developed their own.

Everyone is intuitive to some degree. Those who follow earth traditions, natural healing methods, and spirituality tend to be more intuitive because it is more acceptable to develop their abilities than it is in many religious traditions. Intuition is not magic; it can appear that way to someone who has not acknowledged their own, yet if you ask those very same people if they've ever had a weird and inexplicable feeling knowing that they shouldn't get on a certain plane or turn down a particular alley at night or go into business with a certain person, only to find out later that something awful happened in that location or situation, they will have one of those brilliant "aha!" moments and realize that gift existed within themselves all along.

Listening to that still, small voice within can mean a lot fewer regrets later from choosing to instead listen to external voices....

Writers and artists of every ilk know that intuition is the greatest gift of creativity but often shun it for the professional advice of others (or the unprofessional advice of friends and family) to their later career detriment. Listening to that still, small voice within can mean a lot fewer regrets later from choosing to instead listen to external voices, which are usually louder and more demanding. Intuition is quiet, but it knows what is best for us. Is it the spirits or angels talking to us? Is it the gods or goddesses? The voice of the universe? Or is it just your own inner higher power or knowledge that is tapped into the subconscious and the deeper collective unconscious, a field of information you don't normally have conscious awareness of or access to?

Wherever it comes from, intuition can be developed so that it can help guide your life decisions and choices. Here are some tips to develop that inner knowing:

1. Find quiet time to meditate or just sit in silence and become aware of the small and quiet voice within. Don't force it to talk to you–just listen. The more you do this, the more you will hear it.

2. Trust that your subconscious will understand your intuition and that your conscious mind will fall into place with practice. We are so externally focused; we distract ourselves so much that we drown out that voice and then either underanalyze or over-analyze its messages.

3. Write down or record on your cell phone any intuitive sensations, urges, or messages as you get them. From these writings and re-cordings, begin to journal or at least take notes on what intuitions you followed that panned out and what intuitions you ignored that caused suffering on some level.

4. When you are in silence, check in the ego at the door and stay open and centered on the quieter voice, not the one that yells in your head, which is usually the ego. However, if a voice yells in your head that you are in danger, heed it. It may be your intuition ramping up the volume to get your attention so you don't do something stupid or dangerous.

5. Notice the times in your past when you had an intuition and didn't follow through on it. Did it affect your love life, career, health? How so? It's never too late to listen to it and take the right action.

Over time, your skill will improve, and you will find that you have a wonderful inner GPS or guidance system that you can ask questions to or depend on in various situations. The big difference between listening to the voice of the ego and the voice of that inner guidance is this: The ego wants something now and tends to be fear-ful, doubtful, or even selfish. It often leads to things we think we want, but when we get them, they harm or disappoint us. The ego also leads to decisions based on greed, jealousy, and envy. The voice of guidance will always know what is best for us long-term (the ego is not very good at long-term happiness or satisfaction) and usually leads us to the most enjoyable, fulfilling future, even if it takes longer and doesn't bring us the fame and fortune we begged for in the beginning. Guid-ance knows what we need, not just what we want. Guidance also knows our inner motivations, which may not even be conscious to us. Are we trying to get a lover just to get back at an ex? That's the ego talking. Do we desire a perfect and loving mate to grow old with? That's intuition and guidance talking.

Intuition is tuned in to the field of possibilities our conscious minds may not see, opening us up to ways we can achieve our goals in life, love, and happiness that we never thought of or knew were available to us. Consider intuition your sixth sense, your third eye, and your second gut. Practice getting quiet and undistracted enough to sit still and listen for its voice. Work on cultivating its presence in your life and recording the prompts and knowings it brings you each day. Ask it questions, and be open to any answers that come up, not the ones you want to hear (ego!). Trust in and pursue bursts of inspiration that could lead to incredible things down the road.

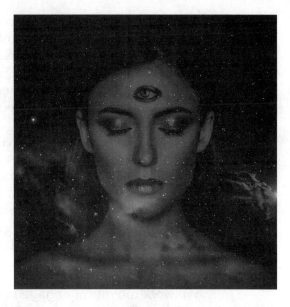

Intuition is like a muscle on the body. You must work it, use it, and make it stronger. If you were lucky enough to be born with a powerful intuition, consider yourself blessed, as most people must work at it. In today's busy, crazy,

Think of intuition as being like a third eye that helps you see beyond the obvious and look at things with a fresh viewpoint.

noisy world, intuition has taken a back seat to Googling information, asking a dozen people on Facebook for the answers to a pressing question, or scouring through podcasts to find one that addresses a need you have. This is all well and good, but it in no way replaces the sharper knowledge you already possess within.

Self-Care

Self-care is important for the body, mind, and spirit, but, like cultivating spirituality, it often gets put on the shelf in favor of more pressing physical and mental concerns. Caring for the self must come first and must be holistic, or you are not going to be healthy enough on any level to care for others or pursue your goals and dreams. We live in a society that makes us feel selfish for seeking self-care. Codependency is rampant, putting the cares and concerns of others above our own. We spend way too much time trying to fix and control the health of others, always to the detriment of our own, and excuse it as being a good person when all it does is bankrupt us of energy, joy, and vitality.

Spirituality is one place where we get to strengthen our bond to our higher self and tune in to the forces that nourish us on a soul level. In the eyes of our Creator, we are just as important as anyone else and totally deserving of our own love and attention. According to Paula Gill Lopez, Ph.D., associate professor and chair of the Department of Psychological and Educational Consultation at Fairfield University in Connecticut, a need for self-care is obvious. "We have an epidemic of anxiety and depression…. Everybody feels it."

We all pay close attention to viral epidemics like the flu or COVID-19, but when it comes to the epidemic—indeed, the pandemic—of illness and general malaise, we fail to grasp how this broad, societal "soul sickness" is harming us all. We work too much, engage in hostility and negativity on social media, watch too much bad news, eat poorly, sleep poorly, rarely get outside or spend time with others, then wonder why we hurt at such a deep level and why nothing we do heals the hurt.

We work too much, engage in hostility and negativity on social media, watch too much bad news, eat poorly, sleep poorly, rarely get outside or spend time with others, then wonder why we hurt….

If each one of us took as good care of ourselves as we do others, showing ourselves the same empathy, love, compassion, healing, and affection, the world would be a healthier, happier place for all. We would collectively prevent more disease from spreading, thanks to stronger immune systems. We would deal with far less violence, thanks to more positive moods and attitudes toward life. We would all feel as though we mattered, thanks to having the time to cultivate the inner world of spirit and not get so caught up in the rules of religions.

Research suggests that self-care leads to more resilience, tolerance, contentment, emotional health, mental health, physical strength, and immunity to illnesses; longer life spans; stronger and happier relationships; greater job enjoyment; and a whole lot more. Exercising self-care also means you are more proactive about your health, what you eat, and how often you exercise, yet it still holds the stigma of being a selfish, narcissistic act. To many, self-care is a luxury they cannot afford as they seek to merely survive another day of poverty, war, and violence.

Even those who are well-off ignore their feelings, symptoms, and inability to cope with life's challenges, big and small, and instead complain about being overwhelmed and exhausted, yet they will readily help someone else who asks for it. We have this weird and unfortunate stigma against taking care of number one. In an article titled "Why Does Self–Care Sometimes Feel So Hard?", Alicia H. Clark, a psychologist writing in *Psychology Today*, lists six reasons why we struggle to give ourselves the same care we are willing give to others:

1. Negativity bias: Knowing all we should do for ourselves doesn't mean we will do it and often makes it hard to see what we are doing that is healthy. Thinking more realistically can help us select strategies that make sense among many choices.

2. Effort: It takes work to take care of ourselves. The last thing we want after a long day of taking care of the house, job, and family is more work. Again, we need to be realistic and set small goals that align with our energy levels.

3. Indulgence is not self–care: We can easily confuse indulging in something unhealthy and passing it off as caring for ourselves. Hot fudge sundaes or sitting on the couch all weekend are okay every now and then but are not great ways to keep up on exercise and healthy eating goals.

4. Shame: Yes, everyone will shame you for wanting to take some time and energy for yourself. Do it anyway.

5. Making good decisions when tired: We don't choose what's best for us when we are exhausted and have no self–control or discipline. Make goals when you feel better and more positive.

6. Too many expectations lead to feelings of failure: Go with the flow. You may decide to take a hot bath with some essential oils, only to find that the tub is clogged. Take a hot shower instead. Had high hopes for running five days a week but got sick and could only run once? It's okay, don't sweat it.

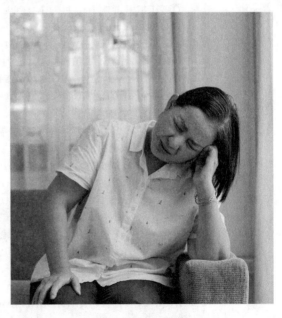

Maybe the biggest part of self–care is continuously cutting ourselves some slack and learning to go with the flow of life. If we don't take care of ourselves, who will? Does it benefit anyone if we are tired, sick, or miserable? Are we

If you spend so much time helping others that you neglect your own health and well-being, then, eventually, you won't be able to keep it up. It's okay to take care of your own needs first.

better parents, friends, lovers, or colleagues if we constantly do too much and give too much? Asking these questions can help you realize how important it is to put yourself and your needs before anyone else's and never feel guilty for doing so.

Vibing Higher

Many spiritual teachings focus on raising your "vibrational frequency" to match those of what you seek to experience. The idea is that if you want love, you must vibrate at the frequency of love, not hate. If you want abundance, you cannot vibrate at the frequency of lack. Paying close attention to feelings and emotions are great indicators of our vibrational frequency; sadly, many of us operate on a default level, then wonder why we are so unhappy and unfulfilled.

Imagine a radio that you want to listen to swing music on. You turn the knob from station to station until you find the swing music channel. You are scanning different frequencies to find the one that you desire. The same concept works on a personal level with your own energy. You must keep tuning the dial until you land on the right station, the right frequency, and the right broadcast because the vibes you feel are the vibes you send out into the world. When you are in a nasty mood, ever notice how others seem to react nastily to you? Or how you automatically notice mean people? You are tuned in to the vibration of mean and, therefore, your brain and consciousness respond like a radio and broadcast that out into the world around you.

Notice how different you feel, and how differently others react to you, when you are smiling and happy. Sure, a few grumpies may be out there who simply don't know how to feel good (imagine what frequencies they are operating from), but you will notice a huge shift in how others respond because you are putting out different vibes. Your radio station is playing "I feel good" tunes instead of "I feel bad" tunes, and it affects everyone you come in contact with.

You can raise your own vibrations by using affirmations, listening to positive music and audiotape lectures, journaling, writing down your blessings every day, taking better care of yourself, putting your peace of mind front and center, and working through negativity and fear to get to the root of it and root it out. This doesn't mean you will always be "vibing high," as you are human, but it does allow you to recognize when you are broadcasting from the basement of life and find ways to raise the vibrations you feel and give off a bit higher.

Human language is so indicative of what is important to us. Look at how we use such phrases as "we had the same vibes" or "she wasn't on the same frequency as I was." We intuitively understand how important the vibratory nature of our thoughts is and how they create an actual physical effect in the external world we live in. People respond much differently to happy people than they do to sad people. They feel more enthused around enthusiastic people and more playful around people who have a great sense of humor.

People respond much differently to happy people than they do to sad people. They feel more enthused around enthusiastic people and more playful around people who have a great sense of humor.

Before you go about your day, check your frequency. How are you vibrating? What station are you broadcasting to the world? These are within your power to change, no matter how bad you feel or what is happening in your life. You can always feel a tiny bit better and climb the vibrational frequency ladder from there. Eventually, you will climb high enough to feel much better, and so will those who interact with you.

Here are some simple ways to raise your vibration:

- Pay attention to your feelings, especially any "gut reactions" and "intuitive hits" you experience. If you meet someone or walk into a room and feel off, that sends you a message. Everyone and everything vibrates and sends you messages, and your "radio station" is tuning in as the receiver. If it feels bad, don't move toward it.

- Be aware of your own energetic frequencies because people will react and respond accordingly. If you walk into a meeting with a chip on your shoulder, the reaction will be toward that chip, not toward what you have to offer in the way of great ideas or solutions to problems.

- Match your vibration to what you want, NOT WHAT YOU DON'T WANT. This cannot be emphasized enough. People go through life miserable, unhappy, and unable to fulfill even the simplest of goals, and it's because of where their focus and energy is directed. Too much time and effort spent on worrying about what you don't want leads to more of what you don't want. Acknowledge your desire, whether it be love, greater prosperity, career success, or a great relationship with your family, then focus on how you can vibrate to the level of having these desires already fulfilled, not on how awful it feels to not have them fulfilled.

- Learn to read the room and avoid people and situations that are draining and make you more negative, doubtful, and afraid. Move toward those people and situations that uplift and empower you, support you, and have the same ... wait for it ... vibe as you.

Think of running a marathon. You are psyched up for this huge goal that means so much to you, but as you go along and the miles creep by, you focus on the soreness of your feet, the aching of your knees, the idiots in front of you who won't move out of your way, the hot sun, the drizzle, the cold, the things you should be doing instead of pursuing a medal, etc. The marathon becomes nothing but a giant negative experience, and you get so angry and feel so miserable and defeated, you are forced to drop out of the race at mile 16.

What would happen if you instead focused on the end result of holding that awesome, shiny medal up to the sky and the pride and accomplishment you would feel afterward? What would happen if you focused on the high energy of the other marathoners, the camaraderie, the fun of being a part of a big event, maybe even for charity? It's a whole different vibe that gives you the motivation and energetic boost to push past that 23-mile wall and cross the finish line.

Same race, different vibe.

The Power of NO!

One of the greatest sources of stress is overwhelm. We do way too many things for too many people. We take on too much and are afraid to pass any opportunity by for fear it might be one that would have led us to success or happiness. We say yes to everything, only to find ourselves too exhausted later to do anything. We have not learned the fine art, and the gift, of saying NO!

Why do we say yes to so many things we would rather not give our time and attention to? It's hard to say no to a request of your time or a favor, especially when the request comes from a friend or loved one. We feel guilty not saying yes, even when everything inside of us screams to say no. We think we are being generous and loving when in fact we are lacking self-love and exhausting ourselves trying to make everyone else happy.

The rules for saying no to things are simple. Don't do anything you don't really want to do. Yes, you should be a helpful, giving person, but only if what is being asked of you will not deplete you in the process. Don't take on anything you do not really want to do, and the trick here is to never say yes to an upcoming event until you have thought good and hard about whether you really want to be there. Too many times we give a knee-jerk yes, then later kick ourselves for having committed to something we don't want to do. Then, we make excuses to cancel or drop out when we could have properly dealt with the request in the first place.

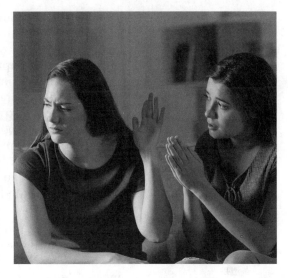

You are not obligated to say yes to everything that is asked of you. In fact, saying yes all the time can prove very harmful to your well-being. Learn to refuse unreasonable or draining requests.

A no doesn't need to be rude, nor should you ever feel you need to explain a no. It might help if you do, but a no should be adequate. However, here are some ways you can say no without saying no:

- I don't have the time in my schedule for that right now.
- I am not ready to do this yet.
- I would prefer not to do this.
- Thanks, but this just won't work for me.
- I am unable to commit to anything right now.
- I need to check my schedule and will get back to you.

Granted, that last one only postpones the inevitable, but these are handy excuses to get out of something or avoid something that will only serve to tire you out, tax your spirit, or just plain not interest you. Our time and energy are so limited these days, and we rarely get any for ourselves, so don't be afraid to say no firmly, but politely, if you need the downtime. In the worst-case scenario, simply ask that you have time to think about the request. Give the person a set day or time when you will get them an answer. They will appreciate your allowing them time to find someone to replace you if you do say no. Here are some tips:

- Just say no: You don't have to embellish or explain. If someone asks you to do something or go somewhere and you don't want to or have a better option, just say, "No, thank you." Many people feel the need to explain and offer an apology for protecting their precious time. If it makes you feel better, go for it, but remember your boundaries and don't offer a long and excessive guilt-based apology. Simply explain why if a why exists, and if it doesn't, just say you can't accept at this time. Feeling the need to explain is not always required and comes from a people-pleasing place that often makes them feel better and you feeling depleted and annoyed because you never stand up for yourself and your time. Not only that, but people can tell when you are weaving an elaborate excuse when a simple "I don't have the time" would suffice.

- Do it with love: You can say, "No, but thank you so much for asking me," and let the other person know how much you appreciate the offer even if you cannot accept. You don't have to be rude or mean. "Wow, that sounds fun, but I just cannot make it." "I really appreciate you thinking of me, but I have another obligation." "I can't commit right now, but how sweet of you to ask me." Unless you feel like offering more, leave it at that.

Our time and energy are so limited these days, and we rarely get any for ourselves, so don't be afraid to say no firmly, but politely, if you need the downtime.

- Ask for time: If you aren't sure, tell the person you must think about it overnight or check your calendar. This will buy you more time to weigh your options. Just be sure to not keep them hanging. If you say you'll let them know tomorrow, let them know tomorrow and not next week.

- Learn to tolerate their reactions: People may not react well to you saying no to them. Learn to deal with it, or you will forever be a slave to the desires and schedules of others. Yes, they will be disappointed for a while, but they will get over it, and seeing you keep your boundaries intact and being respectful of your own time might teach them to do the same. Expect some push-back, especially from those who are used to you saying yes to them. You must cut out all those external voices and listen only to the voice within.

- Don't say no out of fear: Tune in to your intuition and be honest about why you are saying no. If it is something you want to do but have fear around it, this is your chance to get out of your comfort zone and expand your horizons. Be vocal about your fears, and you'll be surprised how supportive the other person will be, encouraging you to go for it with a hearty "yes!"

If the other person reacts negatively, then it truly was not a request you needed to fulfill anyway, as people who really care about us will not penalize us for our own self-care. Saying no also invites others to do the same with you, and you should and must honor that. Get over the initial fear of being rejected, having someone be mad at you, or feeling guilty and learn to only say yes to the things that you really want to spend your time doing with the people you want to spend time doing it with. This is how you live a life of joy, purpose, and well-being.

Dealing with Death

One of the most important purposes of spirituality is to strengthen our connection to something grander and greater, something that is eternal and infinite, something that suggests that a part of us continues long after our bodies turn back into ashes and dust.

So much of our time and effort goes into finding ways to stay alive longer. We have such a fear of death despite it being a natural part of the cycle of existence. All living things are born, live, and die. Humans have a dreadful time accepting the final part of the cycle, yet so many humans live as if they don't care about death by eating unhealthy foods, not exercising or moving their bodies, taking pills with dangerous side effects, developing addictions to drugs and alcohol, overworking, living in a constant state of anger and division, and overwhelming their minds and bodies with a never-ending list of things to do before they die and doing many other things that cause stress and illness, not realizing that these very things will bring death to their doorstep a little sooner than they might like. It's almost as if we have a death wish.

Our ancestors may have been afraid of dying, but as we can learn from other cultures and the traditions they

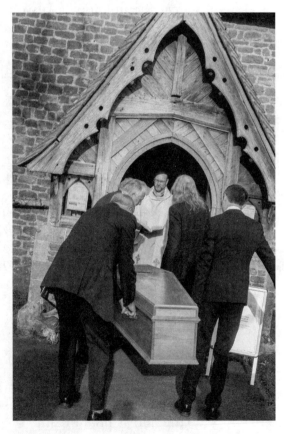

Most people dread the idea of their own demise while simultaneously behaving in ways that are likely to shorten their lives.

formed regarding death and dying, many different perspectives exist regarding the end of life. Some see it as an end, others as a beginning. Many people are uncomfortable discussing death, but until we come to some form of acceptance of it, our resistance to it will rob us of the joys of living in the now, today.

We may never want to die, or fully come to not have any fear associated with the great unknown that death is, but we can work toward strengthening our perspective of it through a closer connection to the unseen, the world of spirit, or God, if we choose. Spirituality helps us deal with the unknowable and find ways to open our awareness and consciousness to the interconnectivity of all life and how some part of us may not cease to exist.

If we are energy, energy never dies; it simply changes form. We fear the unknown, so we seek out ways to know more about death and whether or not something comes after it. We may get comfort in seeing how the world's traditions surrounding death are similar to our own or different. Does every culture fear dying? Do some cultures embrace it? The cycle of birth, life, and death is the same all over the world, but the ways people face the final curtain differ widely.

How the World Views Death

What is death? According to the 31st edition of *Dorland's Illustrated Medical Dictionary*, "death (death) (deth): the cessation of life; permanent cessation of all vital bodily functions. For legal and medical purposes, the following definition of death has been proposed–the irreversible cessation of all of the following: (1) total cerebral function, usually assessed by EEG as flat-line (2) spontaneous function of the respiratory system, and (3) spontaneous function of the circulatory system...."

If you ask most people, death is their greatest fear, yet in some places, death is a time of transition, as necessary to the path of a soul's progression as birth and life. It is not so much an ending as a beginning. Just as a new life is celebrated with baptisms, blessings, and birthdays, many of the world's people engage in rituals designed to celebrate death and the vast unknown that the soul will enter upon the body's final breath.

Death rituals go back as far as mankind, and we have the remains of once sacred sites to prove it, sites such as the pre-Stonehenge megaliths recently found in Dartmoor, England. These nine megaliths pre-date Stonehenge and have been carbon dated to approximately 3500 B.C.E. The standing stones mark the rising midsummer sun and setting midwinter sun. Mass quantities of pig bones found near the site suggest that some type of death ritual occurred here, a kind of feast that marked the passage into the darkness of the underworld, according to archeologist Mike Pitts, one of the key figures in this amazing discovery. Another stone mound called Cut Hill appears to have been a burial place and the site of accompanying rituals and ceremonies.

To the ancient Maya, death was also considered a transition. The good souls would be taken directly to heaven, while the evil would be transported to Xilbalba, the underworld, where they would suffer for all eternity (much like the Judeo–Christian heaven/hell). To the Maya, some individuals upon death became deities. Maize was used to symbolize rebirth and was often placed in the mouths of the dead, who might also be buried with whistles, stones, and engravings designed to help them navigate the spirit world. Lavish tombs were built for the revered, usually at the bottom of funerary pyramids consisting of nine steps to symbolize the nine platforms of the underworld. Temples were often built with 13 vaults to represent the 13 layers of heaven of Maya cosmology.

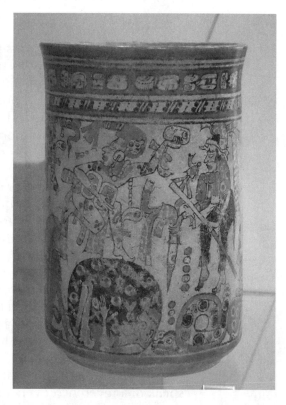

A Maya piece of pottery depicts the underworld known as Xilbalba, where evil souls were sent for eternal punishment.

The Egyptians also built pyramids as death chambers, and their elaborate rituals, including mummification, spoke of a solid belief in the immortality of the soul. To the ancient Egyptians, the protocols of mummification involved magical spells and burial rites designed to re-animate the dead. Burial chambers, though, were often reserved for the highest members of society and even involved access to funerary literature, such as the Book of the Dead, which was "taken" into the afterlife so that the dead could cast the appropriate spells ensuring a safe passage.

Like the Etruscans before them, the Romans cremated their dead and kept the ashes in urns and pots but eventually turned to inhumation, the burial of unburnt remains, which were kept in elaborate graves or sarcophagi (if one could afford them). The catacombs were carved through volcanic rock called tufo, soft enough to create the large, sub-terranean burial chambers, sometimes built under roads named for martyrs thought to be buried below.

Around 380 C.E. when Christianity became the state religion, the practice of catacomb burial declined and was replaced by the church cemeteries we still bury most of our dead in today. Inhumation re-placed cremation in most cases, with burials taking place in coffins, pots, and even vaults. The Roman middle-class dead were often bu-ried in pots partially buried in the ground, which allowed families to leave offerings and libations at the graveside (something we still do today, usually in the form of flowers). Above the ground, giant, elab-orate mausoleums were designed to hold the urns of the dead, usually those of the imperial Roman families and emperors.

It's easy to see where the modern burial and death rituals prac-ticed today have their roots in ancient times. Other cultures have dif-ferent ideas about how to treat the dead. In the Solomon Islands, a state of Oceania east of Papua New Guinea consisting of nearly 1,000 islands, the dead are laid out on a reef and left as food for the sharks. The Aboriginals of Australia would leave the dead bodies in trees, much like the Parsees of Bombay (now Mumbai), India, who left their dead on the tops of towers to be eaten by vultures!

The Maoris of New Zealand place their dead in a hut in a sitting position, wearing nice clothes. The dead are viewed first by mourners wearing green wreaths, who cry out and cut themselves with knives. Then, they hold a feast and burn the hut.

Alaskan Eskimos often make small igloos over their dead, leav-ing them forever frozen in time. Other Native traditions hold feasts with the dead present, then burn or bury the body in a secluded area. It's almost as if once they figure the soul of the dead has passed to the other side, the body is to be cast off as irrelevant.

Native American tribal traditions involve a variety of rituals that speak of a reverence, even a fearful one, of the spirit world. The Navajo destroy the hut of the dead person and then allow relatives to burn the body, being careful to not take a direct route home should the spirit of the dead follow them. The Aztecs deliver a formal speech, much like today's eulogy, over the dead to assure them a safe passage. The Iroquois bury their dead in shallow graves that are later exhumed so that the bones, along with gifts for the spirits, can be brought to a central burial site after a mourning feast.

The Mexican people have a special reverence for death. It may seem quite morbid to those of us outside their culture, but death is something to be observed, celebrated, and honored with art, dance, parades, and even bullfights that symbolize the life and death cycle. Jamaicans celebrate the dead for nine nights to support the relatives and give the body of the dead a safe passage to the other side, with dancing, singing, and eating ... even some good rum, signifying a less fear-based belief in the finality

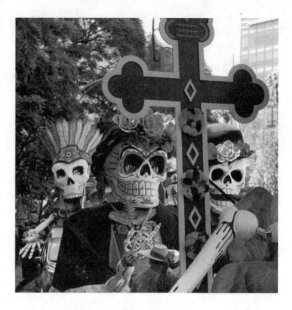

In Mexico, the Day of the Dead is a colorful celebration honoring all those who have passed into the afterlife.

of death. Forty nights later, the relatives return to sing again, symbolizing the completion of the passage of the departed's soul.

If this seems elaborate, Muslim tradition requires that the body of the deceased be placed on its sides and washed with soap and scented water. They wash the body an odd number of times, and the teeth and nose must be cleaned out in a spiritual cleansing rite called ablution. The body is perfumed and wrapped in a white cloth. Prayers are said facing Mecca, and a silent procession delivers the body to the burial grounds. Jewish tradition is similar to this.

Pagan traditions also wash the body with scented oils and herbs, offering a special blessing for the spirit of the deceased. Incense is also used for cleansing the body of impurities. The body is then wrapped in a simple cloth, and a funeral service follows.

Buddhists call in the services of a priest on the first day of a family member's death to come and recite a sutra, a literary narrative based upon Buddhist scripture or teachings. Incense is burned on the second day in front of a butsudan, or family altar. On the third day, the body is burned at a funeral hall, and the ashes are returned to the family home. The actual funeral is presided over by the priest as the family burns incense, then the ashes are laid to rest at a graveyard. The family of the dead will visit the graveside once a week for seven weeks and, on the 49th day, hold a customary feast called the Shiju-ku-Nichi for friends and neighbors.

Hindus believe that death is part of the continuation of the cycle begun at birth: birth, life, death, and rebirth as the soul of the dead simply transfers to another body upon death.

Hindus believe that death is part of the continuation of the cycle begun at birth: birth, life, death, and rebirth as the soul of the dead simply transfers to another body upon death. Hindus cremate their dead, first bathing the body and adorning it with garlands, then wrapping it in a pure, white cloth. The body is burned upon a pyre and, in the days to follow, mourners often remain inside and away from festivals, marriage ceremonies, and other public events.

Tibetans once practiced something called the Tibetan sky burial, where a corpse was sliced up atop a mountain and left for the birds. Called *jhator*, this giving of alms to the winged creatures involved monks with axes chopping up bodies into birdworthy parts, laughing and joking all the while.

No matter how the people of the world envision death or how they treat the body once it has died, one thing remains clear: the vast majority consider the process of dying to be of critical and profound importance. The belief that life goes on in some form other than the physical is as old as humanity itself and permeates every tradition and religion. Knowing how other cultures deal with death can help us find ways of coping with the unknown by opening our minds to the different ways people around the world view this part of the cycle of existence. Whether we then choose to fear death to the point where it negatively affects our life is up to us.

Dealing with Change

"Change is inevitable. Change is constant."
—Benjamin Disraeli

Aside from fearing death, we fear change, and if you think about it, isn't death the biggest change of all? Our ability, or lack of it, to accept and navigate changes, especially big life changes, will dictate much of the happiness and well-being we experience in life. Whether we turn to religion or spiritual pursuits to find truths to help us deal with change or we use the power of our minds and bodies is up to you. Big changes can be worked through in many ways, whether it be a divorce, a new child, moving away from family, a new job, the end of a relationship, an illness, or anything else that removes us from the bubble of the safety of our routine.

Some change is gradual, such as aging and raising children. Other times, change hits us over the head like a falling boulder: unexpected and unplanned for. Learning to be resilient, resourceful, and accepting is a must because life is change, and we cannot avoid or outrun it. We change as we grow physically, mentally, and intellectually. We experience spiritual growth and outgrow old ideals and perceptions. We end up in careers or locations we never imagined in our original plans for our lives. Change is the only thing that does not change, so it behooves us to learn how to approach life from a positive mindset with a combination of spontaneity and planning, able to adapt to anything that comes our way, even as we continue to move forward toward specific goals and dreams.

The most powerful way to navigate change is with mindfulness. When you keep your focus on the moment at hand … problems and challenges become easier to deal with.

Dealing with change begins with how you think and controlling the thoughts going through your mind. Positive thinking has gotten a bad rap in the past, labeled as New Age mumbo-jumbo (usually by those of a negative mindset), but without a positive mind, you will fall apart at the first sign of change, unable to figure out how to process it and move through it, especially when it is a painful experience involving loss or grief. The most powerful way to navigate change is with mindfulness. When you keep your focus on the moment at hand or, as they say in 12-step programs, one day at a time, problems and challenges become easier to deal with. Removing the past and future from a problem eliminates so much of the worry and fear involved and releases the grip of choices we made that cannot be unmade. Then, with the day before us, we can more readily find ways to survive, adapt, and eventually overcome and thrive again.

Imagine losing a loved one. The grief and pain are unsurmountable at first. Life goes on, and we must as well. Overcome with memories of the past with this loved one or dread of a future without them, we remain stuck in a quicksand of despair and fear. Once we can begin to bring our focus back only on the present, even if it is only from minute to minute, then day to day, we make our way out of the quicksand and begin to move forward, even if only in tiny increments. Then, we begin to let time do its healing upon us as we move through the phases of grief and come out on the other side. If we get stuck too long in one phase, we can turn to family, friends, and support groups or therapists to help pull us out and up. We can repeat to ourselves, "This, too, shall pass" because it will pass. The pain will pass, just as joy will pass when things are going great. It all passes, and it all changes.

If change didn't happen, we would never evolve from infants to teenagers to adults. We would also never die. It often feels empowering to sit down and think about, even write down, all the ways we have changed since our earliest memories of childhood. Our whole lives have been about changing and growing. Think about what would have happened if we had stayed stuck at one age, in one job, or with one person. We may miss the past, but we cannot relive it, and we could not have stayed there.

Parents often grieve their children growing up and becoming independent, just as they once did. Imagine your child not changing and being an infant forever. It would be exhausting, and you'd never know the joys of watching them go off to kindergarten or learn to talk. Imagine your child never becoming an adult. You would never know the pride and joy of seeing them go off to college or get the job they wanted. You yourself would never stop being the parent of a teenager and never become the parent of an independent adult. Imagine how no change would create a complete breakdown of all these natural cycles and passages of time, not to mention how no one would ever grow up again to reproduce and perpetuate the species!

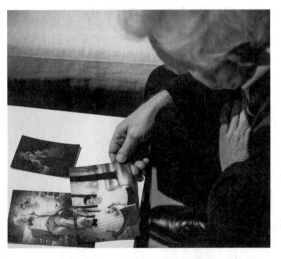

No matter what we do, change is inevitable and the past slips away into the distance. There comes a point where we need to accept this and be agents for positive change rather than always reminiscing about what once was.

We do all grow up and we do all change, though, and the sooner we can learn to be a successful "change agent," the more we will be able to move through each phase and each challenge, even with the pain and suffering, to get to the next phase, with all the new gifts it has to offer.

Here are some tips to cope with change:

- Don't avoid or try to escape change. You can maybe put it off for a while, but it will happen eventually, and the sooner you begin to find ways to cope that are healthy, the sooner you can adapt to the change.

- Understand that you will move through the stages of grief and shock, which include initial disorientation, anger and emotional response, depression, coming to terms with the change, and, eventually, acceptance. Each of those stages will present its own challenges, but if you are moving through them, you are coping well. Expect to fall back a few times into despair, shock, or anger, but keep working toward a forward trajectory, no matter how long it takes.

- Try not to lash out at others in your anger or despair. Ask for help when you need it, but also honor the need to be alone.

- Give yourself an hour each day to cry, scream, yell, ruminate, or freak out, then move on to more constructive uses of your time.

- Write out your fears and feelings in a private journal. Getting things out of your head and onto paper often serves to dissipate their negative energies so you can better cope. Writing down your fears can make them appear smaller and less powerful as your brain finds ways to challenge the fears and work through them.

- Find the help of a support group or therapist if you feel you cannot work through the change. Many parents fall into despair when they become "empty nesters," especially single parents. Support groups exist on social media and in local groups in person for every type of change, but if nothing seems to be helping you cope and feel better over time, don't hesitate to get help. This is about your mental well-being here. Vent if you need to, but don't stay in the venting phase too long.

- Step away from the news or social media if the negativity and drama make you feel worse. Take a news fast or break from talking heads to clear out your own mind and listen better to your intuitive guidance. Turn to nature, close friends or family, or the love of a pet to give yourself some needed downtime to process the changes.

- Eat a healthy diet, get outside and move your body, and do things to increase your sleep quality. Keep to a routine if the structure helps you feel more grounded during the external shifts and changes. Make time for self-care, no matter how crappy you feel.

• Acknowledge that life is all about change, flux, and flow, and find the positives in that. Put it in writing. Think of all the good things that have come out of the changes you've dealt with, even the painful ones. Recall ways you ended one phase and began another and how that new phase became your new normal.

Even positive changes can derail your planned-out life and cause chaos to the structured ways you thought your life should play out. The more resilient and resourceful you become with healthy coping mechanisms, the more you will be able to meet change head-on and find the silver linings on the other side.

Activating a Positive Mindset

We've come so far in the fields of science, medicine, and technology that it's truly possible to live longer than ever before, but the real questions are: Are we prospering? Are we happy? Life seems to be a constant struggle to work, pay bills, deal with other people, and maybe, if we are lucky, have a few moments to ourselves to relax or pursue a dream. Learning to think positive may sound like pie-in-the-sky talk, but the power of the mind is unlimited. What you think, you tend to manifest. In fact, do you want to know the results of your thoughts? Look around at your life: what works, and what doesn't? These external indicators are proof of where most of your thoughts are directed and what you truly believe is possible or what you deserve.

Learning to think positive may sound like pie-in-the-sky talk, but the power of the mind is unlimited. What you think, you tend to manifest.

So, why not try thinking thoughts of abundance and wealth, happiness, and health instead of scarcity and deprivation? Try it for 21 days to set it as a habit. When your mind returns to negative thoughts or you find yourself engaging in negative talk, gently cancel those thoughts out and replace them with positive ones. At the end of the 21 days, see if you feel any different about yourself and your life. If not, you can always return to being negative, whining, and complaining.

Writing out affirmations helps to build a mindset of abundance and prosperity by enforcing the ideas of success, even when it hasn't shown up yet in the external world. Affirmation must be written in "I" language and in the present tense because your subconscious mind listens and obeys everything it is told, especially when something is repeated. Your brain's reticular activating system (RAS) kicks in, which is the filter of the brain that eliminates information that is not directly related to survival or of importance to you so that you can focus on what is. The RAS then goes on to find examples of what is important to you. It seeks out opportunities related to what you have directed it to by your affirmations and repetitive programming of the subconscious.

An example is going to buy a new car. You want a pink Cadillac because none are on the road and you want to be different. Once you put down the big money for a pink Caddy, you drive it off the lot and suddenly notice them EVERYWHERE. Is this some kind of hoodoo magic to make you mad? No, it is your RAS noticing something that is now important to you that was always there, but in the past, before you decided you wanted a pink Caddy, it was not worth noticing. Your brain filtered out all pink Caddys until it became of importance to you. Now, you see them everywhere.

When you repeat positive affirmations in the present tense, using the "I" word, such as in the phrase "I am prosperous and healthy," your subconscious takes it as truth and begins new programming to draw those things to you. Meanwhile, your RAS gets to work noticing all the things you once ignored that can now lead to more prosperity and good health. However, if you say, "I will be prosperous and healthy," you send the subconscious and the RAS the message that someday in the future, you will be wealthy and healthy, but not today. The more you repeat this, the more you push the very things you want into the future, never to manifest.

Keep affirmations in the present tense, as if you already have the things you want. Speak them out loud for even more effectiveness, and do them several times a day to reprogram the subconscious and override blocks, obstacles, and patterns ingrained from your childhood. They need to be cleared out and replaced, just as you would clear out old contacts from your cell phone to replace them with new ones. Affirm that "I am in the career of my dreams and having a blast" instead of saying, "I will find the career of my dreams and have a blast." One leads you to the people, things, and circumstances needed to make the affirmation a reality; the other continuously puts off what you want into some vague future date.

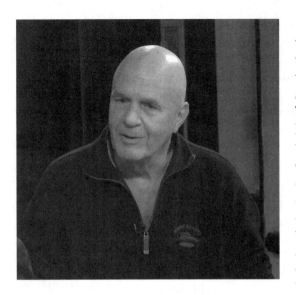

Motivational speaker and author Dr. Wayne Dyer (1940–2015) promoted his theories about self-actualization in his best-selling 1976 book, *Your Erroneous Zones.*

You'll be amazed how your thoughts and words can change your attitude and life when you direct them toward what you want to manifest and away from what you want eliminated. The late motivational author and speaker Dr. Wayne Dyer was famous for saying that if you change your mind, you can change your life. We are what we think about all day long, and we tend to think a lot of negative thoughts: fear, lack, anger, annoyance, and resentment. We think about how tired we are and how sick we are, not realizing that our subconscious mind takes what we tell it as truth. The more we say we are sick and tired, the more sick and tired experiences we attract, and the more sick and tired we become.

Before we look at natural remedies for health and well-being, we need to get our minds focused on how great we will feel when we incorporate these ideas into our lives. Our bodies may be ready for a positive change, but if the mind is still in the complaint zone and our spirit is tired and weary, nothing we do physically will work.

Well-being is about holistic health: body, mind, and spirit. When one is out of whack, the others tend to follow.

Visioning Your Future

In addition to doing affirmations, journaling, writing down goals, and visualization exercises, making a vision board is one way to begin attracting what you want into your life. It's all about focus and using the power of visualization to create a large board filled with images that reflect the essence of what you want.

Vision boards are usually made up of pictures cut out of magazines along with words and phrases that describe what you want to manifest in your present and future. This can be the home of your dreams, the kind of car you'd love to drive, the relationship image you'd most like to emulate, the way you'd love your body to look, and places you hope to travel to. It can be anything you can find a visual representation for of something you truly want.

You can get specific with vision boards, such as using a dream house or car that you really want, but remember that the universe has a strange way of often delivering something better to you that you did not imagine or envision, so while it helps to get somewhat specific on physical items, always write at the bottom of your board "this or something better." Also, never dictate on the board how something will come to you, only what you want. Let the universe deliver the "hows" to your "whats."

Keep the vision board somewhere you can see it every day and spend time looking at it and getting into the feeling and essence of what it will be like having those things. In fact, it's more powerful if you feel what it is like to already have them. It's the power of your imagination working to convince your brain that it's a done deal, which then activates the brain's RAS to look for opportunities, people, and situations to help manifest things physically.

One caveat with vision boards is that they are a one-shot deal, so when your dreams change, you need to change the images on your board or update it once a year.

One caveat with vision boards is that they are a one–shot deal, so when your dreams change, you need to change the images on your board or update it once a year. Perhaps you can create a digital vision board on your computer or cell phone, with images, music, and video clips that represent what you want in life and watch it every morning before you start your day and again at night before you go to sleep. Make your own little YouTube movies, or use a great company called Mind Movies to create your own in any area of life from health to wealth to relationships. You just load up the images you want, choose the music, and voila. You have your own set of powerful mind movies to use as visualization tools. Some apps also allow you to load up pictures and add music clips to create a personal visualization video.

Keep your mind primed on the things that you seek to manifest, especially on those days when you are feeling down or defeated. Don't deviate from your vision, and put your feelings behind it to speed up the manifestation energy. Seeing what you want, and feeling what it is like to have it, is a powerful way to align your imagination, intellect, and intuition to seek out and identify the necessary actions needed to move you toward making all those images a reality. It's important to stay mindful and present because once you put it out there, you want to be ready for insights, aha moments, and synchronistic events that you might otherwise miss if you aren't living in the moment.

You may not manifest everything on your board in one year. It does require some work and action on your part, and knowing what inspired actions to take will come to you if you stay open minded, but you might be surprised to find that as you increase your attention and focus on the things you do want and take off what you don't want, no matter your current circumstances at the time, you will manifest some of them.

This or something better.

The Power of Forgiveness

Forgive and forget, we are told. These short sayings are wise because forgiving others and forgiving ourselves is one of the fastest ways to live a life of well-being. When we are tied to past regressions, resentments, and events and filled with anger and pain because of the behaviors and actions of those in the past, we carry with us a heavy weight that keeps us from truly being free.

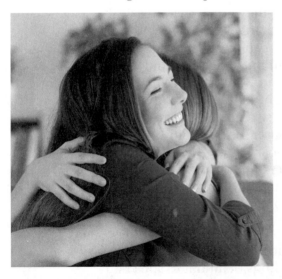

Forgiving others not only helps them but also you, freeing you of negative emotions and stress that will inevitably make you feel better.

Practicing forgiveness gives you the opportunity to cut the ties binding you to the past and the negative emotions associated with it and move forward without being held down by the shackles of the past. It is as much for you as for the person you are forgiving because when you forgive, you set a prisoner free, and that prisoner is you. Forgiveness is not saying that what someone did to you was okay or that you condone it. You don't. It is saying that you will not be confined by it, or defined by it, for another precious moment of your life. It is the conscious decision to let go of negative emotions and patterns holding you back so you can live your best life moving forward.

Zig Ziglar, the famous motivational speaker, once said that you cannot drive a car looking in the rearview mirror. It would be dangerous. Yet, that is what we do when we don't or cannot forgive ourselves or others for past mistakes and hurts. We risk crashing our lives because we cannot look at the road in front of us, as we are still resentful and angry over the road behind us. Learning to forgive leads to better mental health because it gives us permission to stop feeling the ongoing grief or anger we have been attached to. We cut all attachments to the people and things that hurt us, and we are no longer being pulled back into the quicksand of reacting to something or someone who isn't even in our lives anymore.

We have all seen stories on the news or social media of parents forgiving the killer who took their child's life or a woman forgiving her rapist. This takes incredible courage and strength; these people are not saying that what was done to them is okay and not that the killer or rapist shouldn't meet with punishment but that they simply cannot be pulled back down into the deep despair and suffering anymore. It is time to move on and live again.

Before forgiveness can occur, you must grieve and allow yourself to feel the anger, rage, or attending emotions and work through them, with a therapist if needed. Processing the feelings out is critical because they will come back to haunt you if not directly dealt with.

Make the decision to forgive those who have wronged you. You don't have to contact them and become friends unless you feel called to do that. Remember, this is about you freeing yourself from the shackles and showing yourself compassion and love. It sometimes helps to understand that hurt people hurt people and that those who wronged you are dealing with their own kind of punishment, but that isn't what forgiveness is about.

It is an act of liberation that transforms pain and suffering, anger and despair, into healing and peace of mind. It is saying goodbye to the past, taking the lessons from it, and moving on with your life so that you can experience love, joy, and happiness again, which you cannot do if you are emotionally or physically tied to who and what hurt you. It is especially important to forgive yourself for bad choices and decisions of the past, regrets and disappointments, and actions and behaviors that hurt those around you. You may be a lot harder on yourself than you imagined, but you must realize you did the best you could at the time. Let it go now and become better from it.

When you decide to forgive, make sure it is thorough. Any residual anger or resentment must be dealt with and let go of as it arises, so you don't once again become bogged down by the past. It may not be a one-and-done act, but the more you practice forgiveness, the easier it becomes. You are not forgetting or condoning the bad behaviors of others or of yourself. You are freeing yourself from their weight, so you can once again soar.

You are not forgetting or condoning the bad behaviors of others or of yourself. You are freeing yourself from their weight, so you can once again soar.

Finding Your Inner Peace in a Chaotic World

The years 2020 and 2021 were filled with fear, anxiety, chaos, and turmoil as a global pandemic unfolded, adding on to the usual political and economic instabilities of modern life. Social media was filled with attacks, shaming, and cancel culture, and the mainstream media was all about scare tactics and only showing the bad, not the good.

Keeping a center of inner peace during such times is possible, but it does require work and focus. You always have a calm center within to go to and a variety of methods to get there, as this book has offered, yet so many people still claim they cannot find peace at all amid the worries of their health, loved ones, jobs, and communities.

Here are some tips for protecting inner peace:

- Filter: Filter out the negative, the fear mongering, and the uncertain, and focus on the moment. If you seek information, avoid mainstream news and talking heads engaging in debate and negative discourse and look for news sources you trust. Be open to all sides of a story, including those you don't see right away, and stay involved and interested but detached enough to live through each day without being crippled by fear and immobilized by anxiety.
- Keep going within: You can't ignore the external world, but if you stay engaged in it, you will suffer physically, mentally, emotionally, and spiritually. Keep turning inward and checking in with yourself and your center. Tap into that intuitive voice for guidance. Meditate and clear the clutter from your mind and open your heart to find that sense of connectivity to others and the world around you.
- Project love: In a world that projects hate and points the finger of blame outward rather than inward, do you want to add to that

kind of dark energy? Try projecting love from your heart outward to everyone you meet and all situations. You are not being igno-rant of the realities of life, but you are choosing the level of energy you wish to add into that reality. Add love because the world sure can use it.

- Find a routine that works: Sometimes, having a routine or adding some structure to your day removes anxiety. You know what you will do when and where you will do it and don't have to make so many choices at a time when your mind feels frightened and weak. Follow a healthy routine that includes exercise, inner work, good sleep, and a healthy diet, and put aside more challenging goals and ambitions until you feel stronger and more centered. It's okay to slow down life a bit when you need to catch up.

- Face some fears: While it isn't wise to go stand at the edge of a cliff to face your terror of heights unless you feel inspired to do so, facing fears often dissipates the energy they hold on to us to the point where we feel we can not only handle them but get rid

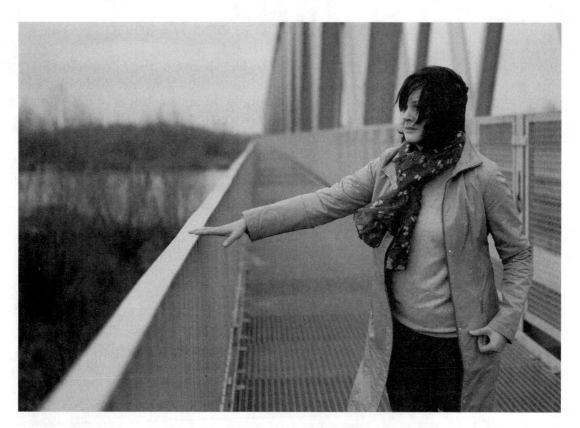

Facing your fears is the best way to overcome them. For example, if you have a fear of heights, slowly exposing yourself to high places can gradually dissipate this fear.

of them. Write down all your fears in a journal, and list ways you can meet those fears head–on if they were to come true. Not only does this make you feel more empowered, but you begin to realize, looking back, how many of your fears never manifested to begin with.

Protect your inner peace, and you will meet life from a higher, more centered energy that will affect those around you, especially your children. They see you operating from a strong center and will be more inclined to find their own. Adding to the negativity and chaos of the world never makes the world a better place. It may feel like your ranting, shouting, debating, and fighting against injustice help because you are doing something, but they're just adding fire to fire, and rarely are others inspired to change when they are burning. Be water. Find your peace, and others will be inspired to find theirs. Can you imagine the outcome if enough people did this?

Finding Purpose and Meaning

One of the greatest paths to well–being of the body, mind, and spirit is having purpose and finding meaning in life. Without these two things, it's easy to feel as though you are a robot or zombie going through the motions with little investment in what is happening around you. Having a purpose itself gives life meaning because it gives life depth and richness. That purpose doesn't have to be big and grand, like saving the world from hunger or finding a new planet. Purpose can be anything. It can be loving your children so they can go off to be happy adults or working at a food bank a few days a month to help those less fortunate. It can be using your job or career to fully express your gifts and talents to the world or buying local foods and products to help your community thrive.

Purpose and meaning are personal and individual and will be different for everyone. We live in a society that looks down on people who don't have lofty goals and purpose to do something on a global, splashy scale, but that is not what everyone is called to do. Not everyone wants to run a marathon, go to college, or feed the poor in a third world country, but everyone has a purpose, even if that purpose is to simply be the best person they can be in the world.

It has been said that the two most important days in your life are the day you were born and the day you find out why. Having a "why" helps you be more resilient through life's challenges because it gives you a North Star to always be aligning with. It's an inner compass that keeps you on track toward the goals you have set for yourself. Again, those goals can be anything that is important to you from scaling Mount Everest to loving your neighbors as yourself. Purpose and meaning can be found in simply living and being alive. Even a monk living on a mountaintop who never comes in contact with anyone has a purpose: to find joy and peace and to express life through his or her being.

Sometimes, we feel like we are here for a reason, but we can't quite figure out what that reason is. That's where things like meditation, prayer, and inner work come into play: to help us quiet down the external voices so we can listen for the whisper of our inner voice telling us what it wants us to know. It might also help to pay attention to what makes you happiest, even if it seems silly to others. Think back to things that brought you joy as a child.

The events and circumstances of your life take on meaning when you look back and see patterns and how one thing led to another to get you to where you are today.

Don't force yourself to find a purpose. It won't be authentic. Perhaps you are already fulfilling your purpose and don't even realize it. You may already be helping others, doing something that gives new value into the world, or just being you in a way that spreads love and good energy in a world that so desperately needs it.

Meaning is what you make of it. The events and circumstances of your life take on meaning when you look back and see patterns and how one thing led to another to get you to where you are today. Meaning also comes from contemplation and looking for connections, cultivating intuition, and experiencing synchronicities. Think about how different the world would be if you were not here, how many other lives would be changed. You may be surprised to find that your being alive has touched more people and altered more circumstances and lives than you ever imagined possible.

Practice mindfulness and be present to the moment at hand, which is where synchronicities occur and intuitions arise. You'll never see or experience them if you are constantly worrying over the future or regretting the past. Try journaling in order to uncover hints as to your purpose and how you can find more meaning in your day-today existence. Focus on your gratitude list, for starters, because those are the things that give life meaning: family, friends, pets, careers, community. Start with what is right in front of you and expand outward, and soon, you will see that your life means something, that it is important, and that you have a grand purpose in the scheme of things.

You Are Enough!

Such a peace comes to us when we realize that we don't have to strive to acquire and achieve things to prove our worth. Knowing that we are enough just because we are here can lessen some of the pressure we put on ourselves to always be on the go and allow us to just be. Society has a way of making us feel as though we are unworthy unless we discovered a cure for cancer, achieved massive wealth or fame, or broke some world record. A great emphasis is placed on achievement and having things to show for our talent and hard work, especially on social media, where it's all about one-upmanship. We spend our lives acting like performing circus animals trying to impress others, only to come to the end of our lives and realize that we didn't have to impress anyone but ourselves.

So much pressure is placed on us to be the best at this or that or at least be better at it than most, even if we don't like what we are doing or it has not succeeded in making us happy, healthy, or wise. We are bombarded with messages telling us that someone else has more than we do or has done more things, traveled to more countries, written more books, expressed more love, had more sex, eaten at more gourmet restaurants, or owned more houses and cars. It's a nonstop barrage of messages telling us we are less unless we have more.

We don't need to become famous for something to have worth and influence in this world. Our sheer presence touches everyone we come in contact with. Our value is who we are and being honest and authentic about it so others will feel that they, too, can be that way around us. No rule anywhere says that people who achieve stardom or massive wealth are better than those who don't. They are just different and have a different path to follow.

Finding value in our existence doesn't come from external things; it comes from within. It is not something we can buy, save up for, or achieve. It is already there from the moment we are born. We are all pebbles in a pond with ripples that extend outward to touch those in our lives, but we are the pebbles, and no pebble is better than any other just because it looks different or is a different size, shape, or weight.

Know that you are enough, and find peace in that so you can stop striving to be, do, or have more to impress someone else, who is probably doing the same to impress someone else. The buck stops here. You are enough as is, right now.

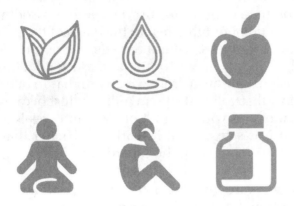

Healing Remedies

Remedies that heal are not all hundreds or thousands of years old. A false assumption exists that all-natural remedies are ancient, and though many are, many are also the result of more current research and knowledge. Just as science is never settled because of new discoveries, natural remedies are never fixed and locked into the past. The more we learn about our planet and the rich resources she provides, the more healing possibilities we must work with.

Many herbs and plants are just now being studied in scientific and clinical settings, which opens the door to potential treatments and therapies even our wise ancestors knew nothing about. Individual creativity and imagination, with people coming up with their own remedies and sharing them on websites and social media, also expands the already massive body of natural remedies available.

Natural remedies come in every form, shape, and size from teas to recipes for detoxing; from ways to overcome pain and get better sleep to lowering blood pressure with a plant-based therapy; from old tips our grandmothers and great-grandmothers passed down through the generations to modern Twitter and Instagram accounts devoted to healing; so much information is available to pick from and experiment with that it boggles the mind.

Whether you insist on some scientific research done in a lab setting before you try a remedy or trust the age-old wisdom of your ancestors, we must point out that before the dawn of the pharmaceutical industry in the early 1900s, natural remedies were considered normal and acceptable. Today, they carry a stigma usually attached by Big Pharma to push people away from what Earth has to offer and toward a pill or product that will make them millions. Just because something is new and shiny and you see a lot of TV commercials about it does not mean that it is safe or that it works any better than something you found in the woods or an herb garden.

We think we are separate from the natural world, as if we are dominant and superior, yet as a species, we are sicker than ever.

The huge disconnect between humans and nature is to blame for our moving away from natural remedies. We think we are separate from the natural world, as if we are dominant and superior, yet as a species, we are sicker than ever. Perhaps the pharmaceutical industry has made us all so tired, weak, and sick that we just don't have the time and energy to mix up an infusion or brew up a tea. It's easier to pop a pill and listen to what the doctors tell us. Natural remedies don't have to be complicated. Many are quite simple and only involve a few steps or a few ingredients. A simple tea or remedy can achieve the maximum effect on our bodies with minimal effort. You don't even need to make the remedies yourself anymore; we have companies, websites, and health stores that offer plenty.

Something is incredibly powerful and deeply profound about snipping herbs from your own garden and mixing them into a tea or blend that will heal your cold or calm your anxious spirit. The hands-on nature of working with nature is inherent in us. Long before technology made our lives so easy and separated us from the processes by which we get our water, food, clothing, shelter, and medicines, we knew what to do and derived pleasure from getting our hands dirty in the soil and feeling the warmth of the sun on our skin as we planted seeds or gathered fruits and vegetables.

Natural healing, remedies, and the quest for true well-being for the body, mind, and spirit bring us back to Earth and back to what truly matters. Our connections to nature, to each other, to ourselves, and to the web of life are things we no longer see or care about as we bury our heads in technology and allow "others" to do for us what we once did for ourselves. Try some of these remedies and be bold and courageous in making some of your own. Share them with family and friends, even as gifts, for a personal touch and to show how much you care about the well-being of others.

Always be safe when using herbs and other products and do allergy testing if you will be putting anything on your skin. Check in with your doctor if you are pregnant or nursing and do your own research beforehand to see if any contraindications exist with medications that you are already taking. Get in the habit of using your own brain cells and discernment when you are reading or learning about anything involving your health, whether it comes from a book like this or an advertisement on TV for a new drug or pill. Don't assume your doctors know everything just because they went to medical school and got a degree. Not every doctor goes on to keep up with the latest discoveries in medicine and healing often simply because they just don't have the time between seeing so many patients and dealing with insurance companies.

If you find something of interest, feel free to show your doctor and discuss it. Bring up natural methods and remedies and how you would prefer these to synthetic, allopathic treatments. If you have a doctor who shames or bullies you or is condescending toward your desire to learn for yourself, GET A NEW DOCTOR. Medical error is the third cause of death in the United States. Some doctors out there are wonderful and can be a partner with you for your best health, will encourage you to ask questions and bring them new research studies they may not have seen, and understand that medicine is ancient and that modern science is forever changing. Don't let "medical ego" derail your health; be your own health advocate.

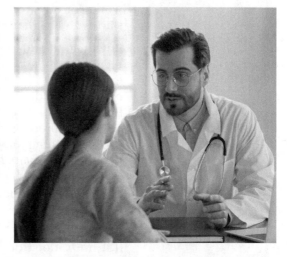

Use common sense, just as our ancestors did when they began experimenting with the natural world's gifts. We have the gift of their successes, as their failures were not passed down through the generations to reach us.

Don't be too afraid or intimidated to talk to your physician openly about your interest in natural remedies. A good doctor will listen to you, and if they don't, you can find a new doctor who will.

Natural Health

Think about that. What failed or harmed us was not passed on to us, so we have some semblance of trust in their methods that we can build upon. Do understand that sometimes, allopathic medicine, treatments, and surgeries are a must, and be open to that. Being extreme either way is not the answer. We can achieve a balance between the gifts of nature and the gifts of technology. Ask questions. Be open.

Here are some great tips to work with on your natural healing journey:

- Know your medical history: Any allergies to food or products? Illnesses that are genetic or run in your family? Issues that may preclude you from trying new things without first talking with your doctor (if you have high blood pressure and are on meds already, you cannot take a natural remedy to lower blood pressure without consulting your doctor, or you will suffer from low BP).

- Start small and go slow: It's a great rule of thumb to try something new a little at a time to see how your body reacts and adjusts to it. Herbs, plants, detoxes, and teas may contain an ingredient you are supersensitive to that causes side effects. Start out with a lesser amount than what might be recommended and work your way up to a higher dosage, keeping a close watch on reactions and how you feel until you reach the recommended dosage. The author of this book tried Ashwagandha and had to cut the dosage in half to get the best benefits. Our bodies are all different, so what works for one won't necessarily work for all. It's always better to start with less than with more.

- Buy the best and forget the rest: Whether you are buying supplements, herbal teas, or premade remedies, always do your due diligence and make sure the products are safety tested and contain no filler ingredients. Sure, this may mean that you pay a bit more, but this is about your health, and it's not a time to be cheap. Read reviews of products and ask people you know and trust if they've used something that worked well for them before diving into the world of "too many choices, not enough time"; at least you'll have a starting point for your own research. Be willing, though, to pay a little more for higher-quality herbs and products. That's not to say that something less expensive is always less effective, just don't be swayed only by price.

- If it hurts, don't do it: Remember the old doctor joke about the guy who goes to see his doctor and says, "Hey, Doc, it hurts when I swing my arm." The doc looks at him and says, "Then don't swing that arm." If you take something that makes you sick or results in a negative side effect, STOP TAKING IT. Don't keep trying it thinking your body will "get used to it." That's not how it works. Side effects may wear off in time but still wreak havoc, and if your initial reaction is a bad one, perhaps the second time you try it, it will be even worse. If you have trouble breathing, your chest hurts, or you experience swelling of the face, tongue, or throat, go to the ER! Use your brain when healing your body. If you had a bad reaction to a pharmaceutical, you would go to urgent care or the ER. This is no different. Even a rash that lasts overnight is an indication that you may have an allergy to something in the product or the herb itself. Move on to something else and keep track of ingredients that trigger a bad reaction.

- Children are not adults: It's important to remember that children are not adults and may not be able to use any adult remedies safely, certainly not in the same dosage. Most natural remedies are safe to use in smaller dosages for children, although it is advised to never try anything without first checking with your child's pediatrician for contraindications and potential allergies. With herbs and plants that you know from research are safe, always dilute the remedy with 50 percent water for a young child. Never give anything to a child under the age of 1, especially if it contains honey, as serious risks exist of bacterial infections with honey that only affect infants.

 If you take something that makes you sick or results in a negative side effect, STOP TAKING IT. Don't keep trying it thinking your body will "get used to it."

You won't overdose from a natural remedy unless you are using some sort of psychedelic or mind-altering ingredient. Most herbs are safe, and the ones that aren't taste awful and result in immediate nausea. The herb list in this book and many others, as well as online, always point out which herbs and plants are never to be consumed internally or used topically, and when buying preformulated products, you can be pretty assured that they don't contain anything you can get sick from and that they can be sued for.

Detoxing

You can't heal a sick body. That may sound confusing but think about it. If your body is filled with toxins and chemicals from the air, water, products, and environments you are exposed to, can you truly achieve healing? If we don't address the underlying causes of many of our ailments, whether physical or mental, we are only putting a bandage on the surface wounds and not excising the poisons down in the wound itself. Then, the same issues return over and over because we only treat symptoms and not causes. We do what we can to remove the physical manifestations of a deeper problem and not the problem itself.

While we may not be able to avoid every toxin in existence, we can certainly cut down our exposure and exert more control over the things we consume and use. Natural remedies can and do work, but we might want to first do some detoxing to prime ourselves for better health. In his book *The Toxic Solution: How Hidden Poisons in the Air, Water, Food, and Products We Use Are Destroying our Health—And What We Can Do to Fix It*, Dr. Joseph Pizzorno states that toxins started entering our food about 60 years ago, and it changed everything. Toxins do damage to every part of our bodies and play a role in all diseases. "They don't act alone. They interact with other factors in our health environment and in many cases magnify the disruption caused by other factors," Dr. Pizzorno said. He presents a list of ways toxins cause and contribute to diseases:

- Toxins poison enzymes so they don't work properly in our bodies.
- Toxins displace structural minerals.
- Toxins damage our internal organs.
- Toxins damage our DNA.
- Toxins modify gene expression.
- Toxins damage cell membranes.
- Toxins interfere with our hormones.
- Toxins impair the body's inherent ability to rid itself of toxins.

While this all sounds frightening, and it should alarm you into learning more and becoming proactive, he also writes that many people believe that nothing can be done about toxins. "But that's not true. Many people don't take toxins into account when they buy food and other products. You can shield yourself and your family by making the right choices." The good news is that you can turn your health around by becoming aware of toxin overload and reducing it when and where you can.

As pointed out in *The Toxin Solution* and other books such as this author's *Toxin Nation: The Poisoning of Our Air, Water, Food, and Bodies: Fact and Fiction* published by Visible Ink Press, a ton of information is out there to guide you into a total life detox and learning what to avoid, and it can indeed be overwhelming to think about doing a complete "toxin life makeover," but you can take small steps to begin. Buying organic; looking for herbicides and pesticides in food products; avoiding things like glyphosate, mercury, lead, and aluminum; checking labels; drastically reducing sugar and high fructose corn syrup; eating less junk food and fewer processed food products; buying from local farmers and butchers; only using products that contain no chemical additives or colorants; checking ingredients in vaccines and becoming an informed consenter; avoiding injected fillers such as Botox that have few long-term studies; buying nontoxic lip balms; and using products without aluminum are all things that can go a long way toward removing some of the negative influences of toxins in the body.

Detoxing programs are all over the internet, and many are run by doctors and researchers with great credentials. Be wary and discerning when following any detox protocol, and if it involves taking one of their products, always check with your doctor about the ingredients and

Toxins in our environment are a major concern for our health, and the author writes about this in another book from Visible Ink called *Toxin Nation*.

potential side effects. If you don't want to go all out with a 10–day or two–month detox program, you can start smaller and still do your body a host of good. Did you know that at night, your body repairs itself and does its own heavy detox? It is one of the reasons people wake up dehydrated. Drinking an 8–ounce glass of water, preferably at room temperature, first thing in the morning on an empty stomach can reduce brain fog, improve alertness and circulation, stimulate a bowel movement, and remove extra waste from the night's detoxing. It also rehydrates you before that morning cup of coffee.

Some of the most toxic foods include anything made with rancid oils. Hydrogenated oils have a negative impact on our cells, cholesterol, heart, and brain and cause inflammation. Oils to avoid include soybean, safflower, sunflower, vegetable, canola, cottonseed, and palm oil. Also, it's wise to keep trans–fatty acid consumption low, so check those labels. Partially hydrogenated oils are a no–no, too, as they are synthetic sources of trans fats. Believe it or not, many of the vitamins and supplements people buy have rancid oils in their ingredient list, especially fish and flaxseed oils.

If you want to assure that the food or supplements you are buying contain little to no toxins, look out for preservatives, additives, artificial coloring, heavy metals such as lead and mercury, aluminum, GMOs, MSG, and yeast. Learning to read a label is a skill you will cherish for the rest of your life. Once you see these ingredients in products you never imagined might include them, you become a more informed consumer.

 Oils to avoid include soybean, safflower, sunflower, vegetable, canola, cottonseed, and palm oil. Also, it's wise to keep trans-fatty acid consumption low, so check those labels.

You can try plenty of simple remedies as well to flush out some of the accumulated gunk, clean up your body, and enjoy improved health and a stronger immune system. Add some of these to your new regimen of eating cleaner, drinking water that is filtered from impurities, buying natural products with no chemical fillers, and becoming as informed as possible about everything you ingest and inject into your body.

Love Your Liver

When it comes to processing toxins, the liver is the king of the organs. It performs over 500 necessary functions to keep ridding the body of waste, metabolize hormones, and aid in digestion. Optimizing liver health is a must for health and well–being. This can include diet and supplementation rich in vitamins A, B, and C; minerals such as zinc, magnesium, calcium, and selenium; and amino acids like cysteine and methionine to prevent oxidation, bind heavy metals, and flush them out of your system.

Antioxidants such as glutathione help to decrease toxins from smoke, exhaust, chemicals, radiation, drugs, and carcinogens. Some of the foods that aid this detoxing powerhouse are garlic; citrus fruits such as lemons and limes; cruciferous veggies; avocadoes; leafy, green vegetables; turmeric; walnuts; and plenty of water to help flush things out. The herb list in this book is filled with plant helpers to assist the liver in doing its job.

How do you know if you need to detox? You feel sick, tired, or weak, or your brain feels foggy. You have digestive issues, allergies, sensitivity to smells like perfumes, rashes and skin problems, dizziness, poor sleep, weight gain, sluggish digestion, constipation, low–grade fever, hormonal disruptions, headaches, congestion, sore throat, body odor, muscle aches, and flare–ups of arthritis. In fact, too many toxins in the body tax the liver and turn down the volume on your entire body as a result because the liver must work extra hard to rid the toxins properly and get them out via urine and feces.

Think of detoxing methods as a bit of rest and relief for the liver to get back to operating at an optimal level, which it cannot do if it's overwhelmed with chemicals and poisons. Think about how many toxins we are exposed to in a single day: the beds we sleep in, the mattresses and bedding that contain flame

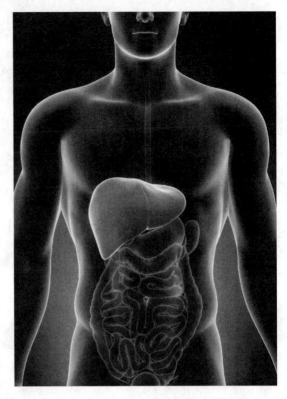

The liver is the key organ in filtering toxins from your body in addition to aiding in digestion and metabolizing hormones. Detoxing your body is a great way to keep the liver running smoothly.

retardants and other chemicals, the toothpastes we use containing fluoride and the antiperspirants we use containing aluminum, the foods we eat and the coffee we drink for breakfast, and the car we drive to work in that exposes us to exhaust outside and benzene coatings on the seats and dashboards inside. We work in buildings made of toxic flooring and paint and walk to lunch amid car exhaust and construction dust, then chow down a meal that may or may not be organic and grown locally. We go back into the toxic buildings, then we drive home again, and, once at home, we quickly attend to our garden with pesticides and herbicides, then open a bottle of wine filled with sulfates and make a dinner consisting of meat containing antibiotics and added hormones and GMO–filled corn and veggies. On the weekends, we clean with products filled with chemicals and inhalants.

Doing this every day for a lifetime means that we are accumulating way more toxic buildup than we are eliminating unless we stop long enough to detox our diets, our households, our workplaces, and our food, even as we struggle with seeing loved ones around us fall to diseases like heart attacks, strokes, ALS, lupus, MS, Alzheimer's, de-mentia, and all sorts of cancers, wondering if we are next. Then, we turn to the medicine cabinet to try to get better, which only fills our bodies with more toxins. A point must come when you get off the toxin train and get aboard the health train.

Simple Flushes

One way to begin is with simple juice or water "flushes" that help move toxins through the body while also aiding in digestion. Water flushes work best when the water is warm. Warm water does not tax the digestive system the way cold or ice water does. Adding a pinch of Himalayan salt or high-quality sea salt to any flush protects the adrenal glands and helps keep electrolytes in balance.

- Take 1 cup of warm water. Add 1 teaspoon of lemon juice and 1 teaspoon of organic apple cider vinegar. Drink this on an empty stomach upon waking up in the morning.

- Another variation calls for one glass of warm water, the juice from half a lemon, and a few mint leaves.

- You can also try adding cucumber slices, a sprig of fresh mint, the juice from half an orange, and 2 tablespoons of lemon juice to 12 ounces of warm water. Cucumber limits the retention of water in your gut and helps alkalize your body.

- You can swap out any citrus, from lemons to limes or from lemons to oranges, in these flushes. Citrus fruits boost the immune system and lower cholesterol levels.

- Try this one before breakfast for a boost. Add 2 tablespoons each of apple cider vinegar and orange juice to a 12-ounce glass of warm or hot water. Mix in ¼ teaspoon of cinnamon, a pinch of cayenne pepper, 1 tablespoon of organic honey, and a dash of ground ginger. Mix and drink immediately. Hot water makes it into a nice tea.

Foods That Detox Heavy Metals

Ridding the body of toxins in the form of heavy metals such as lead, aluminum, mercury, arsenic, cadmium, and barium can often be done by adding a few food sources. Heavy metal exposure causes a host of neurological disorders and health complications and is espe-cially harmful to pregnant women and fetuses. Even a mother's small amounts of exposure to something like mercury can affect the brain development of a fetus in the womb. These heavy metals increase your risk of developing cancers, including those of the skin, liver, bladder, lung, kidney, and colon.

Include the following foods in your diet more often to assist the body in eliminating and fighting back against these toxins:

Heavy metal exposure causes a host of neurological disorders and health complications and is especially harmful to pregnant women and fetuses.

- Cilantro: A natural detoxifier that specifically works to remove neurotoxins such as mercury from the body.
- Lemon: The fresh juice of a lemon is a powerful detoxer and is one of the cheapest and easiest ways to rid the body of toxins. Just squeeze into water every day, and you are good to go.
- Wild blueberries: Blueberries are high in antioxidants, and those found in the wild are even more potent. These help draw heavy metals out of the body and reverse oxidative damage caused by the toxins.
- Chlorella: A nutrient-rich algae that detoxes the body from neurotoxins and protects against exposure to lead.
- Garlic: It doesn't just keep vampires at bay, it also increases the production of glutathione, the most powerful antioxidant found in the body and one that is critical for detoxing.
- Turmeric: Curcumin, the active compound found in turmeric, protects against mercury exposure and even reduces the markers of kidney and liver damage caused by mercury.
- Artichoke: Artichoke extracts contain compounds that protect the liver and support it in its ability to process toxins, including heavy metals, out of the body. It also helps liver cells regenerate.

Many of the herbs and plants listed in the herbal medicine section of this book contain compounds and extracts that help the body detox from chemicals, neurotoxins, heavy metals, pesticides, and herbicides and should be added in some combination to your diet regularly.

Juicing and Smoothies

One of the best ways to consume a lot of healthy and detoxing fruits and veggies is through juicing, which allows you to throw in a variety of items that have different benefits into one meal or snack.

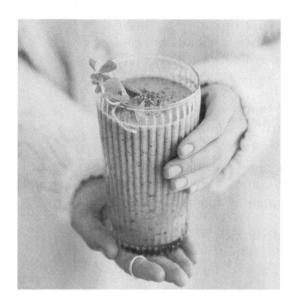

There are a variety of smoothie recipes you can try that are healthy and detoxifying, so experiment with different flavors until you find your favorites!

Green smoothies are one of the best detoxifiers around and also provide the body with vitamins, minerals, and phytonutrients. Green produce contains chlorophyll, which helps to detox and eliminate the heavy metals found in pesticides and pollutants.

A green smoothie or juice is a great way to start off the day and can include things like kale, parsley, cilantro, green apples, and arugula, with a banana, peanut butter, blueberries, or a bit of stevia thrown in to sweeten it up. You can't go wrong with any kind of green smoothie, but a lot of figuring out what works best for you will be trial by fire, or by drinking. Some ingredients may give off a bitter tang, which may require more sweetening ingredients.

Raw juices often contain a variety of fruits and veggies in their whole forms, all blended to taste. You can combine fruits like apples, melon, and berries with carrots, greens, celery, and beets and come out with a refreshing and incredibly healthy blend. It's all about experimenting with raw, organic ingredients to see what you like. Phytochemicals stimulate the immune system, reduce blood pressure, and assist in hormone metabolism while delivering a full day's worth of vitamins and minerals. Add that to the chlorophyll from the veggies, and you have a potent, cancer-fighting drink that you can consume once, twice, or even three times daily (watch out, though, because that's a lot of fiber!).

No need to buy an expensive juicer or blender. A regular blender or older food processor works just fine, but beware of putting in stems and roots that can clog up the blades.

Beet Greens for Detoxing the Liver

Beets are incredibly healthy, and so are beet greens, which serve to alkalize the body and, despite their slightly bitter taste, regenerate and reactivate red blood cells. Beet greens supply oxygen throughout the body and help to detoxify the liver, inhibit the growth of cancer cells, and eliminate constipation, to boot. They contain powerful phytochemicals such as betalains, betaxanthins, vitamins, and minerals that combine into compounds of phytopigments and antioxidants that protect the liver. The amino acid tryptophan is also found in beet greens; 1 cup provides 13 milligrams, which helps produce the feel-good serotonin that boosts mood and helps you sleep better.

Beet greens contain carotenoids such as lutein and zeaxanthin, so they are great sources of vitamins A, C, and K. All these wonderful ingredients clean out toxins and make sure you can eliminate waste properly. Beet greens do contain oxalates, which can be an issue for someone with kidney disease or gall bladder problems, so check with your doctor before eating them. You can put beet greens into a salad, a healthy juice, or a smoothie. You can also cook them by quickly steaming or boiling them for just a few minutes. They can be kept refrigerated for up to three days.

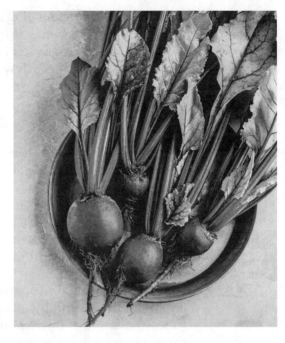

Most people think of beet roots when adding these veggies to their diets, but you can also eat the greens. Just make sure they are not wilted or brown.

Make sure to avoid wilted produce when purchasing at a grocer. The ancient Romans were the first to use beet greens as a medicinal, first eating only the greens, then later learning that the roots were edible and valuable, too.

Lemon Balm Benefits

Lemon balm is a lemon-scented herb and member of the mint family, traditionally used to improve mood and cognitive function, promote better sleep, and detox. Its medicinal use goes back over 2,000 years, and Paracelsus, the chemist known as "the father of toxicology," sang its praises for vitality and well-being, especially for nervous system issues and anxiety.

You can find lemon balm teas, essential oils, and extracts that can be added to smoothies or shakes, or you can apply it topically to the skin for a soothing effect. You can buy the tea, oils, or extracts, or grow lemon balm yourself in direct sunlight. It works equally well in a container, pot, or garden and contains compounds that repel mosquitoes. Try crushing a few leaves in your hand and rubbing it on your exposed skin.

The Many Benefits of Oregano Oil

Oregano is one of the most powerful healing herbs around, and the oil is equally beneficial. Oregano oil has long been considered a remedy for colds and flu bugs in part from compounds called thymol and carvacrol, which are antioxidants, antifungals, antivirals, and anti-inflammatories. The carvacrol aids in better digestion and kills off pathogens such as *Salmonella* and *E. coli* and decreases bloating, gas, and indigestion by stimulating the release of bile and digestive fluids.

The antifungal properties help fight off yeast infections, thrush, and foot fungus, and the antiviral properties remove warts when topically applied (do so by diluting first with a carrier oil and just a few drops of oregano oil, or you can burn the skin) and prevent cold sores, which are caused by the herpes simplex virus. Those same properties and others help heal wounds and reduce scarring and discoloration of the skin. The anti-inflammatory properties of thymol reduce overall inflammation in the body. This oil is currently being researched for its potential effectiveness in fighting off cancer cells, but more study is needed.

You can soak your feet in a pan of oregano oil in water with other essential oils mixed in. You can also take it as a supplement in tablet or capsule form.

Oregano oil can be consumed in many ways. You can drink it by diluting 1 drop of the oil in 500 milliliters of water. You can apply it topically but dilute it first with a good carrier oil to avoid skin irritation or burning. You can soak your feet in a pan of oregano oil in water with other essential oils mixed in. You can also take it as a supplement in tablet or capsule form. Last but not least, you can use it for the ancient Ayurvedic method of oil pulling to remove bacteria from the mouth. You can use 1–2 drops diluted in a carrier oil such as sesame oil, olive oil, or coconut oil.

One word of caution: check with your doctor before administering to a child or pregnant woman. Never use more oregano oil than needed, thinking you will get more benefit. Sometimes, less is more with these powerful oils.

Lime Water

A cup or glass of warm water with lime on an empty stomach first thing in the morning helps dissolve mucoid plaque that is stuck to the intestinal walls. Mucoid plaque is a sticky substance that adheres to your colon wall, and when it builds up over time, it prevents the elimination of toxins from the body. Many allopathic doctors deny the existence of this plaque, but others agree that it is possibly there for a reason and that you shouldn't use an enema to rid the colon of it. They recommend a colonoscopy, but it's not harmful to try this natural lime water remedy first.

Herbal Detox Concerns

Herbal detoxes used in the extreme can make you sick; anything used in the extreme can. Many detox products on the market claim that they will clean out your colon of 20 pounds of "poop," aid weight loss, and clear up all your health issues at once. Maybe they can, but it behooves you to be discerning when trying any product. Check reviews and complaints, and make sure all ingredients are listed on the label. Has the product been tested for safety? Who makes it, and where is it made?

The duration of many toxic cleanse products is usually three to 14 days, but many people believe that "more is better" and continue to use products that shouldn't extend the recommended time frame. Check ingredients to make sure everything is natural and it doesn't contain synthetics. Research is limited as to whether ingredients that have chelating properties, as many products advertise, bind to the heavy metals in the body to eliminate them in waste. Also, check which toxins the product claims to remove and how they can prove effectiveness. Often, they will cite animal studies, and while these can be encouraging, they may not extrapolate to humans.

Detoxes often cause weight loss by the sheer fact that you are eating less during the detox or drinking more fluids to feel full. A lot of the weight loss is water loss because of the diuretic ingredients in many products that cause the body to expel water via the urine and feces. That weight loss may be reversed once the detox program ends.

Keep in mind that your body already has a built-in detox system if you keep it running at optimal levels with a healthy diet, exercise, clean water, and quality supplements. Your liver and associated organs will do what they were meant to do. If you do wish to aid them with herbal detoxes, keep your expectations reasonable and never overdo it or go to extremes where you are not eating food for two weeks or required to have a daily enema. Use your common sense.

Gut Detox Drink

Here is a daily drink for detoxing the gut naturally. You will need three organic apples, a fresh ginger root, one key lime, ½ teaspoon of sea salt, and ½ cup of warm water. Juice the apples, ginger, and lime and pour into a glass. In a small bowl, mix the sea salt and warm water, then add this to the glass with the other ingredients. Stir it up and drink. It works best with warm water, but if you cannot tolerate it, put in a few ice cubes.

Saunas and Sweating

Throughout history, people have used saunas, sauna baths, and sweat lodges for medicinal purposes. The use of heat and sweat comes with many health benefits our ancestors knew about. Heat has a strong effect on the heart, brain, and skin, which is the largest organ in the body. Toxins that build in the cells are released via sweat glands and, other than a long, hot shower, using a sauna regularly is a great way to detox from heavy metals such as lead, arsenic, mercury, and cadmium.

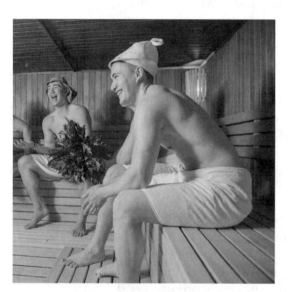

Saunas have been used for centuries by people who long claimed the benefits of steam on everything from skin to internal organs.

According to the article "Some Like It Hot–The Many Benefits of Sauna Bathing" that Dr. Joseph Mercola wrote for his website, sweating in a sauna for an hour can burn as many calories as an hour of intense exercise and has these added benefits:

- Cleaning out pores to prevent acne and blackheads
- Improving blood circulation
- Improving muscle relaxation
- Relieving stress
- Killing viruses and bacteria unable to survive temps of about 98.6°F

•   Expelling toxins and supporting the immune system

Having a good sweat regularly can help keep the body from experiencing a toxic overload. According to Dr. Mercola, many documented research studies show that sweating increases the excretion of heavy metals and exceeds the amount of toxins eliminated in urine and plasma. Sweating in a sauna should be an initial method of treatment for anyone with elevated mercury urine levels.

Sauna bathing can help improve cardiovascular conditions and has been used as a treatment in Japan and Korea, where it is called Waon therapy. This usually involves FIR saunas, or those that use far infrared radiation, which is a subdivision of the electromagnetic spectrum that has been studied for its positive biological effects. The body absorbs FIR–wavelength energy, which penetrates a gentle heat about 1.5 inches beneath the skin and is particularly of benefit for patients with chronic heart failure and peripheral arterial disease. Infrared saunas work by penetrating your tissues with infrared rays using lower temperatures, so you get hotter, and it occurs on a deeper level without the room getting as hot as other types of saunas.

In one German study, patients with rheumatoid arthritis showed a marked reduction in inflammation and pain after using FIR saunas, and articles in the *Journal of Hypothermia* and *Medical Hypothesis* both stated that FIR sauna therapy helps children with autism. It is reported that autistic children do better when they have a fever, showing fewer symptoms, and this could be linked to when glutamine in the blood and brain is low. During a fever, more glutamine is released and metabolized by the intestines, which improves autistic symptoms.

Many athletes favor infrared saunas because they get greater recovery from their strength and training sessions.

FIR sauna therapy assists with the detoxification of toxic debris from the body and was used as part of the protocol on September 11, 2001, to help firefighters after the attacks on the World Trade Center. They had been exposed to many solvents, smoke, chemicals, and toxins that led to mood disorders, depression, and anxiety, and this type of therapy was used to help them recover from the toxic overload.

Two different types of saunas are on the market: wet heat and dry heat. A wet sauna uses air heated by water, which produces steam and high humidity. A dry–heat sauna does not produce humidity but still heats the room and your body. Choosing which sauna to use is really based on your tolerance to heat and humidity or if you prefer the lower temps of infrared saunas. Many athletes favor infrared saunas because they get greater recovery from their strength and training sessions.

Sauna therapy, as the article continues, demonstrated benefits in research studies for those with asthma, COPD, and bronchitis and other respiratory diseases and reduce the risk of death from all causes. Detoxing benefits the entire body, but the heat itself works to improve the circulation of blood, dilate blood vessels, and increase relaxation of the smooth muscle lining the blood vessels.

If you can't afford to buy a home sauna or don't want to use one at the local gym, consider a hot shower–but not too hot. You don't want to scald your skin. Before exposure to heat, always drink plenty of water to get hydrated. Don't use a sauna, hot shower, or hot tub when you have a headache. If you want to have children, you may also want to avoid the heat because as your body heat rises, so does the temperature of your testicles, which reduces fertility and sperm count and mobility.

Our bodies are meant to function best at about 98.6 degrees Fahrenheit. Raising your core temperature above 104.8 degrees Fahrenheit is a medical emergency, so keep the heat below that, and don't stay in a sauna any longer than you should, or you risk dehydration, fainting, and even death. It might be best to avoid public saunas for cleanliness issues and perhaps sign up for sauna therapy at a health facility where they have rigorous cleaning protocols and know what they are doing.

Epsom Salt

Epsom salt baths are a great way to increase your levels of magnesium, which helps to detoxify cells, removes metals from the body, and assists in the functioning of your body's enzymes, which boosts the immune system. The sulfate in Epsom salts aids many bodily functions, including the removal of toxins. They also strengthen the digestive tract walls, which makes eliminating toxins easier.

The salts also soothe sore muscles and body aches and soften rough, dry skin. You can even use the salts to exfoliate dead skin cells.

People with inflammatory diseases can find relief from soaking in an Epsom salt bath, especially those with gout, psoriatic arthritis, and rheumatoid arthritis. The magnesium's toxin-ridding effects contribute to the reduction of inflammation and swelling from a good soak. Magnesium also boosts neurotransmitters in the brain that bring about calm, reduce stress, and induce sleep, so a bath after work or before bed can work wonders.

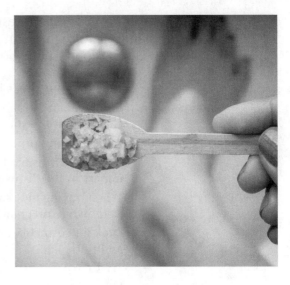

Epsom salt is a salt formed by combining magnesium cations and sulfate anions. It has many uses ranging from preparing cement and as a soil amendment in agriculture to a soothing additive in foot baths.

If you have athlete's foot, you can do an Epsom salt foot soak by adding 1 cup of salts to a footbath full of warm water. Drinking highly diluted Epsom salt with added lemon in water can battle constipation, too. For a bath, add 1–2 cups of Epsom salts, which can be purchased in most stores in the toiletries section, into a tub full of warm water. To better dissolve the salts, add them to the running water as you draw the bath. Soak in this for between 12–20 minutes three times a week.

For additional skin-soothing benefits and to relieve stress, you can add olive oil and essential oils such as vanilla, lavender, peppermint, eucalyptus, and frankincense to the salt bath, but make sure to dilute the essential oils with a carrier oil before adding them to the bath. You can try 3–5 drops of essential oil per ½–1 ounce of carrier oil (olive, coconut, almond). Adding baking soda boosts the bath's antifungal properties.

Epsom salt baths are safe for everyone, but don't take them without checking with a doctor, and do not give epsom salt to a child or pregnant woman for oral consumption. If you have existing kidney problems, check with your doctor about detoxing in salt baths, as the salt could tax your kidneys.

Tips to Avoid Toxins and Chemicals

Find small ways to eliminate toxic exposure with these suggestions from the *NaturalHealth365* website. Toxins in the environment, food, air, water, and products we buy and use all contribute to infertility and lower levels of testosterone in men, so this is important if you plan to get pregnant anytime soon or are already; we can all use less toxic overload in our bodies.

- Take off your shoes before entering your home.
- Buy local and organic produce and wash thoroughly before you eat to reduce pesticide exposure.
- Avoid buying processed, canned, and junk foods.
- Do not microwave food in plastic containers or put plastic containers in the dishwasher and use glass or stainless steel instead.
- When buying new carpeting, furniture, curtains, or bedding, especially while pregnant, avoid flame retardants.
- Look for cosmetics and beauty products that are free of fragrances and phthalates.
- Try to avoid touching the ink on cash register receipts.
- Use air purifiers and vacuum cleaners with high-quality HEPA filters and change them often.

Fighting Colds, Viruses, and Bugs

Elderberry, King of the Virus Fighter

When it comes to fighting the symptoms of colds, flus, and viruses, the elderberry is the best warrior out there. The berry-producing *Sambucus nigra*, also known as the European elderberry and the black elder, is a beautiful tree native to Europe. It has been used in healing remedies since ancient times in Egypt and is known for its antiviral properties and for boosting the immune system to better support good health.

Once cooked, elderberries make wonderful syrups, teas, popsicles, jams, spreads, and wines.

The elderberry is a dark-hued, almost deep purple/blue-colored berry that grows in large bunches and must be cooked before it is consumed safely. Raw elderberries and the bark and leaves of the tree are toxic. Once cooked, elderberries make wonderful syrups, teas, popsicles, jams, spreads, and wines. They have a tart flavor that can be sweetened with natural sweeteners, but most people find that they can tolerate the taste.

The mighty elderberry is packed with nutrients and antioxidants that protect the body from free radicals and oxidative stress. They are also high in the flavanols quercetin, kaempferol, and isorhamnetin, which are all anti-inflammatories with properties that can reduce the symptoms of colds and allergies, protect the brain against neurodegenerative disorders, fight cancer, prevent cell adhesion and maintain barrier integrity, prevent infection, and kill toxic microbes.

Ample scientific research exists behind the use of elderberries to improve cold and flu symptoms as well as upper respiratory infections. One such study found that taking elderberry syrup cut symptom duration from seven to eight days down to two to four days and reduced the severity of symptoms. Other studies show elderberries to work as well as Tamiflu for lessening the impact of cold and flu symptoms. Elderberries contain unique phytochemicals that block viruses from entering and attaching to healthy cells and can be taken as a preventative measure right when flu season begins. One study in 2019 showed that elderberry syrup was not only effective if taken early on but worked even stronger well into a virus or infection.

The high antioxidant levels provide extra support to the immune system and increase white blood cell count and overall immune system functioning. The FDA has regarded the elderberry as a safe treatment, and studies prove it to be safe and effective. The only danger, again, is in not cooking them, which would cause the cyanogenic glycosides in the berries to form hydrogen cyanide in the gut, so make sure that any recipe you make involves cooking them before you consume them. You can buy a variety of elderberry syrups, teas, and other items in the health food section of your grocery store or online, but always look out for added sugar and fillers and buy from a reputable company.

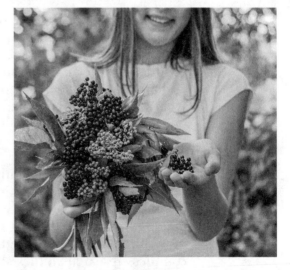

Garlic and Onions Work, Too!

Garlic and onions are also great medicinals for colds and viruses, with garlic being more effective. Both contain compounds that boost immunity and enhance your body's own antiviral white

Even the FDA has declared elderberries a safe and effective treatment for boosting the immune system.

blood cell response. The allicin in garlic is the immune–boosting compound that forms when the garlic is crushed or chewed.

Bee Pollen for Season Allergies

Bee pollen has been used since ancient times for its health benefits. It reduces fever and heals wounds as a topical medication with its antiseptic and disinfectant properties. Bee pollen is made from an enzyme–rich mixture of honey, wax, bee secretions, and flower pollens and contains many essential amino acids and vitamins, including flavonoids. Bee propolis is similar to bee pollen; it is a resinous substance made by bees that is a popular supplement around the world for its ability to ward off upper respiratory infections, colds, flus, and seasonal allergies. Bee pollen and propolis extracts don't leave you with the usual side effects of over–the–counter antihistamines and provide seasonal or year–round relief from allergy symptoms.

Honey

The healing wonders of honey never cease. If you want to ward off colds or lessen the severity of symptoms from an upper respiratory tract infection, organic, raw honey works as well as any OTC medication and has been found as effective as OTC cough medicine for children.

The honey you get at the local store may not be pure and contain impurities, so your best bet is to buy local and organic. Try visiting a farmer's market in your area and get to know your local honey producer. You can ask them all about how they make their product and are much more likely to get pure, organic, real honey there than what's in the watered–down versions sold in teddy bear containers.

Echinacea

Other ways of preventing colds and viruses and lessening their impact when you have them include staying hydrated with water, increasing your intake of vitamins C and D, getting plenty of rest, and taking echinacea at the first sign of symptoms. Echinacea is one of the most popular antiviral herbs around and has been the subject of countless research studies showing it as effective against respiratory tract viruses. One study in 2015 found that echinacea was just as effective as oseltamivir in treating the flu when taken early on and had no side effects. It is key to start taking it as soon as you notice symptoms. You can take capsules, tinctures, sublingual drops, or chews or drink it in tea form, and, as always, look for products with no fillers or added sugars.

 One study in 2015 found that echinacea was just as effective as oseltamivir in treating the flu when taken early on and had no side effects.

Inhaling Steam

Because dry indoor air can make a respiratory infection worse and help spread flu viruses easily, try using a humidifier when you're sick. The increase in humidity makes the indoor area much less hospitable to viruses and pathogens. Warm, moist air soothes sore throats and inflamed nasal passages and helps loosen congestion in the sinuses, chest, and lungs.

Run the humidifier overnight while you sleep, and in the morning, try steam therapy. Heat water in a pot or bowl and hold your face over it with a towel draped over your head to trap the steam. Keeping your eyes closed, breathe in the steam deeply for about five minutes, being careful not to get too close to the pot or water itself. You can also add in herbs such as oregano, sage, cinnamon, and thyme for more healing properties, as they assist in loosening congestion in the sinuses and lungs.

Certain essential oils have antiviral properties and can be used with a diffuser to help you get over a flu or virus. Try diffusing tea tree oil, lemongrass, cinnamon, lavender, thyme, bergamot, peppermint, or eucalyptus, or combine a few of them for an extra boost. You can also dilute eucalyptus oil with a carrier oil such as olive oil and rub on your chest for relief from a stuffy nose and sinus congestion.

Skin Savers

People spend a lot of money for injections to make their skin look plumper and to eliminate fine lines. Hundreds of creams and serums are on the market to tighten skin, many of them way too expensive for the average buyer. When it comes to improved skin, natural skin–tightening and antiaging options are available, such as essential oils that also reduce acne, dark spots, and large pores and lighten scars.

Some of the more popular oils for the skin include:

- Frankincense: Reduces acne blemishes, prevents fine lines, closes large pores, lifts and tightens the skin, and can even be used under the eyes. Combine it with a good carrier oil such as olive oil or grapeseed oil for more effectiveness.
- Myrrh: Soothes dry, chapped skin and prevents signs of aging. It smells nice, too!
- Coconut: You can use coconut oil by itself on your skin as a moisturizer, which also helps to prevent signs of aging and keeps skin super soft. It is an antifungal and antibacterial, so it keeps your skin clean, too. Go light, so you don't end up with shiny skin. Use on the face and body, especially dry spots like elbows and feet.
- Sandalwood: This essential oil is high in antioxidants that fight signs of aging on the skin. It also reduces the damage from free radicals.
- Neem: Neem oil reduces acne, eczema, and psoriasis and heals insect bites and bee stings.
- Buckthorn: This oil eliminates acne, reduces scars and fine lines, heals wounds, and regenerates skin cell growth. It also evens out skin tones.
- Vanilla: An essential oil containing vanilla not only smells nice, but the high levels of antioxidants fight off environmental stressors that can show on your skin.
- Argan oil: Argan treats acne, moisturizes skin, and softens hair while giving it a shine.

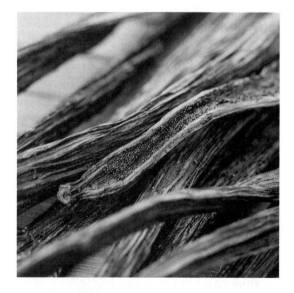

Vanilla is not just a lovely bean for flavoring ice cream; it is also a great antioxidant for the skin.

- Lavender: A calming oil to soothe skin and tighten up fine lines while also making you smell nice and natural. Try a blend with chamomile, which is also great for soothing dry and irritated skin.
- Rose hip oil: Reduces fine lines and wrinkles, protects skin from UV sun rays, evens out skin tone, and fights acne and rosacea.
- Jojoba oil: This oil is a great moisturizer and skin cleanser and can be used as a makeup remover for all skin types.

Castor Oil

Other skin savers include the all-purpose castor oil, which comes from castor beans. Castor oil has been used for decades to assist in hair growth, even eyebrows, and to cleanse the pores of the face.

Try a gentle cleanser of castor oil mixed equally with jojoba oil. Massage into skin and leave for 10 minutes before washing it off your face with a warm washcloth. You can also apply the mix while in the shower, as the steam will increase the cleansing effect on the pores. Castor oil contains a fatty acid called ricinolein acid, which helps heal and prevent cystic acne. You can apply a few drops right onto the acne and leave on overnight, then rinse off in the morning. This same fatty acid allows castor oil to penetrate the top layer of the skin to fade and heal stretch marks and scars, and the biochemical known as unde-cylenic acid heals fungal growth such as athlete's foot and ringworm. Rub castor oil right onto the affected areas until healed. It works even better if you mix the castor oil with coconut oil.

Rubbing castor oil into your hair can create incredible shine and luster, and its humectant properties make hair look thicker, too. Rub just a pea-sized amount into your hair when you get out of the shower and let it dry naturally.

Got stung? Castor oil's antibacterial properties soothe stings and bites and reduce itching. Just apply a tiny amount to the bite or sting until healed.

Acne Fighters

Natural ways to fight and prevent acne include garlic, which is used in Ayurvedic medicine. Grind up a couple of garlic cloves into a paste and apply directly to the acne and affected areas until healed. You can also try a remedy of turmeric and coriander to heal acne. Grind fresh coriander leaves and extract the juice. Mix it with turmeric powder to create a paste that can be applied directly to the acne area.

Tea tree oil has been a mainstay for healing acne for decades. It can often rid the skin of acne overnight.

Aloe vera oil applied directly to the acne area is another great Ayurvedic method. If you have a plant at home, break off a small piece and use the leaf to apply the gel directly onto the acne twice a day until it disappears. Tea tree oil has been a mainstay for healing acne for decades. It can often rid the skin of acne overnight. Take a cotton ball and dab a few drops of tea tree oil onto it, then gently pat the acne. You may feel a tightening or tingling of the skin, but this is purely natural. Other oils to try for acne include jojoba oil, which works wonders to rid the pores of dirt. Apply 2–3 drops onto a cotton ball and pat the acne directly. These methods also work to lighten and heal preexisting acne scars.

Another widely used remedy involves lemon juice, honey, and almond oil. Take 1 tablespoon of each and mix with 2 tablespoons of milk (or water if you don't have milk). Apply directly onto the acne and leave on overnight, then rinse with water in the morning. These are natural remedies for cleansing and healing the skin, so don't follow them up in the morning with chemical–filled creams and lotions that add more toxins into the skin and clog up pores. Keep it natural from cleaning to moisturizing to healing.

Eczema responds well to oatmeal, which can calm itchy and inflamed skin and soothe rashes. The phytochemicals in oatmeal are anti–inflammatory and stop swelling. Try making a paste of ¼ cup of oatmeal with a little bit of water and apply to the affected areas for 10 minutes, then gently rinse off with warm water. You can also put ⅓ cup of plain oatmeal in a blender and grind into a fine powder. Put the powder in a warm bath and soak.

Sea salt can be used as a scrub for rough patches of skin and areas like elbows, knees, and feet. Sea salt is a great exfoliator that rids the dead skin cells and reveals fresh skin. Try making a scrub with 1 cup of sea salt and ½ cup of a light oil such as melted coconut oil or a scented massage oil. The texture should be like that of wet sand. Do not use on the face or sensitive skin areas, as it may be too rough.

Got puffy eyes from lack of sleep or too much partying? Cool a cucumber in the fridge, then slice it up and put a slice over each eye. The cold temperature will cause the blood vessels to constrict and reduce swelling and inflammation. Replace with fresh slices when they get too lukewarm until the puffiness is gone.

Borage seed oil treats everything from eczema and seborrhea to dermatitis and skin rashes. Spread the oil lightly on the affected area as needed.

Herpes sores can be treated with garlic paste, ginseng, comfrey, echinacea, or lemon balm until they clear up.

Get rid of warts by rubbing aloe vera gel on them for a few weeks, or try rubbing the warts with the inside of a banana peel. You can bandage the banana peel in place and replace it every few days for best results. In about a week, the warts should be gone. A salve made with milk thistle will also remove warts naturally.

Balms and Healing Salves

Balms contain shea butter or cocoa butter as extra ingredients and are fairly easy to make. They also contain more volatile oils and are usually more aromatic than salves. Balms can be a little creamier in texture. Salves are easier to spread on the skin for treating sore muscles and in chest rubs. Salves have a more liquid consistency, especially when you introduce the essential oils or flowers, which make it easier to stir; pour into the jar or container while it's still liquid so the volatile oils don't evaporate. Once you seal the jar or container, the balm or salve will harden once it has cooled, but you may need to check it a few times to make sure it isn't too soft and runny or too hard to spread. A nice chest salve can be made out of olive oil you may already have in your cupboard mixed with the wax of your choice and about 5 percent of a favorite essential oil or oil blend. That's it!

Some of the most popular herbal salves include:

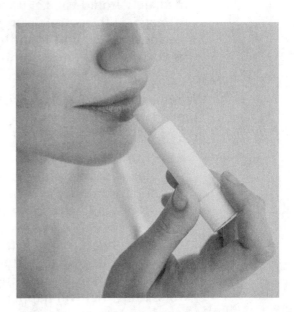

- Arnica flowers
- Calendula flowers
- Chamomile flowers
- Chickweed
- Comfrey
- Echinacea root
- Ginger root
- Lavender flowers
- Myrrh
- Nettle leaf
- Plantain leaf
- Thyme leaf
- Yarrow leaf/flowers

Beeswax comes in white and yellow forms. The yellow is best, as it is not processed or bleached. Candelilla and car-

When someone says "balm," you might think of common, petroleum-based lip balm, but there is a world of natural balms and salves out there you can buy or make that do wonders for the skin.

Natural Health

nauba are harder waxes but are vegetable based. Some people refuse to use beeswax unless they can guarantee that the product comes from a reputable and ethical producer of bee-based products, so if that is a concern, do your research before buying. You can buy beeswax in pastilles or pellets, which melt down more easily than chunks or blocks.

Vegan salves can include infused oil mixed with candelilla or carnauba wax instead of beeswax, but carnauba can be hard and takes longer to melt down to get to the right consistency. When making a lip balm, be sure that all ingredients are edible. You can make in large batches and store for future use or to give as gifts. It's easy to find fun, little containers for salves and balms online or in craft stores. You can also buy an emulsifying wax that comes from natural fat and ester sources and is processed into flakes. This works best for making creams, lotions, and more fluid products with higher oil and water contents.

If you want to avoid the waxy texture altogether, think about making a body butter. You can add in drops of infused or essential oils to cocoa butter, mango butter, or shea butter. Simply melt the oils you choose along with the butter, then add the oils and remove immediately from heat. Let it cool, fluffing it up with a spoon or spatula to keep it at the easy-to-spread butter texture. Cocoa and shea butters are inexpensive and found in most drugstores or warehouse stores, so you don't have to hunt for them.

 Balms are the hardest in consistency, followed by salves, ointments, and butters. Always try these out on a small patch of skin first to test for allergic reactions.

Balms, salves, ointments, and butters are all nontoxic as long as you don't introduce a toxic herb or plant. Balms are the hardest in consistency, followed by salves, ointments, and butters. Always try these out on a small patch of skin first to test for allergic reactions. Use clean fingertips or a cotton swab to apply lip balms, so germs and dirt on your fingers are not introduced to the rest of the product. You can do a lot of experimenting with ingredients and textures, and the worst thing that will happen is that you toss out a bad batch. Just remember a few simple tips:

- More beeswax means firmer product, less means softer product.
- More shea, cocoa, or mango butter means fluffier product.

- Use any essential oils you like for lip balms as long as they are edible.
- Use any oils or herbs for salves, butters, and ointments applied to the skin, but watch out for allergic reactions.

Lip balms from the store or cosmetics aisle often contain fillers and additives that end up being swallowed the more you use them. Try this simple recipe for making your own lip balms. The main ingredient behind a lip balm will be beeswax (or candelilla if you are vegan). To make a simple lemon lip balm, for example, you would need 2 tablespoons of coconut oil, ½ tablespoon of castor oil, 1 tablespoon of shea or cocoa butter, and 3 tablespoons of melted beeswax. Put this all into a bowl, then place into a pot with a few inches of water in it. Put on low heat to melt down the beeswax just enough so that you can mix all the ingredients thoroughly. Add in vitamin E oil (you can open some capsules) and your chosen essential oils: in this case, lemon. Stir until completely mixed, then pour into tubes, tins, or small containers and cover. Let this sit before using, so it solidifies to the proper consistency. If you want a firmer balm, heat it all up again and add a little more beeswax until you get the desired result. For chapped lips, you can use a little tea tree oil or comfrey oil. For dry lips, focus on coconut oil for the extra moisture. For an easy-to-make, two-ingredient lip balm, combine five parts warm olive oil to one part beeswax and follow the same technique as above.

To make a salve, follow the above technique but add a little extra shea or cocoa butter to get the right consistency. Once you master the basics of making salves, you can really mix and match and get creative on your own.

For a great muscle salve for aches and pains, mix 3 tablespoons of dried calendula flowers with 1 cup of olive oil and 1 ounce of beeswax. Add in 12–15 drops of chamomile and/or lavender essential oil.

Dry skin salve: Mix 1 cup of coconut oil with dried lavender, rose, and chamomile and add 1 ounce of beeswax. Add in 12–15 drops of an uplifting essential oil like peppermint.

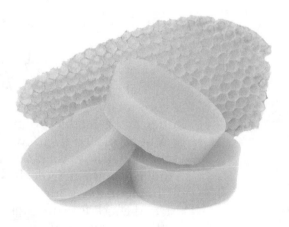

Beeswax serves as a great base for homemade balms and salves.

Calendula/marigold salve: Great for healing bruises, burns, breakouts, rashes, diaper rash, dry skin, eczema, and chapped skin. Make an infusion of 3 cups of dried calendula/marigold flowers and 1 cup of olive oil or other carrier oil. Make sure the oil is organic! Add in a few drops of chamomile essential oil or tea tree oil. After you make the infusion, heat the infused oil in a pot or double boiler and add in 2 ounces of beeswax (shaved or pastilles); melt it down, mixing often with a spoon. Pour it through a clean cheesecloth into your storage container and seal. Let it cool before applying to skin. Keep it in a cool, dark place when not in use.

Try mixing peppermint and lavender for getting rid of headaches. Rose and chamomile soothe the skin and the spirit. Rosemary added to anything does wonders for healing skin issues such as acne, rashes, and an itchy, scaly skin and scalp and also energizes and uplifts. Lemon balm cools and relaxes. Arnica soothes muscle pain and bruised skin. Plantain heals wounds and cuts.

Comfrey salves and balms are good for just about everything that ails you. Jojoba oil is a great addition to a lip balm. The only thing to keep in mind is that you will be licking your lips, so make sure the products you use are edible.

Lemon Lip Treatment

Combine a carrier oil, such as almond or avocado oil, with beeswax and melt down to a salve. Add in pure, organic honey and mix until fully blended. Remove from heat and add 7–8 drops of lemon essential oil. Pour into container and cover.

Lemon Balm Lip Saver

Make an infused oil with lemon balm, then add 2 tablespoons of coconut oil, ½ tablespoon of castor oil, 1 tablespoon of shea or cocoa butter, and 2–3 tablespoons of melted beeswax (or candelilla if vegan) in a bowl placed in a few inches of water inside a larger metal pot. Use a low heat to melt down the beeswax and mix thoroughly, then remove from heat. Quickly stir in any essential oils and the vitamin E oil. Immediately pour into tubes or tins and cover. Let them sit before use and check for consistency. If you want it firmer, heat up and melt a little more beeswax to add to the mixture. To turn this recipe into a salve or body butter, just add more shea or cocoa butter to get the fluffy consistency you want.

Comfrey Healing Salve

Combine comfrey with coconut oil and your choice of wax in a pan or double boiler. Heat to melting, then pour into a jar to let cool. Just before it cools, add in a few drops of tea tree or lavender oil, then cover and store.

Plantain Salve

2 c. olive or almond oil

¼ c. beeswax pastilles

1 tsp. echinacea root (optional)

2 tbsp. dried comfrey leaf

2 tbsp. dried plantain leaf (herb–not banana!)

1 tbsp. dried calendula flowers (optional)

1 tsp. dried yarrow flowers (optional)

1 tsp. dried rosemary leaf (optional)

First, infuse the herbs into the olive oil in one of two ways: you can either combine the herbs and the olive oil in a jar with an airtight lid and leave for 3–4 weeks, shaking daily, OR heat the herbs and olive oil over low heat in a double boiler for three hours until the oil is very green. Strain the herbs out of the oil by pouring it through a cheesecloth. Let all the oil drip out and then squeeze the herbs to get the remaining oil out. Discard the herbs. Heat the infused oil in a double boiler with the beeswax until melted and mixed. Pour into small tins, glass jars, or lip balm tubes and use on bites, stings, cuts, poison ivy, diaper rash, or other wounds as needed.

Herbal Healing Lip Balm

1 tsp. chosen wax or body butter

4 tsp. infused oil or oil blend

Your choice of herbs or flower parts

3 drops skin-protective essential oil, such as chamomile

This natural balm keeps lips moist and prevents cold sores. You can double these amounts for more product. This should make enough for two small 12-milliliter containers.

Put the wax or butter into a pan or double boiler. Melt it down, then add your infused oils. Stir until everything is completely blended and to avoid solidification. Add in essential oil drops and stir again, then remove from heat. Pour into your clean lip balm containers and let it cool before use. Ideally, you want to let it cool for an hour or two before putting on the cap and storing or using the balm. Hot balm on dry lips hurts! Use your fingertip to test. This recipe can be stored for a year or more, but ideally, you want to make sure you identify the expiration dates of the ingredients themselves and go from there. Variations of the above include using lavender essential oil, hemp oil, vitamin E oil, peppermint oil, or raspberry seed oil for extra lip protection and soothing.

Marshmallow Root Lip Balm

2 tbsp. marshmallow root infused oil (use almond or sunflower oil as the carrier oil)

1½ tbsp. coconut oil

1½ tbsp. shredded beeswax or pastilles

Put all the ingredients into a pot or double boiler and melt them on low heat until completely mixed. Remove from heat and pour into your lip balm tubes or containers to let sit until the right consistency for use.

Pine Resin Salve

¼ c. pine resin

½ c. infused oil or carrier oil of choice

1 oz. grated beeswax or pastilles

Put the pine resin and oil into a pot or double boiler and let the mixture simmer until the resin melts. Strain out the mixture using cheesecloth or a coffee filter and put the liquid back into the pot, adding the beeswax. Melt until the beeswax is fully mixed in, remove from heat, and pour into glass or metal containers for use. Store in a cool, dark place.

Honey Hand Balm

¼ c. coconut oil

¼ c. almond oil

¼ c. olive oil

5 tbsp. beeswax pastilles

1 tbsp. shea butter

1½ tbsp. raw honey

Essential oils

8-oz. glass jar or several small tins with lids

Combine everything except for the raw honey in a microwave-safe bowl. Microwave on high in 30-second increments for two minutes until the oils and beeswax have completely melted. Whisk in the raw honey and 10–20 drops of the essential oil of your choice and immediately pour into a glass jar. Let cool to room temperature before testing. If you would like to adjust the texture, remelt the balm and add either more beeswax or more oil until the desired texture is reached.

Multipurpose Balm

2 c. olive oil with lemon balm infusion

1 c. olive oil with calendula infusion

¾ c. beeswax or candelilla wax

2–3 drops of your favorite essential oil

Combine the infusions over a low heat, then add the beeswax, stirring until it's melted down. Remove from heat and stir in your favorite essential oils. Immediately pour into containers and cover them. Let them cool before using.

Pain Salve

1 c. dandelions

2 c. carrier oil of choice (sweet almond, olive, coconut)

This salve can soothe sore muscles and joints and moisturize skin. You can also make it into a balm form for chapped lips.

Pour the dandelions into a jar and cover with the oil. Seal jar and let sit for one to two weeks in a cool, dark place. Strain out the dandelions through a cheesecloth, pressing them with a spoon or spatula to get most of the oil back into the jar.

To make the salve: Take the dandelion infusion and put into a saucepan or double boiler with about 2 inches of water. Let this heat to a boil and add in 1 ounce of beeswax. Lower the heat and let the beeswax melt, stirring often. Mix in 1 ounce of shea or cocoa butter, blending well. Add 10–20 drops of lavender oil or other favorite essential oil. Stir until mixed thoroughly. Remove from heat and pour into prewarmed jars or tins. Let mixture sit until it reaches salve consistency. Cover and use or refrigerate the unused salve for later.

If you are using your own infusions and don't want to cook them, you can put your herbs in a jar; cover it with oil, leaving 1 inch at the top; seal the jar; and leave it in direct sunshine for four weeks. Gently shake the infusion once a day. Use cheesecloth to strain the oil out of the jar while pushing down on the herbs with a spatula.

Salves in larger containers make great gifts, and you can find containers and tubes online or at your local crafting store.

Some tips to remember:

- Always sterilize containers before pouring in your salves, balms, etc.
- Use enamel or stainless-steel pans and measuring tools. You can stir with a wooden spoon.
- A harder salve or balm requires more wax; a softer salve or balm requires more oil.

Experiment with the amount of beeswax to get the texture you want, and have fun putting the balms into containers and tubes for your own use or to give as gifts. Salves in larger containers make great gifts, and you can find containers and tubes online or at your local crafting store.

Make Your Own ...

Mouthwash

Mix 1 cup of hydrogen peroxide with 1 cup of water. Add 8 drops of peppermint or tea tree oil. Swish in mouth for two minutes, then spit out.

Bath Fizzies

Baking soda combined with citric acid creates bath fizzies that are great fun for kids and adults. The tiny carbon dioxide bubbles formed when the baking soda and citric acid are combined help to oxygenate the body and heal.

Mix ½ cup of citric acid with 1 cup of baking soda and 2 table-spoons of bentonite clay. Add 10 drops of desired essential oils for scent and healing properties, such as chamomile and lavender for relaxation, eucalyptus for respiratory problems, tea tree oil for fungal issues, or peppermint oil for a mood lift. Mix the above ingredients in a bowl while wearing protective gloves. Spritz in some water and/or witch hazel and mix it well. When it gets to an almost sandlike consistency, pour into your prechosen molds or cupcake tins with paper liners and allow them to dry overnight for at least 24 hours.

You can add a bath fizzie "ball" or "bomb" into the bath when ready. These can also work great in a foot bath, too, although you may not need as big of a bath fizzie and can cut the ingredients in half. The fizziness will remind you of a hot mineral springs bath, which has been used for centuries for its healing properties.

Dryer Sheets

Cut up cotton fabric into squares about the size of a washcloth. Add 3–4 drops of your favorite essential oils. These dryer sheets do not stop static cling, but they will add a special boost of aromatic scent to your clothes.

Body Wash

Mix 1 cup of water with ⅓ cup of honey or castile soap; ⅓ cup of essential oil, such as lavender, rose, orange, or mint; and the contents of one or two capsules of vitamin E. You can use any essential oil with a scent you love, including patchouli or sandalwood for something a bit more earthy.

Body Scrub

Try blending ¼ cup of raw, unsalted almonds with ¼ cup of rolled oats until it has the consistency of sand. Add in ½ cup of olive or coconut oil and mix into a paste. You can throw in a few pinches of ground rose petals, lavender flowers, chamomile, or peppermint leaves. Mix it all together and apply to the body in the shower. Apply to damp skin and rub all over the body, then rinse off with warm water. You can store any extra scrub mixture in the fridge for a week in a closed container.

Sunburn Relief

Mix coconut oil and lavender essential oil with aloe vera. Spread thinly over sunburned area.

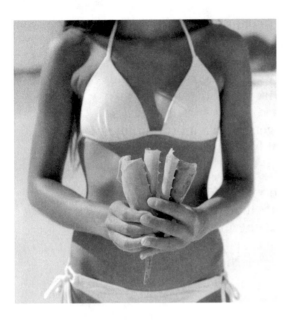

Combine aloe vera with lavender and coconut oil for a soothing treatment for sunburn.

Honey Lavender Mask

Mix 1 tablespoon of honey with 4 drops of lavender essential oil. You can substitute chamomile for the same healing effect. Once stirred, use your fingertips to apply a thin coating as a mask over the face, avoiding the undereye area. You can leave this on for half an hour or up to two hours, then rinse off completely with a clean washcloth and warm water, especially around the hairline. The antimicrobial properties in the honey and lavender will help clear up acne and support healthier skin.

Charcoal Acne Spot Healer

You can buy activated charcoal in capsule form for this treatment and to make your own toothpaste (see recipe in this section). In a small bowl, open one capsule of charcoal and shake out the contents. Add to this ⅓ cup of aloe vera gel and 2 drops of tea tree oil. Mix this thoroughly and apply with your fingertips to the acne. Avoid the area underneath the eyes. Leave on for at least 20 minutes, then wash off with clear, warm water. If it doesn't come off easily, remove with a warm washcloth, then rinse skin. This should help heal the acne and reduce swelling and redness.

Deodorant

Mix 6–8 tablespoons of coconut oil with 4–6 tablespoons of baking soda. Add about 3 tablespoons of shea butter. For women, you can add lavender or lemon essential oil; for men, maybe cypress or frankincense. You may add some arrowroot essential oil for more potency.

Around the House Sanitizer Spray

Mix 1 cup of water with ¼ cup of vinegar or rubbing alcohol. Add 1 teaspoon of liquid castile soap or regular dish soap and 10 drops of essential oil such as eucalyptus or mint. Put in a glass spray bottle and shake to mix.

Household Cleaner

Mix 2 cups of water with ½ cup of distilled white vinegar. Add about 20 drops of essential oil blend such as lemon or eucalyptus. Put in glass spray bottle.

Bug and Mosquito Repellents

Did you know that mosquitoes are drawn to people for various reasons? They are naturally drawn to people who sweat a lot, perhaps because of the salt released in sweat. They also love people who drink alcohol. They are drawn to carbon dioxide, which is why they tend to buzz around your mouth since you breathe the stuff out. If you have Type O blood, they favor you as a juicy treat.

You can defend yourself against these pests in many ways without resorting to toxic lotions and sprays. Here are some ideas:

- Black pepper: Sprinkle some black pepper around your food table if eating outside, and spread a little black pepper oil diluted with a carrier oil such as jojoba, olive, or avocado oil on skin. It can cause irritation to the skin if too strong, so try an allergy test first.

- Anise: Try anise essential oil on exposed skin, or sprinkle it around the areas where you hang out outside.

- Cinnamon and cinnamon essential oil: The oil is pretty powerful stuff and can cause allergic reactions, so try sprinkling a little cinnamon near where you are sitting outside or on the food table at a picnic.

- Geraniol: This is the alcohol extracted from citronella and roses, two plants that mosquitoes hate. It smells nice, too.

- Mint: Mint oil or mint plants around a picnic table or porch can fend off the pesky buggers.

- Lemon eucalyptus oil: The CDC approved this oil as a mosquito

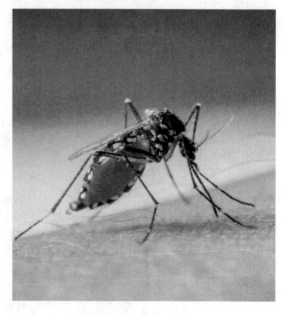

Mosquitoes are not only annoying, but they can also be dangerous. Keep them away with repellants made from natural spices and oils you can find around the house.

repellent; it is one of the best for longer protection, up to several hours.

- Catnip: You can try growing some of this in your yard to repel mosquitoes as long as your kitty doesn't get to it first.
- Garlic: Eat more garlic, and get bitten a lot less. Mosquitoes hate the taste of garlic.
- Cedar oil: Any essential oil with cedar in it will repel mosquitoes. It is potent, so do an allergy test first, and always dilute it with a carrier oil or water.
- Cloves: Try wearing a little sachet or cloth bag of cloves. It works on mosquitoes the way garlic works on vampires.
- Lavender: You can apply the essential oil to your skin or grow it around the garden. If you grow your own, crush the leaves and spread them on exposed skin when outdoors.
- Thyme oil: You can cook with it or use the essential oil. A great idea for a firepit: throw in some fresh thyme leaves to keep the bugs away.
- Rosemary: Cook with it, put a few sprigs on the table, or try the essential oil on your skin.
- Eucalyptus: The smell will set you and your skin free, and it's healing to the skin, too.
- Tea tree oil: A tiny bit on the skin goes a long way toward keeping mosquitoes and lice away.
- Marigolds: Mosquitoes hate the smell of these pretty flowers, so plant some in your garden or keep in pots on the picnic table.
- Citronella: The popular and widely known mosquito repellent, which you can burn in candle form on the picnic table, or crush some leaves from the plant and spread them around the outdoor area.

Bug Spray

Mix ½ cup of witch hazel with ½ cup of water or vinegar. Add in 1 tablespoon of rubbing alcohol and an essential oil blend that includes citronella, lemon, rosemary, lavender, and geranium. Spritz on and around plants and backyard areas to protect. Can use on the skin, too, but do an allergy check first.

Natural Pesticide

Mix 1–2 tablespoons of liquid castile soap with 1 quart of water. Put mixture into a spray bottle and spray areas of the home where bugs get in. Can also add essential oils known to repel bugs such as cinnamon, Pashtun juniper, anise, ginger, and rosemary.

Ant Repellent

Did you know that spraying white vinegar on countertops, windowsills, baseboards, floors, and wherever else you see ants coming into your home is a safe and effective alternative to toxic, store-bought sprays? Pour some into a spray bottle and spray around, including existing ant trails in and outside of the home. The powerful smell will also deter new ants from coming back. You can dilute it with a little water if you wish to tone down the scent indoors.

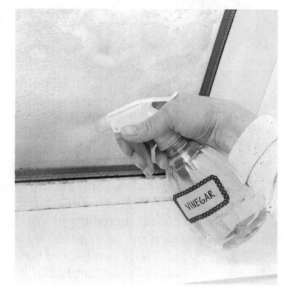

Vinegar is useful not only in cleaning but also as a nontoxic insect repellent.

You can also try blending a few drops of cinnamon essential oil with water in a spray bottle. Focus on spraying the ant trails around doors, windows, and cracks in the walls.

Another natural solution blends about 14 drops of peppermint oil with 7 drops of lemon oil to spray around areas where you prepare food. Peppermint is one scent that ants do not like and will keep them at bay when you spray regularly.

To keep mosquitoes from biting you, try mixing witch hazel with some citronella oil, which bugs find offensive, and rub on exposed skin. This works great on children, and while it may not keep every bug away, it is a lot healthier than the DEET-laden chemical sprays sold in stores.

Yellow Nail Treatment

Treat yellowing nails with a soak made from ½ cup of lemon juice in a bowl. Soak your fingertips for 10–15 minutes daily. Rinse with clean water when done.

You can also try soaking fingertips in a bowl of water mixed with hydrogen peroxide. Just soak for a few minutes, then rinse hands thoroughly with clean water.

Shampoo You

Mix 1 tablespoon of baking soda with 1–2 cups of water for a quick shampoo alternative. You can also try mixing one egg, fresh lemon juice, 2 tablespoons of olive oil, and 2 tablespoons of apple cider vinegar for a shampoo without any chemicals or aluminum. Try blending cucumber and lemon juice into a paste and using for a lovely smelling shampoo.

One of the oldest "DIY conditioners" involves using a cup of mayonnaise spread through the hair and kept on for at least two hours. Rinse it out well, though, as it can leave a greasy feel, but the result is incredibly shiny hair. You can also use coconut oil, jojoba oil, argan oil, or avocado oil as a great "leave-in" conditioner to smooth out frizzies and leave hair shiny and healthy. Put a few drops in the palm of your hands and rub your palms together, then run them over your hair. Put some extra oil on split ends to smooth them over.

One of the oldest "DIY conditioners" involves using a cup of mayonnaise spread through the hair and kept on for at least two hours.

Pain Relief

For back pain from strain and overuse of back muscles, try this soothing tea. Add 1 tablespoon of cramp bark (*Viburnum opulus*) to 1 cup of boiling water. Steep for 10 minutes, then strain and drink the tea. Try this three times daily to relax muscles.

You can also try valerian root, which blocks the transmission of stress from the brain to the body and can relieve a backache. You can take valerian root in capsule form and use it for the duration of the pain. You might even begin taking it beforehand when you know you may be doing some heavy lifting, such as helping someone move.

Got sinus pain? Eat some horseradish.

Got an earache? Eat some garlic.

Other natural pain relievers with plenty of science behind them include arnica, which can be applied topically to relieve symptoms of osteoarthritis; omega-3 fatty acids, which indicate palliative effects equal to ibuprofen; cinnamon, which is as effective as ibuprofen for alleviating menstrual cramps; thyme extract, which reduces the severity of pain and spasms, especially for menstrual cramps; turmeric extract, which relieves knee osteoarthritis as well as ibuprofen; and ginger, which helps with general pain.

Ginger also improves blood flow and reduces muscle inflammation in the uterine area, where menstrual cramps originate from. A study in the *Journal of Alternative and Complementary Medicine* found that ginger was just as effective as ibuprofen for relieving period cramps. You can try ginger chews, capsules, or a cup of warm ginger tea. Ginger in all its forms also fights motion sickness and nausea, including morning sickness. You can drink ginger tea or take supplements and chews. Try making your own tea because it will be stronger than the teas you purchase from a store. Grate half an inch or so of raw ginger and set aside in a cup. Boil 2 cups of water and pour over the ginger. Let this steep for about 10 minutes. Add a little lemon juice and a natural sweetener such as honey or stevia to taste.

For a headache, try an essential oil blend or balm made from lavender and peppermint. This combination is especially soothing for stress-related headaches. You can also find tea blends of lavender, peppermint, and chamomile for soothing pain and relaxing the mind and body. Lavender and chamomile also work together to relieve anxiety. Try making your own aromatic tea from 2 teaspoons of dried lavender, 2 teaspoons of dried chamomile, and 1 cup of hot water. Let the mixture steep for about 10–15 minutes, then strain out the plant parts and drink the tea with a natural sweetener to taste.

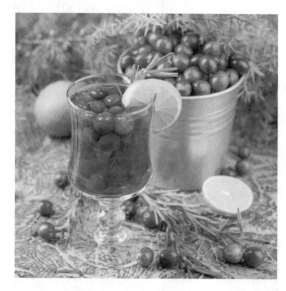

Painful urinary tract infections can be cured with cranberry juice or, even better, eating real cranberries. Cranberries contain proanthocyanins, which fight urinary tract bacteria. This substance keeps bacteria such as *E. coli* from attaching to bladder walls and triggering a UTI. If you already have a full-blown infection, cranberry juice may not be strong enough to stop it, but consuming it daily if you are prone to them does prevent further infections. UTIs can also

Cranberry juice is a common treatment for urinary tract infections. The key is the proanthocyanins contained in cranberries that kills bacteria.

Natural Health

be treated by adding more garlic and vitamin C–rich fruits and veggies to your diet. Garlic's antibacterial allicin, produced when garlic is pressed or chopped, is a powerful tool to fight UTIs. One 2009 study showed that garlic blocks urinary tract and kidney infections caused by bacteria associated with catheter use. Garlic is an antifungal, antibacterial powerhouse that you can easily add to foods or take as a supplement.

Vitamin C makes urine more acidic, which prevents the growth of bacteria in the urethra. You can also try supplementing with grapefruit seed extract, which has been shown in studies to be as or more effective than an antibiotic. One 2005 study in the *Journal of Alternative and Complementary Medicine* treated subjects with grapefruit seed extract for two weeks, and all showed significant relief from symptoms, including suppressed growth of bacteria that had before been resistant to antibiotics.

Chili peppers can stop pain and soreness, thanks to the capsaicin, which has a warming and numbing effect on skin. You can buy capsaicin patches for sore muscles or make a cream yourself. Mix 3 tablespoons of cayenne powder with 1 cup of coconut oil. Melt this over a low heat, stirring constantly for five minutes. Remove from heat and pour into a bowl, then allow it to firm up at room temperature. When cool enough and almost firm, massage into skin.

Natural Migraine Remedies

For those who suffer from migraines, the pain and symptoms can be debilitating. Migraines are neurological diseases that cause nausea, dizziness, fatigue, and extreme sensitivity to light, sound, and smells. Many powerful pharmaceuticals are available for migraines, but if you're looking for something more natural, try the following:

- Magnesium: Adding a magnesium supplement in doses of 400–500 milligrams a day can help prevent migraines, according to the American Migraine Foundation, by averting the occurrence of aura, a type of sensory disturbance. Check with your doctor if you are pregnant, as too much magnesium can cause diarrhea and stomach cramping.
- Vitamin B2: A small 2015 study found that 400 milligrams of vitamin B2 daily reduced the frequency and severity of migraines with minimal side effects.

- Caffeine: While some migraine sufferers find that caffeine increases the severity of migraines, others say about two cups a day helps stop them from happening.

- Peppermint oil: The menthol in this oil can treat migraines when applied to the forehead and temples as soon as you feel one coming on.

- Melatonin: Three milligrams per day can help stop migraines while also regulating your sleep schedule.

- Lavender oil: A 2012 research study showed that people who inhaled lavender oil during a migraine for 15 minutes experienced quicker relief than those who were given a placebo. You can also apply a few diluted drops to the temples.

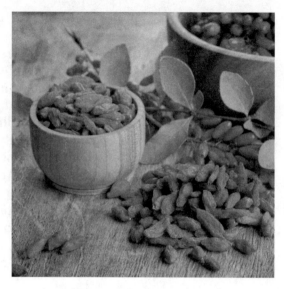

Melatonin can be found in fish, milk, eggs, nuts, tart cherries, and these goji berries (wolfberries), which are often dried and used in baked dishes.

- Feverfew: A few drops on the temples can alleviate the symptoms of a migraine.

- Ginger: Taking powdered capsules or chewing on ginger chews can alleviate nausea from migraines.

Calendula Flower Power

The common marigold, also known as *Calendula officinalis*, has multiple healing properties for skin rashes, wounds, burns, diaper rash, and soreness. It possesses anti–inflammatory, antiviral, antifungal, antispasmodic, and antibacterial properties. In addition to healing wounds, calendula also increases the flow of bile and cleanses the lymph system. For skin issues, it has been shown to regenerate skin. It also stops itching, burning, and the lesions that often erupt on the skin. You can rub the flower right on bee stings and wounds to reduce swelling and pain or make a compress for rashes, burns and scalds, and other skin wounds by chopping the flowers and moistening with water, then applying directly on the skin. Even the stem's sap can be used to get rid of warts, corns, and calluses.

Mouth Sores

Cold sores are recurring fever blisters that appear inside the mouth or on the lips. They cannot be cured, but they can be treated with the amino acid L-lysine, which can also prevent further out-breaks. You can also take L-lysine capsules if you carry the herpes virus that causes mouth blisters. Start with 1,000 milligrams of the amino acid three times daily as soon as you feel or see a blister out-break coming on. Check with your doctor first if you have high cho-lesterol, blood pressure, or heart disease.

Boil 50 fresh sage leaves in distilled water. Gargle the liquid several times daily or make into a sage tea. Sage leaves are full of natural antioxidant, anti-inflammatory, and antimicrobial properties.

Gum Disease

Here are some natural ways to prevent and heal gum disease:

- Turmeric paste and garlic: Turmeric is a natural anti-inflammatory herb, and garlic is an antibacterial agent. You can rub cloves of garlic on irritated gums or make a turmeric and garlic paste to use as a toothpaste. Rinse your mouth for a few minutes after using.

- Sage leaf: You can make a liquid decoction out of sage leaves to fight gingivitis and gum disease. Boil 50 fresh sage leaves in dis-tilled water. Gargle the liquid several times daily or make into a sage tea. Sage leaves are full of natural antioxidant, anti-inflam-matory, and antimicrobial properties.

- Aloe vera gel: Break off a piece of the plant if you have one in the home and rub on gums for its powerful anti-inflammatory effects.

- Mustard oil: An age-old remedy to destroy bacteria in the mouth that causes gum disease. It also reduces pain because of its anti-bacterial and antimicrobial agents.

Eye Puffiness

To reduce undereye puffiness, dip two black tea bags into a cup of hot water for a few minutes. This activates the beneficial tannins in black tea. Cool the bags in the fridge and apply when still damp as a compress on each eye. Be sure, of course, to close your eyes first. Do this for 10 minutes whenever needed. You can also try the usual cucumber slices placed over closed eyes. Leave on for an hour while you relax.

Cooling Sprays and Spritzers

Cool down during those hot, summer months with a spray or spritzer that is good for your skin. Mix herbs with lukewarm or cool water and place into a small pump spray bottle. You can use essential oils, dried herbs, or fresh herbs, or even mild herbal teas diluted with water. Try these or experiment from the herb list in this book.

- Chamomile: soothing, calming
- Eucalyptus: sharp, head–clearing, stimulating
- Lavender: refreshing, relaxing
- Mint: cooling, stimulating
- Rose: relaxing, sensual
- Sandalwood: warming, uplifting
- Peppermint: invigorating, clears the sinuses
- Jasmine: sensual, summery

Avoid the eye area when spritzing the face and always test on the inside of your elbow for potential allergies.

Bad Breath

You can sweeten your foul breath by gargling with a small cup of acidic lemon juice, being sure not to swallow. Then, eat some un–sweetened, plain yogurt, which contains the beneficial *Lactobacillus* bacteria. This combination will neutralize mouth and breath odors for about 12 hours.

Cherry Sleep Aid

Before bedtime, try eating a handful of cherries or drink a cup of tart cherry juice. Cherries contain melatonin, the hormone needed to regulate the body's sleep patterns.

Teeth Whitener

Try crushing some fresh strawberries into a pulp and mix it with 1 inch of baking soda and enough water to make it into a paste. Brush your teeth for a few minutes with the paste once every three months,

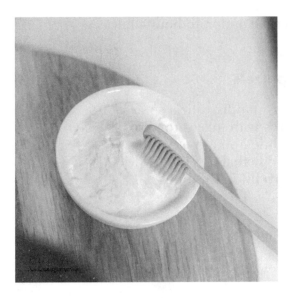

Baking soda both cleans and whitens teeth. You can add other ingredients like strawberries, turmeric, lemon juice, and coconut oil as antioxidants and breath fresheners.

and the malic acid in the strawberries will buff out coffee and red wine stains. Don't use any more often than once every few months, though, because the acid can erode tooth enamel. Always rinse thoroughly with clear water when done.

Natural Toothpaste

If you want to make a natural toothpaste that is free of aluminum and fluoride, here are some simple ideas.

You can brush your teeth with baking soda, which cleans teeth effectively and keeps your mouth's alkaline balanced overnight, to prevent the buildup of bacteria. The taste bothers some, so try putting a few drops of peppermint oil in the baking soda and mix.

Another DIY recipe mixes 1 tablespoon each of black walnut powder, clove powder, and horsetail powder. You mix it up and gently brush your teeth, especially if you have sensitive gums. Use it before bedtime and rinse your mouth thoroughly to prevent buildup of the powder on your teeth after brushing.

Activated charcoal is another great toothpaste that can be used directly on teeth or as part of a blend with a peppermint or spearmint oil for taste. This is also a great way to safely whiten teeth without the chemicals of tooth–whitening kits.

Burns

Honey works wonders on superficial burns and wounds. It is an antibacterial and cleans out the infection. Honey also heals burns on an average of four days sooner than burns not exposed to honey, according to a New Zealand research study. Honey can also reduce swelling and scarring. Put some honey onto a sterile gauze pad and apply gently on the burn or wound as a covering. Change the honey gauze covering every 24 hours until the burn is healed. Try any locally made organic honey, but manuka from New Zealand is highly recommended.

Coughs and Sore Throats

Instead of a cough drop, try eating a little dark chocolate to stop a pesky cough. It contains a chemical found in cocoa beans called theobromine, which calms persistent coughs more effectively than codeine-based syrups.

The *Journal of Alternative and Complementary Medicine* studied 60 adults with inflamed throats and showed that a tea made with marshmallow, licorice root, and slippery elm bark calmed their sore throats by coating irritated membranes and experienced 48 percent less pain than a placebo group. They drank the tea four to six times a day for a week. You can make this tea yourself or buy it in stores under the name Throat Coat. If you have allergies or high blood pressure, check with your doctor first.

Garlic tea may sound disgusting, but it will relieve a sore throat and prevent the secondary bronchial infection often associated with a cold or flu.

Another great tea for a sore throat is mullein tea. Mullein comforts a painful throat and helps alleviate hoarseness. Simply steep 1 tablespoon of dried mullein in 1 cup of hot water for at least 10 minutes and drink as needed. Do not try this tea if you are taking blood thinners.

Garlic tea may sound disgusting, but it will relieve a sore throat and prevent the secondary bronchial infection often associated with a cold or flu. Steep one large, crushed clove of garlic in hot water for 10 minutes, covering the cup with a plate or napkin, then drink. Do not try this tea if you are taking blood thinners.

Try dissolving ½ teaspoon of sea salt in a glass of warm water. Gargle, without swallowing, every three hours. You can also substitute baking soda for salt.

Athlete's Foot

A simple saline solution can help fight athlete's foot. Soaking your feet every day for five to 10 minutes in a mixture of 2 teaspoons of salt per 1 pint of water creates a hostile environment for fungus and decreases foot perspiration. It also softens up the harsh skin of the foot, so if you choose to later apply an antifungal cream, it will absorb better.

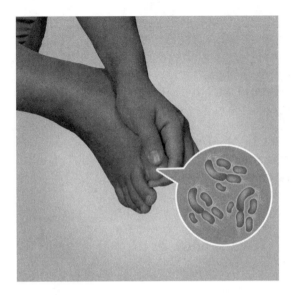

Foot odor is caused by bacteria, and vinegar is a good way to safely kill those little germs. Just soak your feet in diluted vinegar for about half an hour.

Another solution for athlete's foot or other fungal infections of the skin is a tea tree spray. Take ¼ cup of rubbing alcohol and mix with 15 drops of tea tree oil. Put this into a spray bottle that is at least 2 ounces in capacity and spray on the affected area when needed. It can be stored at room temperature for about two months.

Stinky Foot Soak

To get rid of foot odor, try soaking your feet in one part vinegar to two parts water every night for about 30 minutes to kill off the odiferous bacteria, or try soaking them in strong, black tea that has been cooled for about 30 minutes. The tannins in the tea kill bacteria and close the pores on the skin of your feet to keep them drier longer and prevent bacterial growth. One caveat: do not soak your feet if you have any open cuts.

For Sore, Tired Feet

Get a foot tub and fill it with warm water. Add 2 cups of baking soda, 1 cup of Epsom salt, 10 drops of lavender essential oil, and the juice of a squeezed lemon. Soak feet for 30 minutes for best results. Lemon adds a detox element to the soak, too, but you can leave it out if you choose. You can swap out the lavender oil for coconut oil for smoother, softer foot skin. Adding ground orange peel and a few drops of coconut oil soothes, smooths, and scents. Once you remove your feet from the tub, be sure to dry them, followed by a light rub of coconut oil to lock in moisture.

Hemorrhoid Help

Cut 50 grams of oak bark into small chunks and place in 1 liter of water. Boil for approximately three minutes and allow to cool. Pour into a large basin and sit your backside in the solution for 30 minutes. The warm water increases blood flow to the rectal area. The effects may take a few hours, or it may be up to two days until relief is found. This is similar to a sitz bath and promotes circulation of blood in the

Healthy Hair and Scalp DIY Remedies

Banana hair mask: Mix two egg yolks, two ripe bananas, 2–3 tablespoons of honey, ½ cup of conditioner, and 2 tablespoons of olive, coconut, or jojoba oil. You can puree in a blender or mix really well by hand. Rub all over your hair and into scalp and leave on for 30 minutes, then rinse with cool water. It should make hair shiny and healthy looking until your next shampoo. If you have longer hair, you can use a hair cap or net to keep it on top of your head while you wait.

Egg and lemon treatment: Mix two egg yolks with 2 teaspoons of lemon juice and apply from roots to tips. Keep on for 1 hour, then rinse thoroughly with clear water.

Mayo mask: Mix ½ cup of mayonnaise with a splash of lemon juice and 2 tablespoons of banana. Spread on hair, focusing on the scalp, and leave on for a half hour, then rinse thoroughly until hair does not feel slick from the mayo. This is a great moisturizer for the scalp. Can double the batch and apply to the roots, too.

Warm oil mask: Warm up 2 tablespoons of coconut or jojoba oil and massage it into your hair while damp. Put on a cap and sleep on it, rinsing with cool water in the morning. If you have a lot of hair, you may also want to sleep on a towel covering your pillow to keep the oil from getting on your pillow. You can also use avocado or olive oil if you have fine hair.

Itchy scalp fix: Put 3 drops of tea tree oil on a cotton ball or swab and dab onto the scalp. You can dilute it with a little warm water if it stings. Follow up by breaking two vitamin E capsules open and rubbing the oil into the scalp for extra moisturizing.

Deep cleaner: If you want a deep cleaning to rid your hair of excess dandruff and shampoo buildup, try mixing ⅓ cup of your favorite shampoo with 2 heaping tablespoons of baking soda. Massage into scalp. Let it sit for five minutes, then rinse thoroughly.

Volumizer: Mix ½ cup of rolled oats with 2–3 tablespoons of almond or jojoba oil and ½ cup of whole milk. Apply all over hair and leave on for 45 minutes. You can use a cap to keep hair in place. Rinse out thoroughly for extra volume and movement.

Avocado mask: Take one medium-sized avocado and mash it up with one large egg. Apply to hair and keep on for 30 minutes, then wash your hair thoroughly to get it all out and rinse with a conditioner.

anal area to quicken the healing process. The sitz bath is often rec-ommended as a conventional method of treating hemorrhoids. In a sitz bath, the patient is seated in a bathtub with warm water, enough to cover the anal area. This should be done a couple of times a day for 15 minutes each session.

Cold Shower Therapy

Taking a cold shower boosts the immune system, relieves head-aches and asthma symptoms, and cuts anxiety. It also locks moisture and shine into your hair if you end your shower with one minute of cold water.

Hair Color Boosters

In between colorings, you can add a boost to your existing color with a juice rinse. Just rinse through hair unless otherwise indicated, then follow with a quick water rinse and dry hair normally. Hair high-lighters and dyes sold in stores are filled with chemicals and toxins, some carcinogenic, although more natural lines of hair dye are ap-pearing on the market. If you choose to do a permanent dye, do some research and look for dyes that do not contain aluminum or other neurotoxins. Semipermanent dyes are a little better for use, or you can try a henna dye. In between hair colorings, boost your color with these teas and masks.

If you want to bring out your red tones, massage tomato juice into hair, then put on a mask to cover and leave for 30 minutes before thoroughly rinsing. Pureed beets also bring out the red tones in hair, although it will have a purple tone. Apple cider vinegar brings out red highlights in red hair. If you want a little boost of red, use cranberry or cherry juice or try a hibiscus flower and calendula tea or infusion.

Brunettes who want to cover gray can use nettle or sage tea. Sage is a tried-and-true gray-covering remedy and can be used weekly as more gray appears. Brunettes can use coffee or black tea for deeper highlights. If you have light brown hair, try a cinnamon hair mask made up of ½ cup of your normal hair conditioner mixed with 1 table-spoon of cinnamon powder and leave on overnight. You can add more cinnamon for deeper effects.

Blondes can boost their hair color with lemon juice, which is also used to add highlights to brown hair. You can do an overall rinse with lemon juice or apply to strands for a highlighting effect. Cham–omile and calendula tea work better for darker blonde hair, as does a rinse with champagne. Grape juice can rid blonde hair of brassiness.

Herbal Baths

Herbal baths usually use steeped flowers or herbs that can be mixed up on the go or beforehand. You can use a handful of each herb or flower, fresh or dried, in a pot of water. Heat to a boil, then cover and remove from heat. Let the mixture rest for at least 20 mi-nutes to two hours and then strain the plant parts and toss. The liquid can be stored for later in the refrigerator or used immediately in the shower or bath.

An easy way to include herbs and flower parts in an herbal bath without the mess is to put them into a tea strainer or a sachet made of cloth you find at home, preferably a muslin so the herbal goodness

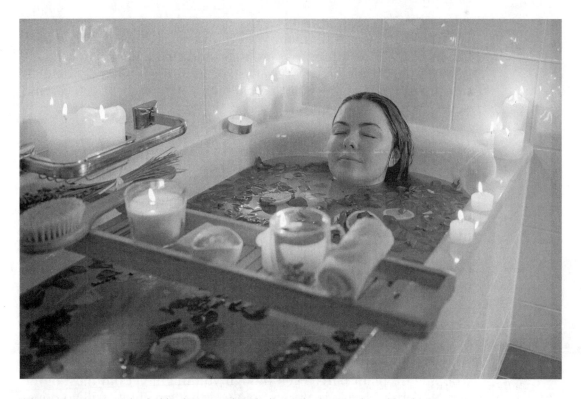

When you picture an herbal bath in your head, does it look something like this? Imagine the cleanup afterwards! You can avoid the mess by putting the herbs and flower parts into a sachet or tea strainer.

passes easily through the mesh of the fabric. Stitch together three sides of the fabric, put in your fresh or dried herbs and flowers, seal up the final side, and drop into the running water. Let the sachet soak in the tub with you to disperse the herbs. You can also put a dry sachet under your pillow to help you fall asleep.

A great sleepy-time recipe includes 2 tablespoons of dried lavender flowers, 2 tablespoons of dried chamomile flowers, one vanilla bean broken apart, and 1 teaspoon of Epsom salt. Mix it all up in the sachet and put in the bath or under your pillow to soothe and relax before bedtime.

In the morning when you need to wake up with an energy boost, try a sachet in the shower made of 2 tablespoons of dried peppermint leaves, 2 tablespoons of rosemary, and 2 tablespoons of rose hips without the seeds. Hang the sachet under the nozzle, so the water can run over it as you shower.

You can also experiment with mint leaves, cloves, orange peel, lemon zest, and anything else aromatic and create blends to keep inside sock and undergarment drawers or in bins of stored clothing. At Christmastime, imagine a hot herbal bath with a sachet of cloves and pumpkin or peppermint oil.

If you don't want to sew up a sachet, try putting herbs or flowers into a muslin cloth bag you can purchase online. Put the bag into a tub filled with extremely hot water and let it steep for a few minutes before the water reaches your desired temperature. You can clean the bags and use them over and over. As a last resort, or if you don't have the time for homemade sachets, you can buy herbal bath infusions and bath "bombs" that can be poured or tossed into a bath. Do check to see what they are made of, so you can avoid any possible allergens that might cause a skin reaction.

A warning note about putting fresh or dried herbs directly into the bathwater: It can be very difficult to clean up afterward, and when you are relaxed from the bath, you most likely won't want to be scooping up plant parts. Even though you might get out most of the herbal "debris," a risk is always involved that small bits will go down the drain and clog it, so it's best to enclose them in a bag, strainer ball, or other method.

Milk and Honey Bath

Add a few drops of essential oils such as lavender, jasmine, or patchouli to about 6 ounces of milk and a few tablespoons of liquid coconut oil. Top off with 2 tablespoons of honey that has been warmed up to a nice liquid texture. Mix it all together and run a hot bath. Add the mixture into the bath and luxuriate in the same beauty method Cleopatra once used in ancient Egypt. For extra moisturizing, add in jojoba oil, avocado oil, castor oil, calendula oil, apricot oil, or sesame oil, or you can rub the oil onto your skin once you have dried off after the bath to lock in moisture.

Relaxing Chamomile Bath

Chamomile baths relieve pain and anxiety before bedtime and are a great way to end a stressful day. You can add fresh chamomile flowers to the water or dried flowers in a sachet or strainer ball. Lavender oil will give you an extra relaxing boost. You can also try hops, steeping the flowers in hot water for 15 minutes before adding to the bath. Hops is known for relieving insomnia, or swap that out for rosemary or orange blossoms for a similar effect.

Dandelion Boost

If you like to take baths in the morning, try adding some dandelion flowers to freshen your skin while also giving you a boost to the spirit. Mix in a little mint with the dandelion flowers for a real pick-me-up. Add a few drops of eucalyptus oil to clear out clogged sinus passages from overnight allergies.

Antiaging Bath

Your skin will love you when you take a bath with ½ cup of rose petals, ½ cup of lavender flowers, ½ cup of dried green tea, ½ cup of jasmine, and a few drops of rose essential oil. Put the ingredients into a bath directly or put the dried ingredients into a sachet or strainer ball and under the running water as you fill the bath, then add the oil into the water directly.

Soothing Bath for Itchy Skin

If you are experiencing itchy, dry skin, try this soothing bath. Take ½ cup of uncooked rolled oats and mix with ¼ cup of dried chamomile flowers, 3 drops of chamomile essential oil, and 2 drops of lavender essential oil. You will need a thin sock or cut-up stocking. Fill the sock or stocking with the mixture and tie off the top. Place the sock/stocking in the bath and soak for at least 20 minutes. You can squeeze the sock to get more of the contents into the bathwater and onto the inflamed skin. Rinse off after use and throw away the sock/stocking. You can also add calendula flowers or essential oil to the mixture. This bath can even soothe the itching from chicken pox and eczema or psoriasis, and it also moisturizes dry skin.

Bath or Shower Body Scrub

You can use this scrub to keep your skin looking healthy and glowing. It works for up to two days after you scrub with it. You will need a small bottle of glycerin, which can be purchased at a drugstore pharmacy or online. Mix 1 cup of sea salt with enough glycerin to just moisten it into a paste consistency. When you are in the shower or bath, leave the mix on a counter until you are ready to use it, so you don't dissolve the salt further. When ready, use it to scrub and lightly exfoliate the dead skin off your body, then rinse for a couple of minutes. If you can tolerate rinsing in cold water, it is better for your skin.

Stop Excessive Sweating

We need to sweat to regulate our body temperature, but some people suffer from hyperhidrosis, a condition that causes excessive sweating beyond what is needed to regulate body temperature. It can occur all over the body or just under the arms or on the face, feet, or palms of hands. Primary hyperhidrosis has no medical cause and can either be hereditary or triggered by nerves. Secondary hyperhidrosis can be caused by a medical issue such as diabetes, heat exhaustion, overactive thyroid, or menopause. Some natural remedies include:

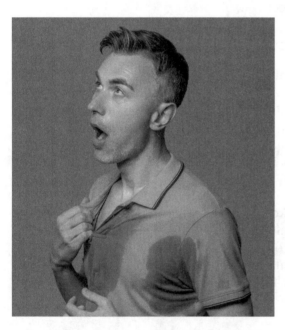

Are you one of those people who can't seem to stop excessively perspiring? Some common plants and fruits such as lemon, apple, and potato may help.

- Lemon: Rub a cut lemon over the affected areas before bedtime. You can also use lemon juice.

- Apple cider vinegar: Mix with a little water and apply with a cotton ball to the affected areas.
- Witch hazel: Apply with a cotton ball to the affected areas.
- Black tea: Place one tea bag in warm water to soak for five minutes, then rub the tea into the affected areas.
- Coconut oil: Very effective in reducing excess sweating; rub coconut oil on the affected areas until it is absorbed by your skin.
- Potato: Clean the potato. Cut into slices, and rub the potato's juices onto the affected area.

Gargles

Sage can help reduce pain from a sore throat when used as a gargle. It can be purchased as dried leaves, an essential oil, or a liquid extract. Pour 1 cup of hot water over 2 teaspoons of dried sage leaves. Let steep for 10 minutes, then add a pinch of salt. Gargle with this a few times a day, but do not swallow it. Keep the extra gargle in the refrigerator until ready for use.

Licorice root is an ancient medicinal for those suffering from a sore throat, viral infection, or ulcers. The demulcent properties found in the root soothe the mucous membrane of the throat. You can purchase it as a tea, capsule, powder, tincture, or extract or as a root, which would need to be boiled in water for five minutes before consuming. Marshmallow root is another demulcent herb that works the same way but is not to be used by diabetics, as it contains properties that can lower blood sugar levels.

Try apple cider vinegar (ACV) with salt as a gargle. In a glass of lukewarm water, add a pinch of salt and a few teaspoons of apple cider vinegar. Gargle with this several times a day to relieve pain and inflammation. Don't drink the mixture; spit it into the sink when done gargling.

 When it comes to sore throats and viral respiratory infections from colds or sinus infections, a saltwater gargle can alleviate pain and prevent infections from getting worse.

When it comes to sore throats and viral respiratory infections from colds or sinus infections, a saltwater gargle can alleviate pain and prevent infections from getting worse. You can give a saltwater gargle to a child over the age of 6, and it only requires two readily available ingredients. Numerous scientific studies prove the benefits of a simple saltwater gargle. It can reduce the severity of sinus infections, strep throat, the flu, and mononucleosis, and one 2013 study showed that flu-prevention methods such as saltwater gargles worked better than the current flu vaccine to prevent reinfection. The gargle also helps heal canker sores and mouth ulcers and improves dental health overall when you gargle daily by lowering the presence of harmful mouth bacteria.

It's easy to make. Take ¼– ½ teaspoon of salt for every 8 ounces of cool water. Sea salt is best. You can use warm water if you can tolerate it. Gargle into the back of your throat for as long as you are able, then swish the water over the teeth before spitting it out into the sink. You do not want to swallow it, as it contains germs and bacteria, and drinking too much salt is a health risk.

You can gargle several times a day until symptoms subside, and if you prefer, you can add a touch of honey, lemon, or mint to taste and for extra healing benefits.

Got Gas?

Try a tea made of peppermint and caraway oils after a large meal to help alleviate gas and aid digestion.

Got Diarrhea?

Believe it or not, a glass of red or white wine was found in a research study to work even better than Pepto-Bismol to relieve diarrhea within a half hour of drinking, thanks to the wine's antibacterial properties. All you need is one 6-ounce glass.

Heartburn Helpers

- Chamomile: A cup of chamomile tea can neutralize the acid content of your stomach.
- Slippery elm: Slippery elm contains substances that can thicken the mucous lining of the stomach to protect against stomach acid. Pour a few tablespoons of slippery elm extract into a glass of water. Drink after each meal and before bedtime.
- Ginger tea: Ginger is one of the oldest remedies for heartburn and nausea. Drink a cup of tea throughout the day or use ginger chews for relief.

- Turmeric tea: Have a cup of turmeric tea three times a day or eat some curry in a meal to help prevent acid buildup and stimulate digestion.

- Baking soda: Baking soda is a known antacid that helps neutralize stomach acid. Drink 1 teaspoon of baking soda dissolved in 8 ounces of water to alleviate heartburn symptoms and acid reflux.

- Bananas: Bananas have natural antacid properties. Eat a fresh banana once or twice a day to restore healthy acid levels in the stomach.

Chickweed Healer

Chickweed is known to herbalists for its skin–healing properties to treat burns, skin rashes and irritations, drying, and itching. You can chop up some chickweed and boil it in lard, then cool to spread as

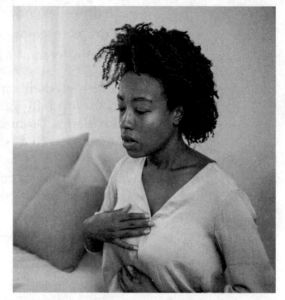

The solution to heartburn might be as simple as eating a banana once a day or drinking some herbal tea. Try these before running to the pharmacy.

an ointment on skin. Use the leaves, flowers, and stems; you can include some organic olive oil if you want to make an herbal infusion, or use chickweed oil alone on skin by applying with a cotton ball. You can also buy or make salves with chickweed oil as the main ingredient.

Household DIYs

Furniture Polish

Coconut oil has so many uses, one of which is a healthy alternative to chemical furniture polishes. Just run a few drops of melted coconut oil over furniture with a dry cloth, and you will coat and protect your furniture while giving it a nice gloss. Orange oil also works as a furniture polish and leaves behind a nice citrus scent.

Bathroom Surface Spray

8 oz. distilled white vinegar

6 oz. distilled water

2 oz. vodka or rubbing alcohol

10 drops lavender essential oil

5 drops rosemary essential oil

5 drops lemon or lemon balm essential oil

Combine ingredients in a 16–ounce spray bottle and shake well before each use on bathroom counters, cabinets, blinds, tiles, sinks, tubs, and fan blades. Do not use vinegar on granite countertops, as it can have an adverse effect on the sealant.

Do not use vinegar on granite countertops, as it can have an adverse effect on the sealant.

Mirror and Glass Cleaner

Fill a glass spray bottle with equal parts distilled water and distilled white vinegar and shake gently to combine. Spray directly on mirror or glass, and use a cloth to wipe in circular motions.

Sink, Tub, and Toilet Scrub

A natural way to clean out the sink, tub, or toilet uses 1 cup of baking soda mixed with 4 drops each of rosemary and grapefruit essential oils. Mix into a paste and scrub with a damp sponge or scrubber brush. You can also use orange or lemon essential oil. Rinse with clear water. It will leave your bathroom smelling great, but it will not disinfect. Also be aware that baking soda is a mild abrasive, so be careful using on certain surfaces.

Easy, Breezy Teas

Herbal teas are an easy way to benefit from a natural remedy without having to do too much work. You can buy them premade, or make them by buying dried herbs and flowers or drying and grinding them yourself. A good rule of thumb is to aim for 2 cups of water to 1 ounce of dried plant parts, which is about 1–2 tablespoons. In general, you take the dried plant parts of your choice, put them into a teacup or small pot, and pour boiling water over them, usually a cup or two, then let it steep for 10–15 minutes covered. Then, remove from heat and strain out the plant parts with cheesecloth or some other strainer. Let the remaining liquid cool enough for you to drink it, adding in any natural sweeteners. You can also put the ground-up plant parts into a strainer ball and steep that in hot water, then just remove the ball, toss out the plant parts, and drink your tea. Unused tea can be stored in the refrigerator in a glass jar with a lid for about three days or pour the tea into a glass full of ice for a tasty, cold drink. If you have a compost pile, toss the used plant parts on the pile, but do not pour down the sink, as they may result in a clog.

Some people really enjoy experimenting with different blends of plants, herbs, and flowers and have a more DIY attitude, but many high-quality herbal teas are on the market. Look for organic and check the ingredients for fillers. Cheaper teas such as Lipton and other mass-market teas contain plastic particulate matter, so be sure to opt for a higher-quality tea. If you want to be sure you are not getting any extra additives or plastic particulate matter, then make it yourself.

Cheaper teas such as Lipton and other mass-market teas contain plastic particulate matter, so be sure to opt for a higher-quality tea.

You can also add herbal teas to your bathwater for a soothing and aromatic bath. You may want to double the concentration of herbs for use in the bath. Focus on herbs that are good for your skin and aid relaxation.

For medicinal and therapeutic purposes, some healing teas should be consumed two to three times a day. Otherwise, you can enjoy herbal tea anytime, as the vast majority do not contain caffeine or other stimulants. Some teas such as valerian, lavender, and chamomile do have a slight sedative effect, so beware of consuming before you drive.

- Ashwagandha: Relieves stress, boosts energy, calms, and soothes. Reduces inflammation and helps the thyroid. Aids sleep.
- Black: Black tea gives a caffeine boost and prevents several types of cancer. It also reduces the risk of heart attacks, regulates diabetes, lowers cholesterol, and has active compounds that treat stomachaches, menstrual cramps, vomiting, and diarrhea.
- Chaga: A mushroom tea that boosts immunity and fights cancer.
- Chamomile: Soothes, calms, and aids in falling asleep. Also aids digestion.
- Cinnamon: Balances blood sugar and lowers insulin resistance.
- Echinacea: Boosts immune system, fights colds and flus, and fights cancer.

- Elderberry: Fights colds and flus and is great for children as a cold ice tea or popsicle.
- Fennel: Relieves coughs and cold symptoms and fights off gas and bloating.
- Ginger: Alleviates nausea and motion and morning sickness and boosts immunity.
- Hawthorn: Naturally lowers blood pressure and aids in heart health.
- Hibiscus: Naturally lowers blood pressure.
- Jasmine: Relaxes and helps you get to sleep; reduces inflammation and fights off viruses.
- Lavender: Calms and relaxes muscles. Aids in falling asleep.
- Lemon: Boosts immunity and detoxes liver, improves digestion.
- Lemon balm: Soothes and relaxes nerves and has a calming effect.
- Lemongrass: Eases pain and reduces digestive discomfort.
- Licorice: Aids digestion and fights off bacterial infections.
- Linden flower: Stimulates the hypothalamus to control body temperature and bring down a fever. Also dilates blood vessels to induce sweating.
- Maca: Boosts energy, relieves stress, and increases libido.
- Marshmallow: Aids the functioning of the digestive system and respiratory tract.
- Matcha: Boosts energy and increases focus and cognitive function.
- Mint: Boosts immunity, fights coughs and congestion.
- Oolong: Supports the malabsorption of fats and protects against free radicals.
- Passionflower: Promotes relaxation and sleep and naturally lowers blood pressure.
- Peppermint: Relaxes muscles of the digestive tract, reduces spasms, aids digestion. Also prevents flatulence.
- Plantain: Wards off bad colds and flus.
- Sencha: Boosts metabolism, regulates hunger and cravings.
- Reishi: Mushroom tea that soothes the nervous system and boosts immunity.
- Rooibos: Aids microbiome health, keeps free radicals at bay, and boosts immune system.
- Rose hip: Boosts immunity with an extra dose of vitamin C.

- *Tulsi*: Also known as holy basil, *tulsi* heals colds, flus, fever, congestion, and sore throats and aids digestion.
- Turmeric: Reduces inflammation and has anticancer properties.
- Yarrow: Calms nerves and soothes the mind for sleep.
- Yerba mate: Stimulant that wakes you up and aids in weight loss. Great when mixed with lemon tea.

When making your own herbal teas, check the list in this book for their medicinal purposes and don't be afraid to experiment. Try a mint–elderberry combo or add some shaved chocolate into mint or peppermint tea. Many of these teas can be made as cold ice teas or popsicles for kids, especially elderberry, lemon, lavender, lemon balm, mint, and peppermint. Elderberry popsicles can help fight off a cold, and your child is a lot more likely to try it than some awful-tasting OTC medicine. Lemon balm soothes children to sleep and is safe as opposed to using an antihistamine like Benadryl with its many side effects. Have your kids make the tea and popsicles with you as a family project. It teaches them about natural health and how Earth has so many wonderful gifts to offer; this is a great lesson for them to learn early. Check with the doctor if you are not sure about using herbal teas for children or while pregnant. Most are perfectly safe, though, and the only factor will be taste, so be sure to keep natural sweeteners on hand, including cinnamon.

Check with the doctor if you are not sure about using herbal teas for children or while pregnant. Most are perfectly safe....

If you do make your own tea, be careful where you buy your tea bags, as they can be made with toxins. Look for a vendor that sells organic tea bags free of fillers and chemical treatments so that you are not adding any unwanted contaminants into your homemade teas. Metal strainer balls are a great alternative because you don't have to keep restocking empty tea bags or worry about how they are made, which can get costly. They are also easier to use with less likelihood of the string getting in the liquid, resulting in burned fingertips. If using a metal strainer ball, be sure to clean it in hot water and watch for any rusting to the metal. Replace it at the first sign of rust.

Last but not least, if you are concerned about making herbal teas as medicinals or even just drinking for your own enjoyment, think about the water you make them with. Use a countertop water filter or one that goes right over your faucet to assure that the water the tea is made from carries no contaminants or heavy metals. It may cost a little more and be a little more inconvenient, but starting off with the purest, cleanest water possible will not only make a better tea, it will also make a better body. Purified and "glacier" water from the local grocery store is usually just glorified tap water, so your best bet is to filter it at home.

Herbal Treats

You will need reusable popsicle molds and a blender. Blend a handful each of elderberries, hibiscus flowers, rose hips, and orange zest. Add 1 cup of frozen berries of your choice and ½ cup of water. Blend until smooth and liquid enough to pour into the popsicle molds. Put in the popsicle sticks if needed, then put in the freezer until firm and enjoy. This blend is high in vitamin C and is a great way to get kids to get their fill of vitamin C while enjoying a cool treat on a hot, summer day. You can also leave out the frozen berries and make an infusion out of the elderberries, hibiscus flowers, rose hips, and orange zest. Put them into a tall glass or jar of water and seal. Leave this overnight to infuse the plant parts, then in the morning, use the infused water to make the popsicles.

Easy Raspberry Peach Popsicles

6 raspberry tea bags
6 peach tea bags
Fresh raspberries and peach slices or chunks

Boil 2 cups of water, pour into a bowl, and steep the raspberry tea bags for six to eight minutes. Boil 2 cups of water, pour into a bowl, and steep the peach tea bags for six to eight minutes. Let the teas in both bowls cool for a few minutes. Add sweetener to taste during this step. Pour into popsicle molds. Add the fruit as desired. Put into freezer. Once almost solid, put in popsicle sticks if they are not a part of the mold. Put back into freezer. That's it. You can use any variety of herbal teas on the market to make all kinds of popsicles.

Elderberry Popsicles

1 handful elderberries
1 handful rose hips
1 handful hibiscus flowers
Tea bag or ball strainer

Put the ingredients into the tea bag or ball strainer. Place into a pot of boiling water. Remove from heat and let the pot simmer. Steep the plant parts for 12–15 minutes. Remove the tea bag or ball strainer and add a touch of honey or sweetener to taste. Put the liquid into the popsicle molds. Freeze. Remove before solid if you need to stick in the sticks! Freeze again and enjoy!

Lavender Lemon Balm Popsicles

4 c. water in a saucepan or small pot
6 whole fresh lavender blossoms
¼ c. fresh lemon balm
2–4 tbsp. honey
1 qt. glass jar

Boil the water and pour over the lavender and lemon balm into a quart-sized glass jar. Steep for 15 minutes, then strain plant parts out with a mesh cloth or sleeve into another clean jar. Add in your honey or sweetener, seal the jar, and shake it up. When mixed, pour into popsicle molds. You can always make herbal ice cubes while you're at it, or get an Icee machine and make herbal Icees for kids. Add some white wine or sangria to make great adult popsicles.

Heart Pops and Cubes

Try this recipe for the blood pressure–lowering effects of hawthorn berries and the antioxidant power of rose hips. Hawthorn berries are one of the most widely studied and used herbal alternatives to blood pressure drugs, which have tons of side effects. You can choose to use fresh products, but you will need twice the amount as dried as a general rule.

Take ½ cup of dried hawthorn berries and ¼ cup of dried rose hips and put into a medium-sized pot with about 4 cups of water. Bring this to a boil, then reduce the heat and partially cover. When it's cooled, strain the tea and put into a glass pitcher that is heat safe. Add in 1 tablespoon of honey and pour into ice cube or ice pop molds. Put in the freezer until ready to use. You can also drink it right away as a warm tea, or let it cool enough to make a nice ice tea.

The Best Healing Herbal Teas for Kids

Before giving any child an herbal tea or something made with herbal teas, make sure they are not allergic to any of the ingredients.

If they are taking any prescription or OTC medications, check with their doctor first for possible interactions. These teas do not have any side effects and can be safely consumed in small doses when needed. Do not give to children under the age of 2 unless indicated, and always check first with their doctor at that age.

- Lemon balm tea: protects against viral, fungal, and bacterial infections. It can also calm them for bedtime.
- Fennel tea: You can give this to younger children, as it is a great remedy for colic and digestive issues and is a natural laxative.
- Ginger tea: Great for a tummy ache; gives relief from a cold, cough, whooping cough, or bronchitis; and tames nausea and motion sickness.
- Cardamom tea: Relieves stomachaches, gas, nausea, and indigestion and reduces phlegm.
- Mullein tea: Relieves coughs, colds, and whooping cough as well as symptoms of bronchitis, the flu, and earaches. It also helps with diarrhea and colic.
- Chamomile tea: Calms and soothes before bedtime and brings relief to stomachaches, gas, colic, colds, diaper rash, and nervousness.
- Rooibos tea: Helps with digestive issues, induces sleep, boosts immunity, and is a great overall health booster for kids.
- Red raspberry tea: Improves kidney and liver functioning but is rich in iron, so check with your pediatrician before administering.
- *Tulsi* or holy basil tea: Fights off colds and flus and clears out the respiratory tract for better breathing and less phlegm. Improves overall immunity in children and even improves their bowel movements.
- Elderberry tea: One of the tastiest and best health teas overall for its amazing list of healing properties.
- Mint tea with honey: This is a stronger tea but is flavorful and aids in teeth formation and relieves stomachaches and tummy troubles.

You can make your own herbal teas for kids as you would for adults, but be aware of the dosage. One cup is enough. If you are uncertain, you can buy herbal remedies for children that are premade and in the proper dosage. Teas are generally mild enough for children, but some herbs can be more potent than others. Never use an herb you have never heard of. Stick with these commonly used herbs when giving them to your children. You can be a little more experimental as an adult. These teas might need a touch of natural sweetener or honey to sweeten to taste.

Herbal Elixirs

> 1 qt. jar or container, preferably glass
>
> 3½ c. water
>
> 2–3 c. fresh herbs of choice
>
> 1 c. sugar, honey, stevia, or natural sweetener (be aware that stevia is extremely sweet, so you will use a lot less; experiment with this)

Elixirs are sweetened infusions of herbs mixed with alcohol, soda, or sparkling water. They are meant to be consumed cold. The process takes about 20 minutes.

Pack the jar full of herbs, preferably fresh. Cover the herbs with boiling water. Steep for 20 minutes. Strain out the liquid through a cheesecloth into a glass jar or container and stir in sweetener until completely dissolved. This should last up to two months refrigerated. You can also infuse dried herbs in brandy or a sweeter alcohol with raw honey. If using brandy or another alcohol, the process takes a bit longer. After you cover your jar of herbs with honey and alcohol, seal the jar and let this mixture brew for at least one month before straining out and bottling or drinking. Shake the jar once daily to keep everything fermenting properly. Make a cold elixir using the above recipe, but cover the herbs with cold, sparkling water and a touch of honey to sweeten. Try the sun method of making elixirs by putting the jar in direct sunlight indoors or out. Instead of adding boiling water, seal the jar and put it in a sunny spot for up to two weeks. Shake the jar once daily. As always, if you are more of a visual learner, many how-to videos are available to help guide you through the process of making elixirs and offer up intriguing herb combinations to try.

Herbal Infusions, Concoctions, and Decoctions

Like teas, herbal infusions and concoctions are steeped liquids that usually use the softer plant parts such as leaves and flowers, where the cell wall can rupture more easily and allow water to enter. The cells of plant bark, berries, seeds, and roots are tougher and require more work to break down the cell walls, which is called a decoction. Infusions and concoctions draw out vitamins, enzymes, and

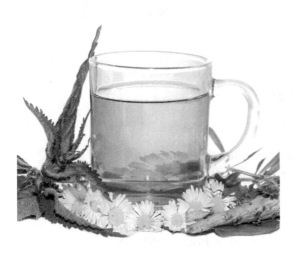

Concoctions use the soft parts of plants, which are then steeped in hot water, typically.

aromas from volatile oils. Infusions and concoctions can include flowers, roots, and leaves in their dried or powdered form or as essential oils. Making tea to drink is an act of creating an infusion, and infusions can be refrigerated as a cold drink or frozen into ice pops.

Infusions and concoctions are normally consumed as hot or cold teas or frozen as popsicles or ice cubes, but they can also be topical healing agents or used in an herbal bath or wash. A hot infusion of herbs and plant parts draws out the healing properties of flowers, leaves, aromatic roots, and dried herbs. Herbs can be mixed and matched to create any number of infusions in the form of teas or hot drinks. The longer the plant parts or herbs are steeped, the more powerful the flavor and nutrients.

Water is the usual base for an infusion, but you can use wine, juices, or oils. Some infusions that contain acidic ingredients may react with metal, so use a glass, enamel, or ceramic container. Avoid mixing and pouring infusions into nonstick containers, aluminum, or pewter, as toxins can leach into the mixture.

How to make a hot infusion: Put 1–3 tablespoons of dried herbs or plant parts (chopped or ground) into a tea strainer. Place the strainer in a teapot or mug. Heat water to boil. Pour hot water over herbs/plant parts to cover them. Cover the teapot or mug to allow the volatile oils to remain trapped. Steep for 15–20 minutes, then strain and use. Steep longer for a stronger infusion.

Some herbs will be better cold infused, such as mucinous herbs like peppermint leaf, rosebuds, marshmallow root, freshly harvested herbs, and lemon balm. Cold infusions are made by filling a quart–sized jar with cold water. Take approximately 1–2 ounces of the herb/plant matter and put on a cheesecloth or inside a tea or muslin bag. Wet the herbs in the bag quickly, then submerge them into the jar below the waterline. Cover the jar and allow the blend to infuse overnight. Strain herbs the next morning with a mesh screen or clean cheesecloth, pushing down on the herbs with a spatula or spoon. Cold infusions can be made into juice pops for kids, too, with a touch of natural sweetener if needed and are great for the hotter summer months as iced drinks.

Infusions for Healthy Skin

Half of the fun of making herbal infusions is going over a list of herbs to decide which ones you want to blend together to heal what ails you. When it comes to healthy skin, certain herbs work better than others:

- Acne: Try a peppermint and birch bark infusion with a few drops of lavender oil, or try witch hazel extract infused with lemon balm and tea tree oil
- Dry skin: Try a rose infusion with a spoonful of honey and 1 tablespoon of almond oil
- Rosacea: Try water or vinegar infused with rolled oats wrapped in a bag or sack, and add a little chamomile to soothe skin
- Eczema: Try equal parts chamomile, nettle, and calendula with a spoonful of honey or Epsom salt dissolved into the mix
- Irritated skin: Try equal parts water, comfrey, and calendula or equal parts water and aloe vera gel

Beauty Booster Infusions

For general beauty boosters, always choose fresh herbs over dried. Some herbs known to improve the look of skin and hair or for their detoxing effects to make you look younger are nettle, dandelion, calendula, rose, elderflower, and lavender. You can add them all to one infusion or mix and match. You don't even have to drink the infusion to get the benefits. Take a cotton ball and rub the cooled infusion over skin as a great toner after you wash your face and before applying makeup. Try a facial steam by placing a steaming bowl of your chosen mix on a table and leaning over it, covering your head with a towel. Keep your eyes closed, though. Beauty infusions can also be used to rinse hair after shampooing. Try to use them once made within a few days, and you can keep any extra in the refrigerator.

Herbal Decoctions

A decoction is a strong tea blend made of roots, berries, bark, and seeds. It is simmered to extract the properties of these plant parts and is much stronger and more concentrated than an infusion but not as strong as a tincture. The dictionary definition of a decoction is "an aqueous preparation of plant parts boiled in water for 15–20 minutes until the water volume is halved."

When making a decoction, grind or crush the root, bark, or seeds beforehand to bring out the healing agents and properties. You can preheat the plant parts in a little water for a half hour and then use the liquid as the foundation of your decoction. Break the plant parts or grind them up and place into an earthenware container if you have one. A glass jar will work, too. Cover the plant parts with water, cover the container, then boil it until the water volume is halved. The preparation is then strained, cooled, and either used right away or refrigerated. It can keep for approximately three days.

If you don't have an earthenware container, place the ground or crushed plant parts into a small saucepan with 1 quart of cold water. Slowly heat the water to simmer and cover. Simmer between 20–45 minutes. Strain the water into a quart–sized jar. Keep the herbs in the strainer. The water will not fill the jar, so you can add a bit of hot water over the herbs in the strainer until the jar is full. Once you are ready to use the decoction, usually either as a warm tea or cold drink/ice pops, you can add natural sweeteners such as honey or stevia to taste. This kind of decoction can also be used in herbal syrups or added to juices.

The dictionary definition of a decoction is "an aqueous preparation of plant parts boiled in water for 15–20 minutes until the water volume is halved."

If you want a stronger decoction, use the woody parts of the plant like the stem or bark. However, this decoction should be allowed to sit overnight after boiling before you strain out the herbs/plant parts. Also, press the plant parts into the strainer with a spatula or spoon to get as much of the decoction out as possible. Decoctions are stronger than infusions, so a typical serving size would be ¼–1 cup, depending on the herbs you've chosen.

Some great choices for decoctions include chicory, astragalus, elderberry, burdock root, cinnamon, hawthorn berry, dandelion root, pine needles, rose hips, ginger root, willow bark, chicory, and echinacea root.

Detox Teas

These quick and easy herbal teas are known to help detoxify the body:

- Dandelion root tea: Boil 2 tea-spoons of dried dandelion root in 1 cup of water. Turn off heat, cover the pot, and let it steep for 10 minutes. Strain and drink the tea twice daily, once in the morning and once in the evening, for several days.

- Licorice root tea: Known for clearing out chemical contaminants from the body, it can also cut cravings for sugary foods. Crush licorice root and add 1 tablespoon and 1 teaspoon of ground ginger to a pot with 1–2 cups water. Bring to a boil and lower heat to simmer. Let it simmer for 10 minutes. Strain the mix and drink the liquid with a little lemon juice added once a day for three to five days.

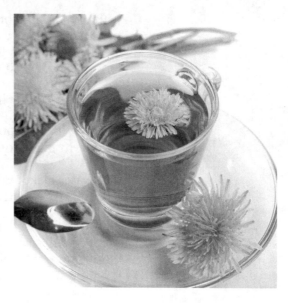

The wonderfully versatile dandelion "weed" can be drunk in a tea to detox your system.

- Turmeric tea: Turmeric detoxes the liver and purifies the blood. Mix 1 teaspoon of turmeric powder with the juice of a lemon, a pinch of cayenne pepper, and organic honey to taste with 1 cup of warm water. Drink once daily for three to five days. You can drink this for two weeks if you feel you need the extra detoxing. You can also add ginger powder instead of cayenne pepper for a different taste.

- Lemon ginger tea: You will need a 3–inch piece of ginger. Peel the ginger and slice very thinly. Pour into a pot of 2 cups of water and bring to a boil. Let it boil for 10–15 minutes with the lid on, then remove from heat and let the mix cool down. When it is warm, put it in a mug and add a squeeze of lemon juice or lemon–flavored stevia for some extra sweetness. Lemon is a known detoxer, but ginger has the added benefit of fighting free radical damage in the body caused by heavy metal exposure.

- Stinging nettle tea: A great blood detoxer, this herbal tea is also a diuretic that helps eliminate waste and stimulates the lymphatic system. Dry and crush some nettle leaves. Add 1 teaspoon to 1 cup of water and boil. Cover the pot and let it steep for 10 minutes. Strain and drink two times a day.

- Green tea: Green tea is one of the most potent detoxing teas. The extracts from the green tea leaves work to remove toxins that are often associated with signs of aging on the face or body. You can make your own green tea by steeping the leaves for 10–20 minutes in hot water, then straining, or buy green tea, but look for organic with no additives or fillers. Green tea can be consumed once or twice a day and because it helps to oxidize fats in the body, it can aid in weight loss, too. The extracts also come in a supplement form for those who don't like tea.

Water Infusions for Health

Try these water infusions, which you can allow to steep overnight, preferably in glass containers, before drinking:

- Rice water makes skin and hair glow and boosts energy.
- Barley water flushes out toxins and cleanses the system.
- Raisin water daily on an empty stomach makes skin glow and banishes acne.
- Cinnamon water balances blood sugar and prevents cravings.
- Fennel water enhances digestion, reduces menstrual cramping, and aids in weight loss.
- Coriander seed water balances hormones and aids digestion and immunity.
- Lemon water enhances immunity, aids digestion, smoothes skin, and flattens the belly.
- Mint water detoxes the body, improves digestion, and clears skin.
- Ginger water reduces bloating, cures the common cold, and relieves headaches.
- Cucumber water flushes out toxins, soothes skin, and helps you have a healthy complexion.
- Lemon/ginger water made with half a lemon squeezed into a cup of water with a few slices of ginger several times a day boosts the immune system and reduces mucous buildup.
- Cucumber/grapefruit water aids in weight loss.
- Cucumber/lemon/mint/ginger water reduces stomach bloating.
- Apple/cinnamon stick water boosts metabolism.
- Cucumber/mint/lemon water clears skin.

Psyllium

Psyllium is an herb from the seed of the fleawort plant that expands when it comes in contact with liquid. People take powdered psyllium as a great source of extra fiber. It scrubs the clogged muck from the digestive system and cleans out the intestines by removing toxins. It must be taken with plenty of water, though, because it utilizes a lot of liquid to do its detoxing magic.

Smell Your Way to Weight Loss

A study done by Dr. Alan Hirsch, the neurological director of the Smell and Taste Treatment and Research Foundation in Chicago, Illinois, found that people who smell banana, green apple, or peppermint several times a day lost an average of 30 pounds in six months. These scents in particular foods curb cravings, so try it and see if your nose can help you drop some excess body fat. It only works if done consistently, but it certainly can't hurt. However, don't offset any benefits by overindulging in junk foods, thinking you can smell your way out of a bad diet.

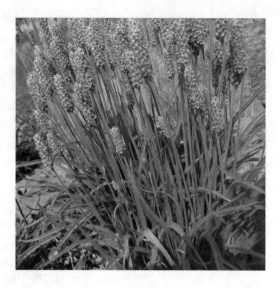

The psyllium plant, which is cultivated in northern India, is a good source of dietary fiber that is great for the digestive system.

Home Remedies for Constipation

Try these home remedies to relieve constipation and get you on a regular schedule again:

- Drink more water! Water helps move poop through the body and keeps it from becoming hard and painful in the colon or intestines.
- Get exercise. Moving the body assists the activity of the alimentary system, which digests food and moves it to the waste organs.
- Drink coffee. It makes you poop!
- Eat popcorn! Three cups of popcorn, without the butter or fake margarine, is a great fiber boost, and fiber is great for regularity. Other pro–poop foods include figs, raisins, and good old prunes. A glass of prune juice can get you back on the throne as well as any OTC constipation medication and is a lot healthier, or eat figs, raisins, or prunes alone for a tasty treat with a sweet touch.
- Try 1 teaspoon of aloe vera gel to get things moving smoothly.
- Honey and molasses are known to move the poop out, so try them in your tea.
- Speaking of tea, try a cup of the following, all known to alleviate constipation: ginger (warms and generates heat, aids digestion); pep-

permint (the menthol soothes an upset stomach to move stool through the intestines); chamomile (relaxes the digestive muscles to easily move bowels along); licorice root (eases digestive issues after a meal); dandelion root (stimulates the liver and alleviates mild constipation); or black or green tea (stimulate the movement of bowels).

- Lemon juice helps you move those bowels, so add some to tea or just squeeze the juice into a warm glass of water.
- Dairy products often cause constipation, but warm milk can stimulate the bowels and works better when ghee is added. Ghee is clarified butter and has been used in Ayurvedic medicine as a healing food for thousands of years. Try adding 1–2 teaspoons of ghee to a glass of warm milk in the evening to have a good bowel movement upon waking up.
- Fennel is a mild laxative. You can roast fennel and add it to a glass of warm water to drink at night. The seeds increase gastric enzymes in the digestive system to move poop through the colon.
- Finally, try some senna, an herb that has been used for thousands of years as a natural laxative. It helps the digestive tract contract and can be taken in capsule form or as a tea.
- You can also try taking more vitamins C, B5, or B6 or folic acid to help keep you regular.

If constipation persists, you can try an OTC medication, but if accompanied by pain, see your doctor right away.

Diaper Cream

Mix equal parts dried calendula flowers, dried Oregon grape root, and dried comfrey leaves in a bowl and place into a quart–sized jar until half full. Cover the herbs completely with olive oil. Cover the jar and place lid on tightly. Store in a warm place such as a sunny windowsill to infuse for two weeks, shaking the jar daily. Strain the plant parts with a cheesecloth or muslin and use the liquid when needed.

Diaper Ointment

1 c. extra virgin olive oil

¼ c. grated beeswax or beeswax pastilles

6 drops vitamin E oil (or three vitamin E capsules broken open)

Put a metal spoon in the freezer. In the top of a double boiler over medium–low heat, combine oil and beeswax. Heat until the beeswax has melted and the mixture is incorporated. Dip the spoon from the freezer into the pot. If the oil no longer drips off the spoon, the salve is ready for containers. If it drips, add a little more beeswax. If it seems too stiff, add more oil. You can pour a little of the oil/beeswax mixture into the spoon and place it back in the freezer for one to two minutes to get a better sense of the final consistency. Remove from heat. After mixture has cooled slightly but before it starts to solidify, stir in vitamin E oil. Pour warm oil into tins or upcycled glass jars with lids. Allow salve to cool completely before placing lids on containers. Remember to label your containers! Store in a cool, dry place. If stored properly, salves can last two to three years.

Remedies for Depression

The herbs listed in this book are chock full of vitamins, supplements, herbs, and plants that help fight depression and anxiety, but here are a few superstars:

- St. John's wort: The herb St. John's wort (*Hypericum perforatum*) has long been used to treat depression, seasonal depression, anxiety, nervousness, and insomnia. Numerous clinical trials suggest that St. John's wort may be effective against mild to moderate depression but not as effective for major depression. St. John's wort is taken mainly in supplement form, and it can take between two to six weeks to notice the full effect. Side effects include dizziness, dry mouth, indigestion, and fatigue. St. John's wort increases photosensitivity, so you should avoid direct sunlight and sunbathing if taking it. St. John's wort can interfere with the effectiveness of prescription and over-the-counter drugs, such as antidepressants, drugs to treat HIV infections and AIDS, drugs to prevent organ rejection for transplant patients, and oral contraceptives. It is not recommended for pregnant and nursing women, children, or anyone with liver or kidney disease.

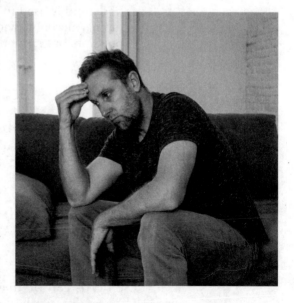

Depression can have many causes, some of which are physiological. You should consult with a professional psychologist or psychiatrist if you have severe or persistent feelings of depression.

- Omega-3 fatty acids: Omega-3 fatty acids such as fish oil and krill oil have been shown in studies to reduce symptoms of depression. Studies have also found that countries with higher fish consumption, such as Japan, have a lower rate of depression. Preliminary studies suggest that omega-3s (DHA and EPA) together with antidepressants may be more effective than antidepressants alone. You can eat more coldwater fish, such as salmon, sardines, and anchovies, all rich sources of omega-3 fatty acids. Fish oil capsules may interact with blood thinners such as warfarin and aspirin and should not be taken for two weeks before or after surgery. Side effects include indigestion and bleeding.

- SAM-e: S-adenosyl-L-methionine (SAM-e) is a compound found in the human body that increases levels of the neurotransmitters serotonin and dopamine. Several studies have found SAM-e to be more effective than a placebo for depression. SAM-e is available in supplement form, and the enteric-coated form offers greater absorption.

- Folic acid: Folate is a B vitamin found in green, leafy vegetables; fruit; beans; and fortified grains. Preliminary research suggests that people with depression who also have low folate levels may not respond as well to antidepressants. Taking folic acid in supplement form may improve the effectiveness of antidepressants.

- 5-HTP: 5-hydroxytryptophan (5-HTP) is produced naturally in the body and is used in the formation of the neurotransmitter serotonin. Anecdotal evidence shows that taking 5-HTP improves depression, but more research is needed.

Herbs for Anxiety

Several different herbs are known to help alleviate anxiety symptoms, relax, and feel calmer. These include:

- Lavender
- Lemon balm
- Chamomile
- Passionflower
- Kava

These herbs can be made into teas, infusions, syrups, and tinctures. They are also available in capsules.

Aromatherapy uses essential oils to reduce anxiety and bring about a state of calmness and serenity. You can use a diffuser, place a few drops on a cotton ball and inhale, or mix your favorite scent in a carrier oil to dab on your wrist or neck. Scents to use for anxiety include:

- Lavender
- Ylang ylang
- Grapefruit
- Clary sage
- Bergamont

Hemp–derived CBD oil can bring about calmness and alleviate anxiety without the high of THC. While research is still in early stages, studies show it may have potential as an alternative anxiety treatment. You can find CBD products in many mainstream stores and in the following forms:

- CBD oil tinctures (liquid drops)
- CBD gummies
- CBD chocolate and candies
- CBD topicals (creams or lotions)

Healing Diabetes Naturally

Diabetes is a serious disease that requires working with your doctor on a plan of action with diet, exercise, and possibly medication. You can look into reducing your blood sugar levels in natural ways but never as a replacement for standard care.

American ginseng shows promise for the treatment of diabetes. A meta–analysis has shown that American ginseng may significantly improve blood sugar control and fasting glucose (a marker of your general blood sugar levels) by increasing your body's insulin sensitivity. Look for capsules with a standardized extract of ginsenosides, the active ingredient.

Chromium is an essential trace mineral that plays an important role in carbohydrate and fat metabolism and helps body cells properly respond to insulin. Studies have found that the incidence of diabetes was lower in people who took chromium within the previous month; a recent review study looked at 20 different randomized, controlled trials on chromium and found that supplementing did decrease fasting plasma glucose levels in five of the 20 studies, while hemoglobin A1C decreased by 0.5 percent in five of the 14 studies.

Magnesium is a mineral found in green, leafy vegetables; nuts; seeds; and whole grains and is needed for more than 300 different biochemical reactions. It helps regulate blood sugar levels and normal muscle and nerve function, heart rhythm, immune function, blood pressure, and bone health. Normal dosage should have few side effects, but taking larger doses is not recommended, as it interacts with medications for osteoporosis, high blood pressure, antibiotics, muscle relaxants, and diuretics.

Cinnamon has glucose–lowering ability and reduces lipid biomarkers including triglycerides, low–density lipoprotein cholesterol, and total cholesterol. A recent triple–blind, placebo–controlled, randomized clinical trial looked at cinnamon supplementation in 140 people with Type 2 diabetes over three months. Study subjects were divided into groups and either given two capsules per day of 500 milligrams of cinnamon powder each or a placebo. After three months, the statistically significant findings included improvements in body mass index (BMI), visceral fat, body fat, fasting plasma glucose, A1C, insulin production, insulin resistance, and lipids as compared to the placebo group. The greatest effects were noticed in those with a BMI over 27.

Studies suggest that the herb gymnema (*Gymnema sylvestre*) lowers blood sugar levels in people with Type 2 diabetes. The herb also reduces fat accumulation and helps with weight loss, thanks to its enzyme–inhibiting properties. It is also a potent antioxidant that can prevent the organ damage that often accompanies diabetes. It can lower blood sugar levels significantly, so never take with another diabetes medication and consult with your doctor first.

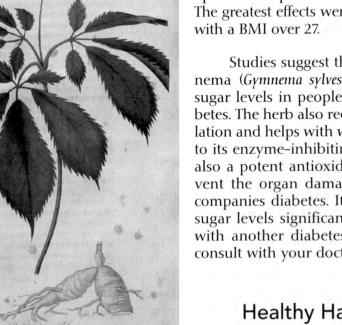

Not all ginseng comes from Asia. American ginseng is native to the eastern United States and has been used for centuries in traditional Native American medicine.

Healthy Hangover Remedies

Hangovers are no fun. In addition to the usual suggestions of sleeping it off, drinking the hair of the dog that bit you, and guzzling buckets of water, these natural plants are great choices:

- Korean pear juice: This is considered an old-school hangover remedy. Research shows that drinking about 7.5 ounces lowers blood alcohol levels and makes hangovers less intense. The catch: you have to drink it before you imbibe, as it won't work afterward. Korean pears break down alcohol faster, so if you know you are going to be drinking, you may want to down a glass ahead of time.

- Ginseng: Chinese medicine reveres the ginseng root and has for thousands of years, thanks to its many properties. It works to alleviate stress, asthma symptoms, and hangover symptoms when used in a drink form. You can try some ginseng tea after you've had a few drinks.

- Siberian ginseng extract: Another herb that improves hangover symptoms such as dizziness, headache, and stomachache.

- *Phyllanthus amarus*: This is a medicinal herb that grows along tropical coasts and is used to treat the liver, kidney, and stomach. Taking the extract twice a day for 10 days can lower blood alcohol levels, ease hangover symptoms, and improve mood all at the same time.

Natural Remedies for Motion Sickness

Motion sickness is the result of nausea and sickness from the sensation of movement that happens on planes, trains, and boats and in cars. Those who suffer from it know the awful feeling of wanting to vomit or faint and often break out in cold sweats and become delirious if they do not get relief in a timely manner. Other than taking prescription meds or OTC meds like Dramamine and Bonine, which come with side effects such as drowsiness, here are some natural ways to combat motion sickness:

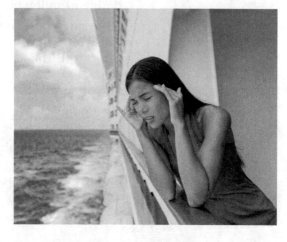

To lessen feelings of motion sickness, try drinking more (avoid caffeine) and try some simple tricks such as breathing exercises or pressing on the pericardium.

- Drink plenty of water and eat small meals before traveling.

- Avoid trigger situations such as sitting backward on a train or subway or riding in the back seat of a car.

- Avoid caffeine and alcohol before traveling.

- Tilting your head into turns may help, according to a study published in *Ergonomics* in 2016. Researchers found that passengers experienced less motion sickness when they tilted their heads into the direction of a turn and kept their eyes open.

- In one small study published in the 2015 *Aerospace Medicine and Human Performance*, participants either practiced slow, diaphragmatic breathing at a rate of six breaths per minute or breathed normally while viewing a virtual reality simulation of a boat on rough seas. The diaphragmatic breathers had a greater heart rate variability and less motion sickness than the normal breathers.

- Do not read or look at your cell phone or computer while traveling, as the balance center of the inner ear senses movement that contradicts the fixed words on the screen and sends your brain mixed messages that result in nausea. Look instead at the horizon.

- Try pressing the pericardium 6 pressure point used in Chinese acupressure. This point is located on the inner side of the forearm about 2 inches above the crease of the wrist between the two tendons. Press on this point with the index finger of your other hand. You can also find acupressure wristbands to wear that do this for you.

- Ginger root is a widely used remedy for nausea and motion sickness. It can be taken in the form of tea, chews, lozenges, capsules, tablets, candies, or ginger ale. If you are on blood thinners, beware of using ginger and check with your doctor first. You can also cut raw ginger root slices to suck on before and while traveling. You can also put a few drops of ginger essential oil onto a hankie or cloth and sniff while traveling.

- Peppermint oil also relieves nausea. Carry a bottle of essential oil with you on travels and pour 2–3 drops onto a cloth to sniff as you travel. The aroma helps stop nausea. Smelling a cut lemon works, too, as the acidic nature of the lemon neutralizes acids that cause nausea.

- Try sipping pickle juice to balance pH and restore electrolytes, which prevent hangovers, vomiting, and nausea.

- Before traveling, take vitamins B6 and B12, which are known to alleviate nausea, or try a cup or two of chamomile tea or licorice root tea to ease nausea and calm you down.

Healing Creams

You can buy these creams at drugstores and online. Look for creams with no fillers and pure ingredients; try an allergy test first on the inside of your elbow to check for a reaction.

- Calendula cream: Use only on superficial wounds, burns, rashes, itchy areas, and cuts to alleviate inflammation and promote healing. This cream can prevent further infection and works even better if it includes comfrey or plantain in the ingredient list. Do not apply to anything deeper than a surface wound or cut because it will quickly heal the surface skin without allowing the deeper tissue wounds to heal first and could trap in microbes and bacteria.

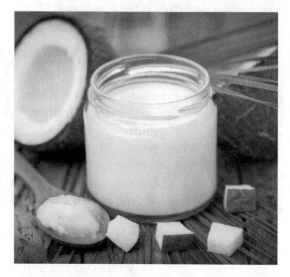

Coconut oil has been gaining in popularity in the United States, both as a healthy ingredient in cooking and also because it is great for your skin!

- Aloe vera gel: A super healing gel that you can get right from the plant itself or buy in a tube form. Heals burns, itchy areas, rashes, sores, cuts, and stings. Keeping an aloe vera plant in a bedroom can help clean the air of toxins, and when you need the healing gel, just snip off a piece and use it. It won't kill the plant.

- Arnica cream: Arnica is an all-purpose healer that comes in a cream or a gel and can be applied to unbroken skin to heal bruises, sprains, bumps, and strains. Do not apply to broken skin or open wounds.

- Coconut oil: Whether it's a bite, sting, cut, rash, or blister, you can rub some melted coconut oil on the skin and let its antibacterial and anti-inflammatory properties do their healing magic. You can also rub some on mouth sores and ulcers. Coconut oil can also be rubbed on white patches on the skin three to four times a day for quick healing.

- Tea tree oil: Rub this potent oil on wounds or acne and watch it heal like magic. It disinfects as it heals and also assists hair growth when rubbed into the scalp. As a powerful antibacterial, it heals athlete's foot, acne, nail fungus, and insect bites and kills lice. It is a traditional medicinal that has been used by the Australian Aborigines for centuries.

- Grape seed extract: Topical application of this powerful antioxidant can speed up the healing of wounds and promote dermal cell regeneration and healing.

The Benefits of Oil Pulling

Around 700 types of bacteria can be found in your mouth. Many of these are harmful and cause tooth decay and gum disease. Because of the heavy bacterial load in the oral cavity, which can lead to inflammation and eventually heart disease, the ancient Ayurvedic practice of oil pulling has become all the rage in modern times as a way of keeping the mouth healthy and clean. This simple and natural detox eliminates toxins and bacteria from the mouth and can reduce gum disease, bad breath, toothaches, *Candida* infections, cold sores, and gingivitis. The antimicrobial effect of the oil has a waterfall effect on the body by reducing inflammation throughout and benefiting digestion and heart health, relieving pain, and improving the immune system.

It is called oil pulling because the oil pulls the bacteria from the teeth and gums. Basically, you swish 1 tablespoon of either sesame, sunflower, olive, or coconut oil in your mouth as if you were using mouthwash. Do this for a minimum of 15 minutes until the oil becomes thinner and foamy. Then, spit the oil into a bag or trash can to dispose of. Do not spit into the sink, as it can clog your drains. Follow this with your regular teeth brushing and rinsing. Do it daily for a few weeks to get the best results. Never gargle or swallow the oil, as it is filled with the bacteria and toxins that have been pulled from the mouth.

The American Dental Association does not endorse oil pulling, citing no credible evidence, but another study with 20 children showed that oil pulling over a two-week period reduced the presence of harmful bacteria and plaque, which causes cavities, as well as any mouthwash.

Oil pulling also helps to increase saliva production, which in turn moisturizes gums and dry sockets. Some say it can also whiten teeth. The key is to use an edible, high-quality oil and only use 1 tablespoon of it each time. Coconut oil has been suggested by many oil-pulling devotees to be the best for getting rid of mouth bacteria. In a 2007 study for the *Indian Journal of Dental Research*, 10 men did oil pulling for 10 days, and 10 men did not. The ones who did showed a reduction of plaque.

The American Dental Association does not endorse oil pulling, citing no credible evidence, but another study with 20 children showed that oil pulling over a two-week period reduced the presence of harmful bacteria and plaque, which causes cavities, as well as any mouthwash. Another study with 60 participants who rinsed their mouths with either mouthwash, coconut oil, or water for two weeks found that those who used the oil had a reduction of bacteria in their saliva. Reducing bacteria not only helps prevent cavities, gingivitis, and gum disease, it also fights bad breath by eliminating the bacteria trapped on the tongue.

Oil pulling is cheap and easy and has been shown to reduce inflammation, which can only add to overall better health throughout the body. It also doesn't contain sugars or aluminum, which are found in most mouthwashes.

Herbal Tinctures

Tinctures are liquid extracts from herbs that are taken orally and often include alcohol. They are a lot stronger as medicinals than herbal infusions, concoctions, or decoctions. They can also be extracted in apple cider vinegar or vegetable glycerin if you are making them for children. Tinctures are easy to make, and the extraction liquid makes the herbal properties stronger and more effective and helps them enter the bloodstream directly. Some tinctures work immediately, but others may require a buildup in the bloodstream over time to work effectively. If you are not the crafty DIY type, plenty of how-to videos are available on YouTube and herbal remedy websites that can show you how to make a tincture step by step.

Tinctures are made like teas but without the brewing and are administered via a dropper as opposed to a spoon like herbal syrups. A dropperful is the equivalent to approximately 30 drops. The general dosage for adults is 2 droppersful two or three times a day. Children under 12 can take 1 dropperful twice a day but check first with their pediatrician to see if it might interfere with medicines they are taking. Tinctures are not recommended for children under the age of 2. You can also add 1–2 droppersful directly to a cup of warm water to make a tea. Pregnant and nursing women should avoid tinctures because of the alcohol content.

Tinctures made with alcohol last for a couple of years if kept in a cool, dark place and don't need to be kept in the refrigerator. Without alcohol, the shelf life is much shorter, and they must be kept in the fridge. To make tinctures, you will need a clean, glass pint-size or

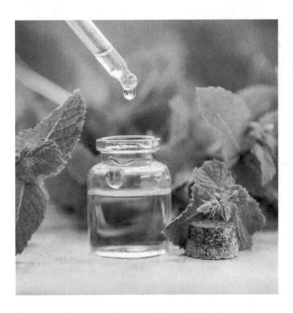

Extract of peppermint, combined with ginger root and alcohol such as vodka or rum, makes an excellent tincture that can help with diarrhea, nausea, indigestion, irritable bowel syndrome, menstrual pain, flatulence, and even muscle and nerve pain and anxiety.

bigger jar with a lid, herbs of your choice, and either vodka, rum, apple cider vinegar, or vegetable oil. You will fill your jar between one-third and one-half full with herbs, then pour in boiling water to dampen them, or just fill the jar to the top with your alcohol or nonalcoholic liquid, and stir the mix.

A general rule of thumb is about 4 ounces of finely chopped or ground herbs to 1 pint of alcohol (or nonalcoholic liquid of choice). Cover tightly with lid and label and date the jar. Store in a cool, dark place because light can destroy the compounds. Shake the tincture every day for the first week or two, then let it sit for four to six weeks. Strain off the herbs with a strainer, cheesecloth, or a very clean T-shirt. Squeeze more of the tincture out of the herbs by pressing down on them with a spatula. Pour the tincture into your dropper bottles.

Here are two recipes that can serve as templates for making your own tinctures.

Peppermint Tincture

½ c. dried peppermint leaves

¼ c. ground ginger root

1 ½ c. boiling water

1 ½ c. vodka, rum, or nonalcoholic apple cider vinegar or glycerin

1 glass jar with lid, quart size

Place the herbs in the glass jar and pour the boiling water in the jar, covering the herbs. Fill the rest of the jar with your alcoholic or nonalcoholic choice of liquid. Cover the jar with the lid and store for two to six weeks. Shake the jar daily. When ready to use, strain out the plant parts and store the liquid in smaller jars or droppers. Adults can take 1 dropperful (or 1 teaspoon) as needed. Children can take

10–12 drops of the nonalcoholic tincture once a day, but check with their doctor first. Use the same process as above but with ½–1 cup of dried chamomile or lavender flowers for a calming tincture that works well for children.

Maceration Versus Percolation

Tinctures can be made using two different methods:

- Maceration: soaking or steeping herbs or plant parts to make them soft and separate the compounds out.
- Percolation: the process of seeping water through the herbs or plant parts by filtering into a liquid via a porous material like a cloth or coffee filter.

Maceration involves biological and chemical processes to soften herbs and allow the active compounds to enter the liquid used in the tincture. Alcohol helps this process along. Maceration takes a lot more time because after you prepare your tincture you must let it sit for at least a month before straining the liquid.

Maceration takes a lot more time because after you prepare your tincture you must let it sit for at least a month before straining the liquid.

Percolation is a lot quicker because once the plant parts are strained out, the liquid sits for about 24 hours maximum. Gravity pulls the liquid down from the plant parts and allows more of the compounds to drip from the bottom of the filter into the jar. The result is a much stronger tincture because the ingredients are fresher and have not been distilled for weeks or longer as you would with maceration, but both are great ways to extract compounds from herbs for your tinctures. It's all a matter of individual style and time.

Tinctures are popular items online and in health stores, but they are easy and inexpensive to make, so make your own and avoid unnecessary ingredients or high packaging costs. They also make great gifts for friends and family, and you can order vials, droppers, or boxes to put them in or make in larger amounts to give in small, decorative mason jars. Though it is often the alcoholic content that adds to their potency, it is not a necessary ingredient. If you prefer something other than vodka or rum, experiment.

Oxymels

An oxymel is an herbal preparation similar to a tincture but made with vinegar and honey. Oxymels have been around for thousands of years and were suggested as medicinals by Hippocrates for their special healing properties. You can make any apple cider vinegar tincture and mix in raw honey to taste, adding more if it still tastes too vinegary. Oxymels are best when using spicy, pungent herbs, as the honey will tone down the overwhelming taste. Garlic, ginger, basil, cayenne, and other aromatics are often used in making oxymels. You can make them both hot as teas or cold with ice cubes and some soda water. The honey will appeal more to children than straight apple cider vinegar tinctures, but don't give honey to children under the age of 2.

Glycerin Tinctures

Like oxymels, glycerin-based tinctures don't add alcohol. A glycerin tincture, or glycerite, is made by adding vegetable glycerin, which has a sweet taste, so you don't need to add honey. They are great for kids because they avoid the sourness of vinegar and the problems of giving honey to younger toddlers.

Bitters

Bitters are traditionally alcoholic preparations that are flavored with plant matter to impart a bitter or bittersweet flavor. They were originally developed as medicinals and are now also sold and consumed as digestifs and cocktails. Most bitters are made with aromatic herbs, bark, roots, fruit, and berries for flavor and healing compounds. Common ingredients in bitters include orange peel, cassia, cascarilla, gentian, and cinchona bark. The alcohol serves as a solvent for the plant part extracts while also acting as a preservative. You can buy bitters premade or learn online how to make them but be prepared for a different taste experience than the milder herbal teas and infusions because they are very concentrated liquid extracts similar to the vanilla extract used in baking.

If you want to try your hand at making bitters yourself, you will need bittering agents, aromatics, and alcohol. Bittering agents can be any edible roots such as burdock or licorice or bark such as wild cherry or sarsaparilla. Aromatics are things like citrus peels, dried fruits, herbs such as mint, rosemary, sage, and various spices, or try coffee beans or toasted nuts. Alcohol should be vodka or grain alcohol, although you can use rye, rum, or bourbon.

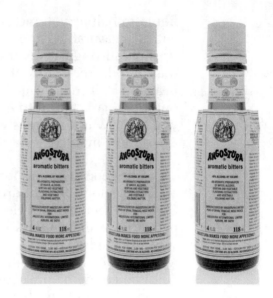

In a small glass jar, put your spice/herb/fruit/etc. at the bottom: 1–2 teaspoons, coarsely chopped. Cover with about 4 ounces of alcohol. Cover the jar tightly, and make sure to label what herbs you used. Shake the jar once a day to mix up the ingredients. Taste and/or smell the infusion daily; some ingredients will be infused within one week and others several weeks. To taste the tincture as it ages, add a few drops into a small glass of sparkling water. If you taste it directly, the flavor may taste too intense. When the mixture is ready, strain through a cheesecloth into smaller jars or receptacles. Use a medicine-type dropper to combine flavors and put into your cocktails. Keep bitters in a cool, dry place, and the mixtures should last indefinitely, thanks to the alcohol.

You might be acquainted with aromatic bitters, which are sometimes added to cocktails to put some zing into the flavor of the drink.

Herbal Syrups

It's a lot easier taking medicine when it doesn't taste like chemicals. Making herbal medicinal syrups is easy, or you can buy them already made (just watch for sugar content). They work especially well with children who refuse to take traditional liquid medications because of the bitter taste. To make an herbal syrup, you can follow a simple, basic recipe and add in the herbs you choose for their healing benefits.

Start out by getting a slow cooker or nonreactive pot, a teaspoon, a tablespoon, a spatula, honey, some cheesecloth, and glass jars with lids for storage. Some common medicinal herbs used in syrups are elderberry, lemon, peppermint, ginger, rose hips, lemon balm, *tulsi*, fennel, echinacea, astragalus, hawthorn berry, dandelion root, and marshmallow root. For sweetening, you can use stevia, monk fruit, cloves, cinnamon, or cardamom.

Take 1 ounce of herb per 16 ounces of water and put them into the pot. Warm the water to a simmer. Cover the pot to reduce the liquid to half its volume, so the mixture thickens. When you are left with 1 measurable cup of liquid, add in 8 ounces of honey, then re-warm it, stirring frequently. The temperature should never get hotter than 110 degrees. Once the honey is integrated, take the pot off the heat and let it cool. When cool, pour it through a cheesecloth to strain out plant parts and into a clean, sterile glass jar. Cover and label, so you know which syrup is which. You can store in the refrigerator for up to three months.

The general dosage for herbal syrup is 1–2 tablespoons for adults and ½ teaspoon for children three times daily until you feel better. Children can have allergies to an herb or honey, so check with their pediatrician first. Adults may want to add a little alcohol to their syrup. If children don't like the taste, you can add their syrup dosage to a smoothie or some juice to mask the flavor or sweeten it a tad with something natural. You can even mix it into a bowl of ice cream or yogurt. Do not give herbal syrups to children under the age of one.

Children can have allergies to an herb or honey, so check with their pediatrician first.... Do not give herbal syrups to children under the age of one.

Fresh herbs are best for syrups, but you can use dried in a pinch. Honey should be raw and organic.

For colds and flus, try elderberry or elderflower. Both reduce the duration of the illness and lessen symptoms. Echinacea, goldenseal, ginger, and astragalus are also potent immune boosters for colds and bugs. You can blend a few herbs together in a syrup for extra benefits.

Syrups with elecampane will fight off a sore throat or pesky cough. Try 2 tablespoons each of elecampane, licorice root, ginger, and elderberries in 1 quart of water with 1–2 cups of honey as a potent remedy. Adults may enjoy this blend with a little shot of brandy.

If you want a syrup that calms and soothes anxiety, try hawthorn berries, chamomile, lavender, valerian, and ashwagandha root together.

A nice healing syrup with a more liquid texture combines 1 tea-spoon of fresh ginger juice with 1 teaspoon of raw honey. You can add a few drops of lemon juice. Take by spoon three times a day to fight off colds and flus, aid digestion, and stop a cough. The antimicrobial and anti-inflammatory ingredients can also act as an expectorant.

Dandelion syrup makes use of those pesky weeds that grow everywhere. This recipe takes more time but is worth the effort. Take 3 cups of water; 2 cups of clean dandelion flower petals; 2½ cups of organic sugar; ½ cup of raw, organic honey; and ½ teaspoon of lemon grind. Put the flower petals, water, and lemon grind into a pot and let it boil, then remove from heat. Cover and let this mixture sit overnight. In the morning, use a cheesecloth to strain out the plant parts. Take the liquid and add the sugar, honey, and a little cinnamon if you wish in the same pot and let it simmer for an hour and a half, stirring frequently. Check for consistency. When it has a syruplike consistency, remove from heat and let it cool. You can store it in glass jars with lids in the refrigerator until ready to use.

Elderberry syrup is a favorite for kids and adults alike and is a powerhouse against colds and flu bugs. This recipe will yield 3 cups of syrup. You need 1 quart of cold spring or distilled water; 2 cups of dried, organic elderberries; 3 teaspoons of dried ginger root; 1 cup of raw, organic honey; and a cinnamon stick to taste. Pour the water into a pot and add the herbs and berries. Bring to a boil, then let it simmer for about 45 minutes. Remove from heat and let it steep in the pot for one hour. With a cheesecloth, strain the plant parts from the liquid, which may still be quite hot. You can press the berries down with a spatula to get as much juice out of them as possible. Take the remaining liquid and cool until it is room temperature, then add in the honey to taste. Pour this liquid into clean jars with lids for storage. You can take 1–2 teaspoons a day during cold and flu season as a preemptive measure, too. Store the rest in the refrigerator.

An easier version combines 1 cup of dried elderberries with 1 cup of raw, organic honey and 4 cups of water. Put the elderberries into a pot with the water and bring to a boil. Reduce heat to a simmer for one hour. Take off heat to cool, then when room temperature, strain the berries through a cheesecloth and add the honey to the liquid. Serve as needed and store the rest in the fridge.

Kids love the taste of lemon, so take the above recipe and replace the elderberries with lemon balm for a great calming syrup.

Once you have the basic recipe and ingredients down, you can experiment with different herbs and flowers for the taste and different healing properties. The honey is what gives it its syrupy texture, so if you don't like honey, you can simply make these without it for a more liquid consistency and sweeten with another healthy source. Don't stress over getting the measurements and amounts exact, either. It may take a bit of practice to find the best tastes and consistencies and makes a fun activity to do with kids.

If you cringe at the thought of trying to follow a written recipe, rest assured that you can find hundreds of instructional videos on YouTube on making herbal teas, syrups, tinctures, infusions, decoctions, gummies, bath bombs, and so much more. You can easily follow along and get new ideas on herbal blends to try. TGFTI: Thank God for the Internet.

Herbal Gummies

If you have kids, healing has never been more fun than popping a few chewy herbal gummies. Adults love them, too, and they are not that difficult to make yourself if you prefer homemade to the store-bought kind, which are possibly full of extra sugars and fillers.

The key to making gummies is the use of gelatin, a translucent, colorless food that is derived from the collagen of animal parts. There are vegan substitutes for gelatin, and you can also find gelatin made from grass-fed cattle. You also need ice cube trays or gelatin gummy molds, which can be found online or at a craft store in fun shapes and sizes. You will also need a small saucepan or pot, and a whisk comes in handy for stirring the gelatin.

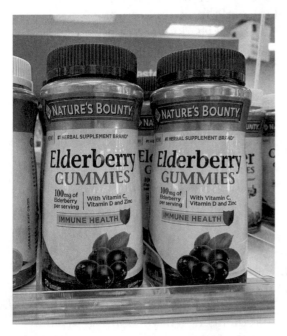

Herbal gummies aren't just an alternate way to get a high from marijuana; you can infuse gummies with all kinds of other, healthful herbs. Buy them in the store or make your own.

Here is a basic herbal gummy recipe: Take 2 cups of water, 1½ tablespoons of gelatin, 1½ tablespoons of honey or sweetener, and two bags of your favorite herbal tea. Bring 1 cup of water to a boil and steep your tea bags in this hot water for about five minutes or so. Take the other cup of water and pour in the gelatin. Mix thoroughly. Now, combine the gelatin water with the tea water in a container and add in the honey/sweetener. Mix it all together and pour into your mold or ice cube trays.

Put in the refrigerator and let it cool for at least an hour before eating. You can use a toothpick to test the consistency to see if it's firm enough.

For an elderberry gummy, take ½ cup of dried elderberries, ⅓ cup of dried rose hips, 3 cups of organic apple or grape juice, 3 tablespoons of gelatin, and a few cinnamon stick chunks. Combine all ingredients except for the gelatin in a small pot with water in it. Bring to a simmer and let it simmer for 20 minutes. Strain the liquid and measure out 2 cups' worth. Add more juice to taste if you need to. Put ½ cup of the liquid into a glass bowl and put in the fridge until it's cold. Sprinkle the gelatin over the cold juice and let it sit for a minute. Take the rest of the uncooled liquid and heat it almost to a boil, then pour it over the cold, gelatin-covered liquid, mixing with a whisk until the gelatin is dissolved. Add honey or sweetener if needed and pour into your molds. Stick in the fridge and eat when needed. They will keep for up to three weeks.

Hibiscus and berry teas are great, as are lemon tea and peppermint. You can add a tiny bit of food coloring to make them more fun and appealing for kids.

Here is a passion fruit gummy recipe. Take ¾ cup of water, three passion fruit tea bags, 6 tablespoons of gelatin, and 3 tablespoons of honey or sweetener. Put the water and tea bags into a small pot and bring to a boil, then remove from heat and let the tea steep for 10 minutes. Take ½ cup of this liquid, transfer it to a glass bowl, and put in the gelatin. Stir and set aside. Heat the rest of the tea and water again to a simmer and remove the tea bags. Add the gelatin mix and stir until it's dissolved. Take the pot off the heat and add your honey, removing any white foam that might rise with a spoon. Let it cool enough to pour into the molds or trays and put in the fridge to set.

The great thing about the above recipe is that you can replace the passion fruit tea with any herbal tea of your choice, and cleanup doesn't require straining when you buy tea bags. Hibiscus and berry teas are great, as are lemon tea and peppermint. You can add a tiny bit of food coloring to make them more fun and appealing for kids. For larger gummies, you can add all kinds of fun stuff like shaved chocolate or candy sprinkles, then pour into regular-sized ice cube trays. Kids can even take these and cut them into cool shapes as a fun treat that also has some health benefits.

Wonderful Witch Hazel

One natural medicinal with a long history of health benefits is witch hazel, which comes from *Hamamelis virginiana*, a small shrub native to the eastern coast of North America. The leaves and bark of the shrub can be used to make teas, ointments, and liquid treatments that have anti–inflammatory properties such as gallic acid and tannins. It also contains antioxidants that neutralize free radicals and is an astringent, which causes the contraction of skin cells and other body tissues, making it a wonderful, soothing topical medicinal for skin issues such as acne, eczema, dandruff, and psoriasis.

You can apply witch hazel directly to affected areas of the skin with a cotton ball. If you have dandruff, apply witch hazel to your scalp right before shampooing. It not only reduces itching from dandruff but relieves the inflammation that causes scalp sensitivity from psoriasis and eczema. Witch hazel has also been used to lighten stretch marks from pregnancy, reduce the swelling and discomfort of bug bites and bee stings, and soothe the discomfort from sunburn when applied with a cotton ball to the exposed skin.

Test tube studies show that the tannins in witch hazel slow skin tumor growth in mice exposed to radiation, but no human studies

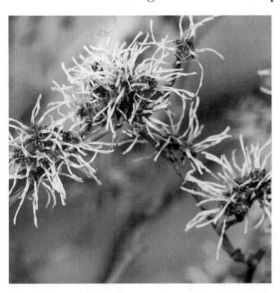

have been done. Other test tube studies show that tannins prevent inflammation, preventing substances from entering your skin cells, and that witch hazel can neutralize free radicals to prevent skin cancer from spreading. Tannins have also been shown to have some antiviral effects at stopping and preventing infections. A test tube study showed that witch hazel extract can inhibit herpes simplex virus 1 from turning into cold sores and showed antiviral effects against influenza A and HPV (human papillomavirus).

Small amounts of witch hazel can be added to herbal teas or ingested, but it is not recommended without first discussing with your doctor. Ingesting too much witch hazel will lead to stomach upset. It is also wise to do a skin allergy

Witch hazel, a common shrub that grows on the east coast of North America, can be used for its antioxidant and anti-inflammatory properties.

test by dabbing some witch hazel on the inside of your elbow with a cotton ball and leaving overnight to see if any rash or irritation develops.

People have benefited from adding witch hazel to a warm bath to heal hemorrhoids, which are caused by inflammation of veins in the rectum and anus, thanks to its anti–inflammatory properties. You can also apply witch hazel with a cotton ball to the affected area to reduce pain, redness, swelling, and bleeding from hemorrhoids. The pain from varicose veins, which are dilated veins in the legs, can be treated by wrapping a cloth doused in witch hazel around the leg for a few hours. Witch hazel's astringent properties, which tighten skin and constrict small blood vessels, also help stop bleeding from minor cuts, scrapes, and nosebleeds.

Healing Heartburn

Heartburn not only burns, it can also cause chest pain. If you think it might be a heart attack and does not go away after a few minutes or if the pain spreads to your arms, jaw, and neck accompanied by sweating, nausea, and fatigue, call 911!

When you eat, your esophagus, the tube that connects your mouth to your stomach, pushes food down in rhythmic waves. Once the food hits your stomach, powerful acids and enzymes break it down for digestion. The stomach has a special lining that protects it from being affected by acid, but when heartburn occurs, stomach acids travel back up into the esophagus, causing the burning sensation known as acid reflux.

Heartburn can be caused by consuming too much caffeine, spicy food, or chocolate or by eating too much too quickly. It can be mistaken sometimes for food allergies or intolerance. If it is indeed heartburn, and you will know by the sensation that your entire esophagus is on fire, then you can take prescription and OTC meds, especially if it is chronic, or try one of these remedies for some quick relief from that nasty burn:

- Baking soda: Baking soda (do not take baking powder) is inexpensive and natural and is probably in the pantries and cupboards of most households. Dissolve 1 teaspoon of baking soda into 1 cup of water. The baking soda will help neutralize acid. Baking soda contains sodium, so consult your doctor if you're on a low–sodium diet.

- Aloe juice: Aloe juice is sold at most grocery stores and, like aloe vera gel, which soothes sunburns, aloe juice soothes irritation caused by acid reflux. Try drinking half a cup of aloe juice before meals to keep your stomach and esophagus soothed.

- Sugar–free gum: Saliva helps dilute acid, so increasing the amount of saliva you produce after a meal is a great way to help prevent acid production. Chew a stick of sugar–free gum for 30 minutes for decreased heartburn.

- Apple cider vinegar: Mix 3 teaspoons of apple cider vinegar in 1 cup of water, then drink before each meal or at bedtime. Add a splash of lemon juice or honey if you need it for the taste.

- Eat a banana: Bananas contain natural antacids. Start eating a banana every day to help counteract acid reflux. If you don't have a banana, an apple will do. A banana a day keeps the reflux away!

- Stop smoking: If you're a smoker and you need yet another reason to quit, here's one. If you've noticed your acid reflux has gotten worse and you're a smoker, the smoking will aggravate your esophagus and make everything hurt. Now's a good time to quit.

- Lose weight: People who are obese have more digestive issues and also experience increased acid reflux and heartburn. Losing weight is a good idea for a lot of things, and alleviating heartburn is one of them.

- Drink water: Drinking cool water often is the only thing needed to alleviate the burning sensation of heartburn.

- Tea power: Try chamomile, licorice, slippery elm, and marshmallow teas to make better herbal remedies to soothe heartburn and acid reflux symptoms. Licorice helps increase the mucus coating of the esophageal lining, which helps calm the effects of stomach acid. Stay away from green tea, which contains tannins, which stimulate more stomach acid and can increase heartburn and cause stomach upset.

Natural Vapor Rub Recipe

½ c. olive oil, coconut oil, or almond oil

2 tbsp. beeswax pastilles (level, not heaping)

20 drops eucalyptus oil (use only 4 drops for use on babies and small children)

20 drops peppermint oil (substitute 4 drops fir essential oil for use on babies and small children)

10 drops rosemary oil (omit for use on babies and small children)

10 drops cinnamon or clove oil (optional; omit for use on babies and small children)

This is a great, petroleum-free version of the classic Vicks rub for clearing stuffy noses and chest congestion.

Melt beeswax with your oil of choice in a double boiler until just melted. Add the essential oils (use half the amount for a baby version, or dilute with coconut oil before using). Stir until well mixed and pour into some type of container with a lid to store. Small tins and small jars work well, or try empty chapstick tubes to keep in your pocket or purse. Use as needed to help reduce coughing and congestion. For babies and small children, many of these oils are not safe, so check first with their doctor. For safe herbs and oils, be sure to dilute them even more so. Play it safe when it comes to any herbal remedy and to your infant or child.

Remedy Creativity

Thousands of healthy, natural remedies and recipes are out there in books, online, or via video tutorials, but much of the art of herbal remedies comes from your own research and willingness to experiment with tastes, textures, and properties. You can't do it wrong because if something tastes awful, you throw it away, but you might be surprised to find that your own unique blends are amazing and work wonders.

If you find you have a knack for creating your own remedies, start up a blog or post about it and share your knowledge and successes with others.

Clearly, not everyone has the time, talent, or inclination to make their own herbal remedies, and numerous options exist for buying premade products in stores, health food outlets, and online. Just do your homework and check labels. It does you no good to buy a natural toothpaste that still contains the neurotoxins fluoride or aluminum. It isn't healthy to buy a natural lipstick that contains fillers that will make their way into your stomach and liver. It is not a health benefit to use herbal syrups that contain half their weight in sugars and high fructose corn syrup. Some products out there will save you time and effort, but buy quality and don't be fooled just because they claim to be "all natural."

Herbal remedies such as balms, salves, creams, lotions, teas, in-fusions, and syrups can be given as gifts, too, for a personal touch that is also productive and useful. You can even gather some friends and have an herbal remedy party where you cook up some interesting bitters or try out some new teas and concoctions. If you find you have a knack for creating your own remedies, start up a blog or post about it and share your knowledge and successes with others. Make your own YouTube videos and instruct others on how to make a yummy syrup kids will love or a great alcoholic popsicle for your next back-yard party.

Natural healing remedies are meant to be shared. Our ancestors often wrote them down in books and passed them down to future generations. Now with computers, it becomes even easier to keep track of remedies and print them out to put into a beautiful scrapbook or binder and give to your children. Men and women who once prac-ticed the "old ways" carried on the tradition of passing down herbal remedies by teaching their own sons and daughters how to make these recipes and keep them in a book for posterity. Whether ancient Chinese medicine, Ayurveda, or old kitchen witchery, the knowledge of the past is now in our hands to work with, experiment with, and add to so that it continues to help and heal others.

May this book continue that tradition.

Nature Heals Us,
but Can We Heal Nature?

Writing about natural health and well-being is a difficult chore because each and every topic can be a book or two in itself. Such a vast body of information and knowledge exists to try to share in the pages of one book that it feels overwhelming to the writer to pick and choose what to include. Let this book be an invitation to you, the reader, to go off on your own journey and do your own research and knowledge gathering in your quest to experience optimal health and well-being.

At this point, we know for sure that for every health problem, nature has a solution that does not include the side effects of something made of chemical components that is synthetically engineered in a lab. While we do not have to shun allopathic medicine and medications entirely because they do have their place, it behooves us to look first at the plethora of natural substances, techniques, modalities, therapies, and products that offer the same benefits, with the added benefit of allowing us to feel good about using them.

This starts with becoming more aware of how the media and health and pharmaceutical industries play upon our fears to sell us a product–for their profit, not ours. Watch an hour of television to see the many ads for this drug or that, each followed by a long litany of horrible side effects, all urging you to ask your doctor about using the drug, even if you don't think you need it.

Drugs and pharmaceuticals can save lives, but remember, they are first and foremost products that make some corporation money. They are profit-based healers, and their makers and manufacturers often have that profit margin as their top priority despite your top priority being better health. The healthcare industry is not much better when it comes to protecting us and making us healthier. It is more oriented toward profits and covering up symptoms rather than taking the time, energy, and effort of getting to the causes and healing them. Maybe it's because curing diseases means far fewer customers, lower profits, and lower stock performances for shareholders.

When it comes to your health, you are your best advocate because for you, it's not about money. It's about quality of life and well-being.

When it comes to your health, you are your best advocate because for you, it's not about money. It's about quality of life and well-being. The focus is on getting better, not just feeling better by covering up symptoms. You want to be healthy for good. It starts with you and your diet and exercise and the things you can do for yourself without the aid of a doctor or surgeon. Natural health comes from making better choices and being aware of where the things you ingest and inject into your body come from. It is not something to leave to chance or to the whims of those who seek to profit off of your ongoing illness.

Going grocery shopping in these times often involves clicking on a cartful of products to be delivered by someone else. Sure, it's convenient, but we miss out on the experience of slowly walking the aisles, reading labels, and choosing products that are best for us, not just what is convenient. Natural healing involves all aspects of life from what we eat to what we do and how we find the time to connect with other living things.

The more oriented society becomes to cubicles and working or schooling at home or sitting on the couch surfing through our phones and binge-watching TV shows, the less time we spend outdoors in nature or hanging out with people in person, enjoying the many benefits of living life to the fullest. We become a little agoraphobic and start to avoid going out of the house and interacting with other people if we can find an easier way, then wonder why we feel so lonely, tired, un-motivated, and passionless. Just because we are human doesn't mean we aren't as much a part of the natural world as a tree or raccoon. We need to get outdoors. We need to do things in person with people and pets. We need to turn more to nature than we do to big corporations in order to make us feel better, smarter, and more energized.

The world of medicine that we are most used to leaves little room for spending a day at the beach with our toes in the sand or having a picnic with our kids at the local park. It rarely prescribes a fun night of doing puzzles with the family or sitting down with the spouse and laugh-ing over a movie together. So much of disease is responded to in ways that alienate us and keep us separate from others: taking pills, having surgeries, going in for treatments, and spending days in hospitals and recovery centers. Often, we don't have much of a support system other than a friend or two, some family nearby, and our doctors, and they tend to have too many patients to sit down to have a long chat with us.

Connection to nature, to others, to life around us, and, most im-portantly, to ourselves has been cut off, derailed, detoured, and den-igrated down the totem pole of priorities. Yet, we all suffer for this disconnection and can't figure out why. Natural health understands that we are a whole unit, and that unit must be treated as a whole: body, mind, and spirit. Imagine a triangle with only one strong side. The other two would collapse the whole triangle in on itself.

When was the last time you went outside and took off your shoes? Wiggled your toes in the dark soil or the cool, green grass? Felt the warmth of the sun blush your skin a bit pink? When was the last time you planted flowers or vegetables, watched them sprout and grow, and harvested them for use with the kind of pride that comes from being a part of the cycle of life, not just going out and buying stuff in a store?

This is a call to action. Earth is a giant, magnificent gift ripe with the things we need to not just survive but thrive: food, water, air, earth, and the spirit of the ongoing cycle of the Wheel of Life. We feel small and insignificant when we look out at the roaring ocean waves but in a good way, a reverent way. We feel empty, hollow, and insig-nificant when we spend most of our time sitting in an office or on the couch at home, our noses glued to our gadgets or watching television, or driving in our cars to places we don't even really want to be.

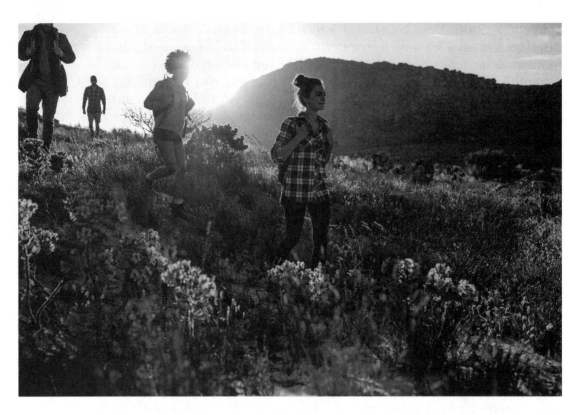

Many of the physical and mental ills experienced by modern-day people are the result of—or exacerbated by—our lost connection to nature. The good news is that you can turn your TV, computer, or iPhone off and reintroduce yourself to the natural world any time you want.

Life can deaden us to the gifts of the natural world. It is our responsibility to stop and set down the distractions that keep us from those gifts. Work can wait 10 minutes. Our bodies cannot wait, and nor can our spirits. We need to get back to nature not in a tree–bark-eating way, unless that turns you on, but as a part of life in general. The large amounts of time we spend working, sleeping, and being inside four walls must be balanced with the expansive freedom of playing, being, and doing nothing more than looking up at the vast, limitless, blue sky.

Without nature, we wouldn't exist. Why, then, have we separated ourselves so much from the very thing that can most save us? Go pick some flowers, grow some herbs, or make something. Stand beneath the light of a full moon, clothed or otherwise, and feel fully present. Go ahead and dance if you want to. Who cares who's watching? Let them judge and talk. Mother Nature doesn't care; she's seen it all! She made you naked, remember? She also sustains you. She provided you with everything you need to be healthy, to thrive, to live. She asks only that you respect her and put back some of what you've taken so that enough will always be around.

She wants you to dance with her and not against her. Don't sit out the dance. Time passes so quickly. Flowers bloom and die. People live and pass away. Generations begin and end. Suns and moons come, go, and come again. Seasons rise and fall. Days turn into nights, followed by a new dawn. The Wheel of Life turns quickly and without distraction, for it must turn. We have the choice to enjoy our part of the dance when we can. Why on Earth would anyone choose otherwise?

Encourage your children to list ways they can help heal the planet. Come up with fun rewards each time they recycle, reduce waste, or plant a tree. We only have one planet, and our children and grandchildren are relying on us to treat it the way we want them to treat it. We are their role models. They are watching our every move, our every action. They are learning from us. It is their duty to make Earth a better place than we left it. It is our duty to leave Earth a better place than we found it.

It's impossible to write a whole book about the bountiful gifts of Mother Nature without asking this question: Can we save Mother Nature? If we hope to utilize her amazing collection of plants and herbs to heal ourselves, it behooves us all to become advocates of the natural world, doing our part to cut back on our own carbon and waste footprints and reduce the amount of chemicals and pollutants we contribute.

Overwhelmed by the state of Earth and not convinced that what you do makes a difference? It does, and it doesn't require a complete overhaul in how you live unless that's your intention.

Overwhelmed by the state of Earth and not convinced that what you do makes a difference? It does, and it doesn't require a complete overhaul in how you live unless that's your intention. Sometimes, tak- ing baby steps is the best way to start. Here are some small, simple things we can do to treat Earth better:

- Reduce our carbon footprint

- Recycle
- Give away what we no longer need or use
- Make pesticides
- Make medicines
- Grow herbs, flowers, and plants
- Compost
- Donate money, food, and time to charities
- Eat local and buy organic
- Attend a beach or park cleanup
- Never take more plants and flowers from natural settings than what you need if you cannot grow your own
- Plant new trees
- Get to know your neighbors
- Check on seniors in your neighborhood
- Become an active part of your community
- Avoid harming wildlife that must share space with humans because of overbuilding and destruction of habitats
- Don't waste electricity, water, paper, food, etc.
- Develop compassion and understanding
- Learn about other races and heritages
- Stand up for the rights of children, the poor, humans, animals, and the planet itself
- Avoid pharmaceuticals when possible
- Enjoy money and use it for good
- Avoid pointless arguing and debating on social networks
- Avoid spreading gossip and bad news
- Live by example
- Teach your children what they need to know that isn't taught in schools such as financial planning, how to open a bank account, how to apply for a job, etc.
- Behave in front of your children the way you hope they will one day behave in front of theirs
- Question your doctors when they automatically put you on a pill or suggest a dangerous treatment
- Do your own research
- Promote healthy diets and exercise
- Meditate and teach your kids how to meditate
- Support Native and indigenous people to own their own land

- Boycott corporations that destroy the air, water, and life
- Buy local and support local farmer's markets and small businesses
- Invest your money in stocks that reflect your beliefs and protect the planet
- Vote only for those candidates who are devoted to putting people over corporations
- Learn about the chemicals in your food and make better choices
- Post on social networks about the things you're learning and be ready for backlash
- Honor the truth, even if others are in denial
- Learn about cognitive dissonance, media manipulation, and political and corporate corruption and support companies that have a record of caring for people over profits
- Stand for something, or you will fall for anything

Nature is a giant treasure chest filled with gifts that we should be cultivating and celebrating. So much is out there to be grateful for, yet we remain blind to it or mesmerized by the distractions of shiny newness and modernization until something happens that thrusts us into the present moment, into the awareness of what has always been there. If we are not careful, those gifts can be taken from us from those who wish to only profit from Earth and from climate change, poverty, and global pandemics, to name a few things. Those gifts of natural healing and fabulous vitality and health are always there and have been for thousands, if not millions, of years, awaiting our attention and rediscovery. Open the treasure chest now and discover the abundance within.

Finally, in the words of Mexican healer and poet Maria Sabina:

Heal yourself with the light of the sun and the rays of the moon. With the sound of the river and the waterfall. With the swaying of the sea and the fluttering of birds. Heal yourself with mint, neem, and Eucalyptus. Sweeten with lavender, rosemary, and chamomile. Hug yourself with the cocoa bean and a hint of cinnamon. Put love in tea instead of sugar and drink it looking at the stars. Heal yourself with the kisses that the wind gives you and the hugs of the rain. Stand strong with your bare feet on the ground and with everything that comes from it. Be smarter every day by listening to your intuition, looking at the world with your forehead. Jump, dance, sing, so that you live happier. Heal yourself with beautiful love, and always remember … you are the medicine.

Natural Health

FURTHER READING

"6 Benefits of Oil Pulling." Healthline.com. https://www.healthline.com/nutrition/6-benefits-of-oil-pulling.

"7 Benefits of Resveratrol Supplements." Healthline.com. https://www.healthline.com/nutrition/resveratrol.

"7 Natural Benefits of Oregano Oil and 5 Ways to Use It." https://blog.paleohacks.com/oregano-oil/.

"Alternative Medicine: The Science Behind 10 Alternative Therapies." https://greatist.com/health/alternative-medicine-therapies-explained.

Alton, Lori. "9 Supplements for Optimal Blood Pressure Management." NaturalHealth365.com, August 15, 2020. https://www.naturalhealth365.com/reduce-blood-pressure-3517-html/.

———. "Gingivitis Can Be Eliminated Naturally." *NaturalHealth365*, December 1, 2019.

Axe, Josh. "7 Adaptogenic Herbs or Adaptogens That Help Reduce Stress." January 20, 2018. https://www.draxe.com/nutrition/adaptogenic-herbs-adaptogens/.

———. "Anxiety Natural Remedies: 15 Ways to Find Relax and Calm." July 17, 2018. https://draxe.com/health/natural-remedies-anxiety/.

Bart, Brian. "10 Edible Weeds Likely Growing in Your Yard." *Modern Farmer*, July 10, 2018.

Bell, Dawn Branley. "Six Tips to Avoid Being Overwhelmed by the News." Berkely.edu, April 7, 2021. https://greatergood.berkeley.edu.

Blasi, Elizabeth. "8 Biggest Health Risks Associated with a Sedentary Lifestyle." Aaptiv.com. https://aaptiv.com/magazine/health-risks-for-sedentary-lifestyles.

Bongiorno, Peter. "Ashwagandha for Anxiety." *Psychology Today*, January 8, 2014.

"Calories Burned in 30 Minutes for People of Three Different Weights." Harvard Health Publishing, Harvard Medical School. March, 2021. https://www.health.harvard.edu/diet-and-weight-loss/calories-burned-in-30-minutes-of-leisure-and-routine-activities.

Campbell, Leah. "Coronasomnia: How the Pandemic May Be Affecting Your Sleep." Healthline.com, March 1, 2021. https://www.healthline.com/health-news/coronasomnia-how-the-pandemic-may-be-affecting-your-sleep#The-coronasomnia-cycle.

Clark, Alicia H. "Why Does Self-Care Sometimes Feel So Hard?" *Psychology Today*, February 19, 2020.. https://www.psychologytoday.com/us/blog/hack-your-anxiety/202002/why-does-self-care-sometimes-feel-so-hard.

Davidson, Katey. "Herbal Detoxes: Myths, Facts, and What to Know." Healthline.com. August 7, 2020. https://www.healthline.com/nutrition/herbal-detox.

Ellison, Shane, M.S. *Over-the-Counter Natural Cures: Take Charge of Your Health in 30 Days with 10 Lifesaving Supplements for Under $10*. Naperville, IL: Sourcebooks, 2014.

Fite, Vannoy Gentles. *Llewellyn's Book of Natural Remedies: Over 400 Ayurvedic, Herbal, Essential Oil, and Home Remedies for Everyday Ailments*. Llewellyn Publications, 2020.

Gillaspy, Becky. *Intermittent Fasting Diet Guide and Cookbook: A Complete Guide to Fasting Strategies with 50+ Satisfying Recipes and 4 Flexible Meal Plans*. Indianapolis, IN: DK/Random House Publishing, 2020.

———. "Apple Cider Vinegar: Science-Backed Benefits for Weight Loss and Health." *Dr. Becky Fitness*, January 4, 2020.

Gordon, Sandra. "7 Natural Remedies for IBS." *Everyday Health*, April 28, 2021.

Halewicz, Julia. "Can White Noise Help You Sleep Better?" *Prevention Magazine*, November 17, 2017.

Hampton, Dr. Tony. "How to Manage Stress for Diet and Health Success." The Diet Doctor. https://www.dietdoctor.com/dr.hampton-stress-less-for-diet-and-health-success.

"Health Risks of an Inactive Lifestyle." MedlinePlus. https://medlineplus.gov/healthrisksofinactivelifestyle.html.

"Healthy Sleep Habits." SleepEducation.org. https://sleepeducation.org/healthy-sleep-habits.

"Here's How Jigsaw Puzzles Can Benefit Brain and Mental Health Conditions." LongevityLive.com. https://longevitylive.com/anti-aging/heres-how-jigsaw-puzzles-can-benefit-brain-and-mental-health-conditions/.

Holland, Emily. "7 Benefits of Owning a Pet." Chopra.com. April 8, 2016. https://chopra.com/articles/7-health-benefits-of-owning-a-pet.

"How Breathwork Benefits the Mind, Body, and Spirit." Chopra.com, October 5, 2020. https://chopra.com/articles/how-breathwork-bebefits-the-mind-body-and-spirit.

Johnson, Joe. "22 Brain Exercises to Improve Memory, Cognition, and Creativity." *Medical News Today*, January 27, 2021.

Jones, Marie D. *Earth Magic: Your Complete Guide to Natural Spells, Potions, Plants, Herbs, Witchcraft, and More*. Detroit: Visible Ink Press, 2020.

Jones, Marie D., and Larry Flaxman. *The Resonance Key: Exploring the Links Between Vibration, Consciousness, and the Zero Point Grid.* Franklin Lakes, NJ: New Page Books, 2009.

Kubala, Jillian. "14 Natural Ways to Improve Your Memory." Healthline.com. March 25, 2016. https://www.healthline.com/nutrition/ways-to-improve-memory.

LaMotte, Sandee. "The Benefits of Owning a Pet–and the Science Behind It." CNN.com, February 20, 2020.

Malhotra, Samir. "A Scientist's Take on the Power of Prayer." *The Wire*, July 29, 2019.

Marti, James E. *Alternative Health & Medicine Encyclopedia.* Detroit: Visible Ink Press, 1998.

McDermott, Annette. "10 Ways to Naturally Reduce Anxiety." Healthline, June 29, 2020. https://www.healthline.com/health/natural-ways-to-reduce-anxiety.

Messonnier, Shawn, D.V.M. *Natural Health Bible for Dogs & Cats: You're A–Z Guide to Over 200 Conditions, Herbs, Vitamins, and Supplements.* New York: Three Rivers Press, 2001.

Mills, Betsy. "Can a Puzzle a Day Keep Dementia at Bay?" *LiveSmart*, July 15, 2019.

Moralis, Shonda. "12 Simple Ways to Teach Mindfulness to Kids." *Psychology Today*, May 2, 2020. https://www.psychologytoday.com/us/blog/breathe-moma-breathe/201605/12-simple-ways-teach-mindfulness-kids.

Patiry, Megan. "Elderberry Benefits for Viruses, Colds, Allergies, and Flu." Paleo hacks.com. https://blog_paleohacks.com/elderberry/#.

Pemberton, Corey. "Cacao VS. Cocoa: The Difference and Why It Matters." Paleohacks.com. https://blog.paleohacks.com/cacao-vs-cocoa/htm.

Petri, Alana. "8 Common Signs You're Deficient in Vitamins." Healthline, November 4, 2019. https://www.healthline.com/nutrition/vitamin-deficiency.

Pizzorno, Dr. Joseph. *The Toxin Solution: How Hidden Poisons in the Air, Water, Food, and Products We Use Are Destroying Our Health, and What We Can Do to Fix It.* New York: HarperCollins, 2017.

Red, Michelle Roya. "The Power of Prayer: Why Does It Work?" HuffPost.com. December 24, 2011. https://www.huffpost.com/entry/power-of-prayer_b_1015475.

Rehman, Anis. "What Is Healthy Sleep?" SleepFoundation.org. January 2021. https://www.sleepfoundation.org/sleep-hygiene/what-is-healthy-sleep.

Sanders, Karen. "Ease Chronic Fatigue with 3 Great Ayurvedic Herbs." NaturalHealth365.com. February 23, 2021. https://www.naturalhealth365.com/chronic-fatigue-syndrome-3740.html.

Santos-Longhurst, Adriennae. "How to Live Your Best Life As You Age." Healthline.com, June 18, 2019. https://www.healthine.com/health/aging-gracefully.

Stahl, Ashley. "Here's How Creativity Actually Improves Your Health." *Forbes Magazine*, July 25, 2020.

Staughton, John. "8 Proven Herbs for Weight Loss." OrganicFacts.net. July 3, 2020. https://www.organicfacts.net/herbs-weight-loss-html.

St. Ours, Melanie. *The Simple Guide to Natural Health: From Apple Cider Vinegar Tonics to Coconut Oil Body Balm, 15+ Home Remedies for Health and Healing*. New York: Adams Media, 2018.

Tinsley, Grant. "How Tryptophan Boosts Your Sleep Quality and Mood." Healthline.com, February 25, 2019. https://www.healthline.com/nutrition/tryptophan.

"The Top 12 Herbs for Weight Loss." Explore.GlobalHealing.com. October 4, 2018. https://globalhealing.com/natural-health/top-herbs-for-weight-loss/.

"What to Know about CBD and Cannabis." *Consumer Reports*, October 2020.

Wilson, Shelly. *Embracing the Magic Within: Choose to Live Your Life with Passion, Presence, and Purpose*. Shelly R. Wilson Books, 2020.

Wong, Cathy. "8 Natural Depression Remedies to Consider." VeryWellHealth.com. June 2020. https://www.verywellhealth.com/natural-treatments-for-depression-89243.

APPENDIX

Herbs and Plants from A to Z

Acacia–Heals wounds and provides relief for a sore and raw throat.

Alfalfa–Consuming the juice can aid in regrowing lost hair, especially if used in a mix with carrots.

Allspice–Comes from a tree in the myrtle family grown in Central and South America. It is called allspice because it has the scents of many species, including nutmeg, cinnamon, cloves, pepper, and juniper berries. Its antiseptic properties make it useful for fighting infections and can even treat depression when used in aromatherapy. Allspice also helps stop indigestion.

Aloe vera–Loaded with 75 active compounds, this plant has been used for thousands of years as a medicinal but also for its nutrition benefits. The sap contains anti–inflammatory and pain–relieving compounds. It's a natural remedy for diabetes and is clinically proven to lower blood sugar and triglycerides. Aloe vera sap applied directly to the skin helps with the healing of cuts, burns (especially sunburn), and wounds and is a potent digestive system detoxifier when taken internally. Aloe vera gel mixed with a few drops of almond oil rubbed into the scalp and left overnight (wash out with shampoo) helps hair growth. It is a great laxative and aids constipation and has even been shown to work much better than a placebo in a study of chronic psoriasis. In spell casting, use it for protection and to attract good luck.

Angelica–This European plant is now grown in the United States for its many medicinal purposes. It can reduce coughs, colds, bloating, menstrual pain, nerve pain, arthritis, stomachaches, and motion sickness. Use the dried roots and seeds in syrups and infusions, but do not give to pregnant women or diabetics because of its ability to raise blood sugar levels.

Apricot–The fruit is not only good for your eyes, stomach, liver, heart, and nerve health, thanks to an abundance of vitamins and minerals, but apricot oil is wonderful for treating skin ailments.

Arnica–A healing herb that when applied to bruises and sprains, the pain and inflammation will vanish. Arnica not only reduces swelling and trauma to skin and tissue but also stops the pain associated with overused muscles from hiking or walking without the nasty side effects of pharmaceuticals. It has been used for these properties as far back as the twelfth century in European countries. The most common type, Arnica Montana, is part of the daisy family, which includes chamomile, yarrow, echinacea, and calendula.

Asafetida–This Indian cooking spice is a gum from a type of giant fennel plant. It has an awful odor like rotten garlic, but it tastes savory in cooking, with an oniony–garlicky flavor. It has amazing healing properties as an antibacterial, antiparasitic, antiviral, antispasmodic, laxative, sedative, expectorant, and carminative. Over history, it has been used to treat asthma, bronchitis, whooping cough, nervous disorders, and gut ailments as well as painful labor and menstruation. It is also a natural blood thinner and can lower blood pressure. In traditional Indian medicine, it has been successfully used to break up gallstones and kidney stones and help in their elimination. It is usually sold as a ground powder mixed with flour, starch, or turmeric, as eating it raw can cause severe vomiting and diarrhea. It works best when first fried for 10 seconds in hot oil to reduce its pungency but is worth the effort for its many health benefits.

Aster–Chinese herbologists use aster for many things, including controlling bleeding, curing hepatitis, and treating snakebites.

Banaba leaf–Comes from a Southeast Asian tree and has been used in medicinals for centuries to improve glucose levels and heal metabolic syndrome due to the active ingredient, corosolic acid.

Basil–Native to tropical regions from Africa to Southeast Asia, basil is used in cooking all over the world and can stop stomach spasms, gas, fluid retention, parasites, and loss of appetite. Topically, it can heal snake and insect bites and reduce warts. Sweet basil provides vitamins, minerals, and many antioxidants. *Tulsi*, or holy basil, is used in therapeutics in Ayurvedic medicine. In India, *tulsi* is considered one of the most important healing herbs, and a study in 2015 for the journal *Ayurvedic* showed that it had a positive impact on the liver health of rats. *Tulsi* tea is sold in most stores, but make sure to buy high–quality organic products to get the most benefits. Basil can also be used as an essential oil to treat colds and reduce inflammation of the nasal passages to improve breathing.

Bay leaves/bay laurel–As a medicinal, bay is taken orally for infections, congestion, allergies, asthma, anxiety, and even psychosis. Bay leaves are used in cooking to add flavor.

Bee balm–The pretty flowers of this plant give a hot and spicy flavor to foods to help flush the sinuses and clear stuffy noses. The thymol found in bee balm is a potent antibacterial, antifungal, and antiviral ingredient that fights off infections, allergies, and illnesses of the respiratory system.

Benzoin–The oil can calm and soothe anxiety and is often used as a scented vapor to soothe the mind from exhaustion and stress.

Berberine–A chemical compound found in several plants, including European barberry, goldenseal, Oregon grape, philodendron, and tree turmeric. It is a powerhouse in supplement form for fighting diabetes by regulating blood sugars, and it has a positive impact on insulin and triglycerides. It has been used for thousands of years in ancient Chinese and Ayurvedic medicine, and a 2014 meta-analysis for the *Journal of Ethnopharmacology* found that it was more effective than making lifestyle changes at improving blood sugar levels. It is also effective at improving mitochondrial health, is an anti–inflammatory, improves gut mobility, prevents hepatic inflammation, and promotes healthy endothelial function.

Bergamot–It heals cuts, bruises, scrapes, and acne when used externally.

Blackberry leaves–Blackberries are powerful antioxidants and anti–inflammatories, and chewing the leaves heals sore throats and mouth sores.

Black cohosh–Well known for its properties that relieve symptoms of menopause, this perennial plant, topped by a long plume of white flowers, is native to North America and part of the buttercup family. It has been studied extensively for reducing hot flashes, cramping, and other "female" maladies, especially during premenopause and menopause, especially for women who were not able to take estrogen. It also enhances energy.

Black pepper–This spice boosts metabolism and increases serotonin production.

Black walnut–Use the nuts and the hull to detoxify the body, especially the intestines. The hull can fight fungal infections.

Bladder wrack–This plant is a type of seaweed that is rich in vitamins A and C and minerals such as calcium, iodine, magnesium, sodium, zinc, and potassium. It is great at reducing mucus and congestion because it has antiviral and antimicrobial properties. It also reduces inflammation, aids in weight loss, and promotes a healthy digestive system. Bladder wrack also helps with eye and heart health and can reduce the effects of radiation. It also helps detox heavy metals out of the system.

Brahmi–Also known as Indian pennywort or *Bacopa monnieri*, this herb is used in Ayurvedic medicine to fight chronic fatigue syndrome and age–related deficits. It has been used in Indian medicine as a tonic to treat Alzheimer's disease. The constituents in the plant include bacosides that relax the veins, allow enhanced blood flow, and increase mental focus and clarity. A 2008 study in the *Journal of Alternative and Complementary Medicine* found that 300 milligrams of extract a day given to elderly subjects for six weeks showed enhanced word–recall memory scores in a battery of tests as well as less depression and anxiety.

Burdock–A biennial plant with roots that can be dried, burdock is considered an antioxidant superpower when it comes to natural healing. Burdock has some diuretic properties. In traditional healing, it has been used to remove toxins from the blood and slow the growth of cancers. It also fights the effects of aging and strengthens the lymphatic system, improves arthritis symptoms, fights tonsillitis, and heals skin ailments.

Butterbur–An herb that rivals any over–the–counter allergy drug. Studies show it treats allergy symptoms as well as the leading ingredient in Zyrtec, cetirizine, without the drowsy side effects.

Calendula/marigold–Calendula is a perennial plant that is a close relative of the marigold plant. It has yellow flowers that look like daisies because they are a part of the daisy family. Calendula is a powerful antiviral, anti–inflammatory herb that is often used in salves and infusions. Calendula salve, cream, and balm heals cuts, wounds, scratches, scrapes, and rashes and treats skin diseases such as psoriasis, eczema, and skin ulcers.

California poppy–A sedating plant that reduces anxiety and stress and can help alleviate insomnia without groggy side effects or the threat of dependency. The roots and aboveground parts of the flower work best in a tincture, with just a few drops providing relief, but you can also make a tea. This plant could cause uterine contractions in pregnant women and is best avoided. Do not give to children under the age of 6 because of sedating properties.

Camphor–Assists in easing spasms, breathing issues, and pain when camphor oil is used in vaporizers and aromatherapy. It can also treat wounds and skin disorders.

Caraway–The seeds made into tea form stop colic and digestive disorders.

Cayenne pepper–These hot chili peppers work wonders to help lower blood pressure and improve heart health, thanks to the compound known as capsaicin, a potent anti–inflammatory agent that gives them their heat. A study in the 2020 issue of *Cell Metabolism* found cayenne peppers to be beneficial for improving heart health by relaxing blood vessels, which allows more blood flow and lowers hypertension. These peppers may also reduce heart damage from a heart attack by protecting the heart muscle itself, and they have other benefits such as fighting cancer cells by causing them to commit cell suicide, raising metabolism due to thermogenic properties to burn fat and assist in weight loss, prevent sinusitis, and relieve sinus congestion, and provide topical pain relief for osteoarthritis pain. Capsaicin has also been shown to kill bacteria that could prevent stomach ulcers.

Cedar–The oil makes a natural insecticide and, as a medicinal, stops breathing issues, congestion, infections, bronchitis, and acne and skin disorders.

Celery–Lowers blood pressure and stops cancer when the stalk is eaten, and the entire stalk, leaves, and heart contain a ton of fiber, vitamins, and minerals. Celery is anti–inflammatory and helps manage diabetes and blood sugar, promotes liver health, boosts the immune system, acts as a diuretic to rid the body of excess water, protects the heart, and aids in a healthy digestive system and weight loss.

Chamomile–The tea is soothing for an upset stomach and aids sleep with its calming properties. The incense form rids the body and mind of stress and anxiety.

Chaste tree–A strong plant for relieving PMS symptoms in women when taken in herb form with minimal side effects.

Cherry and cherry bark/wood–The cherries are an aphrodisiac and work better than most pain relievers, thanks to their anti–inflammatory properties.

Chia–The tiny, black seeds of the *Salvia hispanica* plant are potent antioxidants, and just 2 tablespoons give you more potassium than a banana, more calcium than five times the amount of milk, and more than three times the iron of spinach. High in magnesium, fiber, healthy fats, and omega–3 fatty acids, the seeds of the chia plant can be eaten whole, sprinkled onto salads and meals, or ground and included in juices and sauces. Chia seeds have been considered an important plant since ancient times by Maya and Aztec healing traditions. The word *chia* means "strength" in the ancient Maya language. Today, chia seeds are considered a superfood because of the abundance of vitamins and minerals packed into the tiny, little seeds.

Chickweed–This common plant, found throughout North America, can in a balm or ointment form help relieve dry and inflamed skin with its cooling effect. High in vitamin C, important trace minerals, and potassium, it prevents infection and inflammation. Be aware that paralysis caused by using large amounts of the plant in infusions have been reported; use in small doses.

Chicory–A biennial plant that makes a great digestive tonic.

Chili peppers–Chili peppers are part of the *Capsicum* genus and nightshade family; the capsaicin charges up the body's metabolism, improves red blood cell formation and cognitive function, and clears out sinus and nasal congestion. It also lowers blood pressure and acts as a natural pain reliever.

Chokecherry–Native American tribes use this as an all-purpose medicinal treatment. The berries are pitted, dried, and crushed into a tea or poultice to treat a variety of ailments such as coughs, colds, flus, nausea, inflammation, and diarrhea. As a salve or poultice, it treats burns and wounds. The pit of the chokecherry is poisonous in high concentrations, so remove the pits before using.

Chocolate/cocoa–Dark chocolate is an aphrodisiac and a superfood that, consumed in moderation, lowers blood pressure, and reduces free radicals.

Cilantro–A popular herb that helps expel heavy metal toxins from the body. Contains chelating agents that attach themselves to the toxins and are released through the excretory channels.

Cinnamon–A great spice that, in tea form, helps with digestive issues and headaches.

Citronella–When burned in candle or incense form, it wards off bugs and mosquitoes. Used on the skin, it can aid irritations and improve the look of wrinkles. Rub it on feet to stop excessive sweating.

Clover–White clover grows everywhere and is known for medicinal benefits. Because of its anti-inflammatory properties, it boosts the immune system when used as an infusion or strong tea. Red clover is a highly sought-after weed for herbal medicinals because of its high mineral, vitamin, and amino acid content. It has a gentle detoxifying effect on the body and helps deliver nutrients to the vital organs while ridding the body of metabolic waste. Red clover contains phytosterols, the building blocks of hormones, and helps balance hormonal issues. It can prevent hormone-related breast and prostate cancer. Red clover treats respiratory infections, boosts the immune system, and detoxifies the liver. It makes bones stronger and contributes to heart health. Drink it in a tea or include the dried herbs in food and juices. Red clover salves, balms, and ointments are a popular natural topical medicine.

Cloves–Cloves possess antibacterial, antiviral, antifungal, antimicrobial, and antiparasitic properties that dissolve the eggs of parasites and worms in the intestinal system.

Coconut–The tree that gives us coconuts should be commended for providing us with one of the healthiest foods on the planet in the form of coconut oil. Over 1,500 published studies have shown the positive benefits of coconut oil, and it is considered a healthy fat that promotes weight loss, lowers cholesterol levels, and improves skin and hair. Coconut oil contains about 62 percent medium-chain triglycerides, known as MCTs, which are burned by the body as fat and promote the burning of the body's own fat stores. Coconut oil is the best oil for cooking because it has a high heat stability of 350 degrees Fahrenheit.

Coffee–Coffee is known for boosting energy, mood, and clarity, but space it out to avoid overstimulation from caffeine.

Comfrey–As a medicinal, in small doses, it can aid digestion, ulcers, and bronchitis. Not meant to be consumed in excess.

Cucumber–The plant cools and soothes sunburn. Slice thinly and place on the eyes during meditation to assist in astral traveling. Cucumber slices also heal undereye bags and circles. Hold a slice of cucumber on the roof of your mouth for 90 seconds. The photochemicals found in cucumber kill bacteria that causes bad breath.

Cumin–Roasted cumin seeds heal mouth sores. You can boil 1 teaspoon in water to make a tea that soothes urinary tract issues and promotes a healthy bladder and kidneys. Cumin tea is a natural sleep aid.

Dandelion–This flowering weed comes from the same family as the sunflower, and 1 cup gives you 535 percent of your daily recommended vitamin K and 112 percent of vitamin A. Every part of the plant can be eaten. Dandelion has long been used to fight bile and liver problems. Consuming them in plant form on salads or in tea form helps heal urinary infections, inflammation, eczema, psoriasis, digestion problems, cancer, diabetes, high blood pressure, irritable bowel syndrome, and a host of other issues.

Dates–Dates have antioxidants that boost the immune system and compounds that lower blood pressure, balance blood sugar levels, and help prevent Alzheimer's. Just a handful of dates provides the body with enough magnesium to dilate blood vessels for better circulation. They also contain potassium and help women who have gone through menopause maintain bone mass by reducing the amount of calcium excreted via the kidneys.

Dill–Dill relieves digestion problems like gas and bloating and prevents diarrhea. It reduces the severity of menstrual cramps in women, and its flavonoids and B vitamins can help you get a good night's sleep. Have a bad case of the hiccups? Consuming dill can stop them in their tracks by dissolving trapped gas in the esophagus.

Dogwood–The bark of the tree is an astringent.

Echinacea–This herb boosts a weak immune system and is both antibacterial and antiviral. Topically, it heals stings, wounds, bites, and skin infections, even poisonous bites from snakes and spiders. It also heals toothaches, sore throats, respiratory infections, colds, the flu, herpes, skin ulcers, and swelling of the lymph nodes.

Elderberry–Elderberry is a potent superhealer rich in minerals and vitamins, including vitamins A, B, and C. Used in teas, tinctures, syrups or extracts, the berries and flowers help heal colds, flu bugs, respiratory infections, fevers, stomachaches, constipation, and viral infections. Elderberry, which is part of the honeysuckle family, is one of the best herbal remedies for boosting the immune system. Because of its pleasant taste, it is a favorite herbal remedy for children when made into a syrup form. The elderberry bush blooms in late spring with its pretty cluster of white- and cream-colored flowers and bursts of small black, blue-black, or red berries.

Elder flower–The frothy flowers fight signs of aging when infused in oils and used as a serum on the skin to prevent fine wrinkles and age spots.

Elecampane root–This nutrient-rich root works well as an expectorant to alleviate coughs, chronic cough, bronchitis, colds, and flus.

Elm slippery bark–Use the inner layer of the bark of this tree, found in the central and eastern United States. Also called slippery bark elm, it has a host of properties that help fight sore throats (slippery elm is a common ingredient in throat lozenges), possibly increase bowel movements, and, in small studies, prevent constipation and bloating.

Eucalyptus–The leaves of the tree are anti-inflammatory and great for healing and ridding the body of disease, especially arthritis and muscular pain.

Eyebright–Eyebright is an anti-inflammatory with the ability to stop a cough or sore throat. It also soothes tired eyes and has a cooling effect on the skin.

Fenugreek–This bitter herb helps milk flow in breastfeeding women and lowers fever, reduces blood sugar levels, and has both a laxative and diuretic effect. It has antitumor and antiparasitic properties, and the sprouts promote hair growth. Men can use it to increase libido and prevent premature ejaculation. It is effective at lowering insulin resistance and can be used in tea, spice, or supplement form. One can even use fenugreek flour for making baked goods.

Feverfew–Feverfew tea can help stop migraine headaches, menstrual cramps, arthritis pain, and muscle spasms.

Fig–Figs contain phytochemicals and polyphenols similar to garlic. The milky sap of the fig plant was used in Mediterranean folk medicine to soften calluses and warts so they could be removed and to ward off parasites. Research has shown that figs can lower blood pressure, rid the body of dangerous free radicals, and protect against cancer, diabetes, and infections. Fresh or dried figs contain vitamins A, E, K, and B-complex along with minerals.

Flaxseed–When consumed, flaxseed is one of the best superfoods for the body and immune system. Flax is one of the first domesticated crops known to man, related to the wild form of pale flax, and is also called linseed. Textiles made from flax are called linens, and the oil is referred to as linseed oil, although we now have flaxseed oil, which contains properties for healing menstrual and menopausal discomfort and relieving hot flashes.

Garlic–This herb and spice is antibacterial and lowers fever, reduces blood pressure and cholesterol levels, lowers blood sugar levels, and detoxes the body. It is considered a broad-spectrum antibiotic without the side effects of pharmaceutical antibiotics. As an antiviral, it helps fight bad colds, strep infections, and the flu and fights cancers of the stomach and colon. It is considered one of the most healing and beneficial superfoods. It is also an antifungal and can destroy parasites and fungal infections and kill fleas, ticks, and mosquitoes. Black garlic has twice the antioxidant levels of regular garlic.

Geranium–Geranium is an astringent that can minimize wrinkles on the skin. It is also a potent anti–inflammatory that works wonders to heal wounds. The fragrance is soothing and relaxing and helps relieve anxiety and nerve pain when used in an essential oil massage or bath.

Ginger–A great perennial herb and root for healing stomach issues. Asian healing traditions consider ginger a longevity herb for its internal and external properties. When used as a salve or balm, it heals wounds and skin ailments. Ginger is one of the best medicinal anti–inflammatory plants for stopping nausea, healing morning sickness, controlling spasms and pain, improving circulation and hearth health, and aiding digestion. Ginger can be taken in supplement form or brewed into a tea with 2 teaspoons of freshly grated ginger root per cup of water. Ginger chews are now a popular way to deal with motion sickness while traveling. It is also effective in reducing muscle pain from exercising.

Ginkgo–Sharpens the mind and increases clarity. It is used as a medicinal for improving memory, focus, energy levels, and attention. As *Ginkgo biloba* in herb or supplement form, it aids circulation, dilates blood vessels and bronchial tubes, and even treats impotence in men.

Ginseng–Ginseng soothes anxiety and enhances sexual vigor. It improves physical stamina and helps the body fight disease. A powerful aphrodisiac, ginseng rejuvenates the body, mind, and spirit. According to *WebMD*, American ginseng studies have shown some sugar–lowering effects in fasting and after–meal blood sugar levels, along with A1C levels in diabetics.

Goldenrod–As a medicinal, it is bitter and astringent but reduces inflammation, stimulates liver and kidney function, and has antifungal properties. Many people use it to treat kidney stones.

Goldenseal–The herb is bitter and has blood–purifying effects. It helps with stomach and digestive issues, reduces inflammation and bleeding, and even works as a decongestant for stuffy noses.

Grapes–Eating grapes, especially the red and purple kind, promotes heart health, improves cholesterol levels, aids digestion, supports balanced blood sugar levels, and strengthens bones and eyesight. The resveratrol in red and purple grapes and in wine is a known potent antioxidant.

Gymnema sylvestre–Native to India, Africa, and Australia, it can decrease cravings for sweets and support healthy blood sugar levels, according to a 2007 study in *Biochemical Nutrition*.

Hawthorn–Hawthorn tea made of the leaves and flowers helps lower blood pressure and improve blood circulation. It also calms and aids in treating sleeplessness. Hawthorn berries are used to make tea because it increases blood flow to the heart and is even known to help mend a broken heart.

Hazel–Witch hazel is specifically a favorite natural medicinal and topical for treating insect bites and sunburn and as a refreshing facial spritzer or aftershave lotion.

Heather–Heather treats arthritis and prevents kidney stones. It has been used to treat tuberculosis in the past.

Hemp–Hemp is such an all–purpose plant, it can be made into dozens of products like paper, clothing, fuel, pasta, foodstuffs, bedding, and containers that won't fill landfills and destroy the environment. The root of the hemp plant can remove radiation from soil through the process of phytoremediation, where the natural growth process of the plant absorbs harmful chemicals in the soil while putting back in beneficial nutrients. This process makes the soil fertile again for future growth.

Hibiscus–Tea made from hibiscus can lower blood pressure and fever and provides a great source of vitamin C.

Hops–This plant, which beer is made with, helps with sleep issues. Hops treats anxiety and has hormonal and antibacterial properties. It's a bitter herb and a diuretic. It relieves pain and muscle spasms but is believed to put a damper on sexual energy.

Horseradish–Though it is best known as a condiment, the plant roots are used in medicinals to treat coughs, colic, gout, intestinal disorders, swollen joints, and nerve pain; fight spasms; and kill off bacterial infections. When applied directly to the skin, it eases the pain of inflamed tissues and minor muscle aches.

Huckleberry–The huckleberry is the state fruit of Idaho and has been used in Native American traditional medicine for hundreds of years. The small, round berries are like blueberries but more tart in taste. Medicinals using huckleberry treat pain, infections, and heart ailments.

Hyssop–This bitter and astringent herb can be used as an expectorant, to aid digestion, and to lower fever in a tonic form. It is an anti–inflammatory. The actual mold that penicillin is made from grows on its leaves.

Irish sea moss–This powerhouse provides fiber and trace minerals such as calcium, potassium, iodine, and vitamins A, B, D, E, and K. A type of sea moss, it contains 92 of the 102 minerals the human body needs and has powerful alkalinizing and healing effects. Its iodine levels are beneficial for thyroid function and produce hormones that control metabolism and bone growth. It is a rich source of potassium chloride, which helps dissolve catarrhs, inflammation, and phlegm in the mucous membranes that cause congestion. It also contains compounds which act as a natural antimicrobial and antiviral agent, ridding the body of infections.

Jasmine–Jasmine is a potent astringent, antibacterial, and antiviral herb. It can cool a fever or sunburned skin. It is considered an aphrodisiac but also has calming effects. Studies show that jasmine has a soothing effect and relieves anxiety and stress. You can keep a jasmine plant in your bedroom or use essential oils to get the calming benefits of the GABA receptor modulator found in jasmine, which aids sleep and relieves aggression. Researchers have found jasmine aromatherapy to be more effective than antianxiety medications, sleeping pills, and sedatives.

Juniper–This herb is strongly aromatic and bitter. It is both an antiseptic and a diuretic, which improves digestion and reduces inflammation. It makes a wonderful aromatherapy oil.

Kudzu–A perennial vine used in ancient Chinese medicine for thousands of years. The roots and flowers are nutritious and alleviate vomiting, nausea, fever, and diarrhea. It also eases menstrual cramps, hot flashes, migraine headaches, and psoriasis. Kudzu has been used in ancient Chinese medicine to improve blood sugar levels, reduce cravings, lower inflammation, and balance sex hormones.

Lamb's quarters–This common garden weed is found all over North America and is filled with amazing medicinal properties. It includes the same amount of protein as spinach as well as vitamins A and C, iron, minerals, calcium, and phosphorous. It has properties that improve blood flow, treat rheumatism and arthritis, heal insect bites and stings, lessen the effects of tooth decay, and help relieve constipation. The leaves, flowers, and shoots can be eaten in salads, meals, juices, and steamed. The seeds are not meant to be eaten in large quantities.

Lavender–The flowers make for a sweet-smelling essential oil, lotion, potion, or dried sachet; they bring peace of mind and aid in a good night's sleep when used in dried form in a sleep pillow, a few spritzes of essential oil on your pillow, or in the bathtub to relax and calm before bedtime. Lavender oil calms and soothes bug bites and stings. It has a relaxing effect and helps relieve headaches and ear infections.

Lemon–The sour herbal form can soothe and cool skin and has diuretic and anti-inflammatory properties. It also soothes bites and insect stings and reduces the effects of eczema. Lemon in water helps stop sore throats, and a little lemon juice in the hair lightens and brightens highlights.

Lemon balm–Once used by the ancient Romans and Greeks, lemon balm treats digestive problems, gas, bloating, vomiting, headaches, menstrual pain, and toothaches and has a calming effect that lowers anxiety and stress, yet also uplifts the spirit. It has been used as a part of aromatherapy for treating Alzheimer's, autoimmune diseases, Graves' disease, ADHD, and thyroid issues and lowers blood pressure, fights off tumors, and, when applied to the skin, treats bites, stings, and wounds. Lemon balm extraction and oil are favorite herbal remedy ingredients that our ancestors have used for hundreds of years. The delicate lemon flavor makes it a wonderful addition to salads and meals and as a soothing tea or tincture. Dried leaves can be made into essential oil or soothing salve, balm, or ointment for the skin. Lemon balm tea is a safe remedy for children to calm restlessness and aid in sleep. It can stop teething pain in babies when rubbed on the gums.

Lemongrass–Soothes the nerves and has antimicrobial, antifungal, analgesic, and antioxidant properties. Used in aromatherapy, it restores energy and fights jet lag.

Licorice–Licorice tea fights laryngitis and is also a mild laxative. Use internally with caution, though, because it does contain natural estrogen.

Lilac–The flowers are used to treat kidney issues, but it has no other known medicinal values.

Lily–Lily helps heal irritated, dry skin and treats burns and scalds.

Lime–The juice of the lime is great for stopping diarrhea, and the essential oil is energizing and mood boosting. Lime oil is antiseptic, antiviral, astringent, and disinfectant.

Marshmallow root–The herb controls bacterial infections and can boost cellular immunity.

Milk thistle–This bitter herb is a diuretic that helps restore a healthy liver. It stops a hangover when used in a tonic. It can reduce the negative effects of chemotherapy.

Mint–An energy herb that brings vitality to the body, mind, and spirit. Mint is used to reduce fever and as an antibiotic.

Motherwort–A weed that can improve heart health and lower stress. It relaxes blood vessels and lowers blood pressure to improve circulation. Because of its relaxing properties, it relieves anxiety in teas, tonics, and infusions.

Mullein–As an infusion in tea or added to a salad, this plant has been used by Native Americans to treat inflammation, coughs, congestion, and general lung afflictions. It is quite common and may be growing in your own backyard.

Mustard–Mustard poultices have long been used to help stop respiratory issues and stimulate the immune system. Mustard packs can also relieve pain and sore muscles.

Myrtle–The oil heals sinus infections.

Nettle–The leaves can help stop heavy bleeding, hemorrhoids, gout, and allergies. The roots stop allergies and reduce prostate cancer. Nettle is a known treatment for eczema when used on the skin as a topical. It can also be turned into a pesto sauce and eaten in cakes and soups.

Nutmeg–Taken internally, it stops diarrhea, vomiting, bloating, gas, indigestion, and colic.

Olive–The oil is a superfood. The herbal form is astringent and antiseptic and works well on lowering blood pressure and fever and reducing stress and anxiety.

Oregano–This potent-smelling herb protects against tiredness by giving an added boost to energy and vitality levels. Oregano oil is chock full of phenols and has antibiotic, antimicrobial, antiviral, and antiparasitic properties that can kill viruses and parasites. The oil has been a favorite medicinal all the way back to ancient Greece, where it was used to heal wounds, bites, digestive issues, respiratory infections, and fungal infections. Today, it is used to restore the gut's microbial balance and fight stomach flus, ringworm, sinus infections, acne, warts, allergies, and eczema. Because it is a strong oil, it should be diluted with a carrier oil before placing on the skin. Oregano tea is a traditional medicinal that can help stop menstrual pain, end bloating and flatulence, and relieve symptoms of colds and fevers, including coughing and bronchial irritation.

Painted daisies–Painted daisies contain pyrethrum, a natural insecticide. Plant the colorful flowers in and around gardens as a natural alternative to toxic insecticides.

Parsley–This popular plant can be used as a fresh or dried herb in cooking. It is also useful in medicinals. Eat parsley to draw a lover to you or mix it with jasmine and put in your sock or shoe to attract others.

Passionflower–Passionflower reduces anxiety and calms chaotic situations. It is bitter and has sedative properties and taken internally, can alleviate irritability, insomnia, and even withdrawal from drugs like Valium. It lowers blood pressure and stops muscle aches and spasms. Drink passionflower tea right before bed to calm the mind and help you fall asleep faster. Word of warning: some side effects are associated with passionflower, including vomiting, rapid heartbeat, drowsiness, and dizziness, so talk to your doctor first. Pregnant women, nursing women, children, and people with kidney or liver disease should avoid passionflower.

Patchouli–A distinctly scented plant used in meditation and yoga studios to assist with relaxation. As an oil used on the skin, it balances emotions and stimulates the growth of new skin cells.

Peppermint–Peppermint is a cross between watermint and spearmint. It's a multifaceted plant and a source of menthol. Peppermint essential oil, balms, and salves relieve pain, itching, muscle aches, and nausea. Peppermint tea boosts energy and aids in relieving irritable bowel syndrome.

Pine–The scent of pine oil fights fatigue and relieves tension.

Plantain–A perennial ground cover (broadleaf plantain) that is easy to cultivate in any type of soil with sunshine. Native Americans called it "life medicine," as it has many healing properties and has been used for healing all the way back to ancient times. The powdered root could ward off snakes and heal snakebites and was said to heal leprosy, dog bites, and epilepsy. It has healing properties as an anti-inflammatory, antiseptic, diuretic, expectorant, ophthalmic, cardiac, and antitussive, and it also is a great alternative medicine for respiratory and breathing problems. The plant extract is antibacterial and effectively stops excess bleeding and repairs wounds and damaged tissue. Poultices with ground or hot leaves stop inflammation and heal cuts and wounds and even draw out thorns and splinters. Plantain packs a punch when it comes to vitamins and nutrients. It is high in vitamin K, calcium, and other minerals that have a detoxifying effect on the body, and on top of that, it serves as food for important caterpillars to become butterflies. The young leaves are edible in salads and contain plenty of vitamin B1 and riboflavin. To top it all off, plantain decoction made of the roots can stop smoking, as it causes an aversion to tobacco. It can be made into a tea, salve, balm, or poultice and is found in many backyards in North America. (The larger species of plantain offers bananalike fruit.)

Pomegranate–The fruit is a potent antioxidant and can be eaten as is or in juices and smoothies. Pomegranate has been found in numerous studies to lower blood pressure and prevent cardiovascular disease.

Primrose–The dainty flowers can be put into herbal baths, and evening primrose oil is a powerful medicinal.

Purslane–The leaves are filled with healthy fiber; omega-3 fatty acids; vitamins A, B, and C; iron; calcium; magnesium; copper; and potassium. The plant is a powerful medicinal that has been used for hundreds of years because of its antibacterial and detoxifying properties that treat high cholesterol, skin conditions, digestive problems, and cancer. Purslane can improve vision, aid weight loss, strengthen bones, reduce fever, and rid the body of excess water as a diuretic.

Plus, it gets rid of inflammation and headaches and can be included in herbal remedies for coughs and colds.

Raspberry–Raspberry leaves provide respite from diarrhea and intestinal issues and, when made into a mouth rinse, can stop sore throats. Raspberry leaf tea can be put on the skin to soothe irritation and even tighten loose skin. The raspberry itself is one of nature's best superfoods and is full of vitamins and antioxidants.

Rhodiola–Helps improve brain function, reduce fatigue, alleviate depression, restore sleep, and increase energy and vitality. This plant is known for its ability to improve mental function and cognition and to increase physical stamina and strength and is backed by a body of clinical evidence. It is one of the herbs most utilized for battling chronic fatigue syndrome.

Rose–As a medicinal, the lovely rose is astringent and aromatic and controls bacterial infections. Rose hips treat colds, flus, and scurvy and control digestive problems.

Rosemary–Aside from being a favorite cooking herb, rosemary relieves spasms, stimulates the liver and gallbladder, improves digestion and circulation, and has antibacterial, antifungal, antiviral, anti-inflammatory, antioxidant, analgesic, and other properties that make it a potent all-purpose healing herb.

Rose petals–Rose petals and rosebuds are powerful nervines, medicinals for healing the nerves, relieving sadness, grief, and depression. The petals are anti-infective and anti-inflammatory and are an effective remedy for wounds, burns, sore muscles, and fatigue.

Saffron–Saffron reduces depression, and studies have shown that it helps lessen the effects of Alzheimer's disease.

Sage–A variety of dried leaves can be burned for the smoke used in smudging and cleansing an area of negative energies. Sage can relieve muscle spasms and tension, stop excessive sweating, improve digestion, and even has antidepressant properties as well as being anti-inflammatory. Oil applied to the skin heals sores, acne, dermatitis, and skin ulcers. It also boosts blood health, prevents constipation, and can soothe a sore throat.

Sea moss–Sea moss contains 92 of the 102 minerals your body needs. It is an anti-inflammatory and increases sexual vigor and health. Best to only buy the organic form.

Skullcap–Skullcap contains a flavonoid that has been shown to protect neurons in the brain after a traumatic brain injury and has additional healing properties for heart health. It can be taken as a powdered extract or in liquid form. Do not mix this up with the toxic deadly autumn skullcap mushroom!

Snake plant–The snake plant releases nighttime oxygen. Grow the whole plant in a pot and keep it in your bedroom to help you breathe better.

Spearmint–This herb oil is soothing to the skin, and the herb brings aid to digestive problems, stopping gas, hiccups, fever, and upper respiratory tract issues.

Spider plant–One of the best indoor plants for purifying the air. Removes the toxins benzene and xylene, known toxins.

Stinging nettle–Stinging nettle has been used in ancient Egypt as a medicinal. The tea made from this perennial flowering plant helps fight chronic fatigue and illness. The leaves have anti–allergy and anti–inflammatory properties and help lower blood pressure, boost the immune system, lessen allergy symptoms, reduce dandruff and thicken hair, rid the body of excess water, and treat prostate issues in men. It can be boiled and used in salads or soups or baked into chips with a touch of salt or seasoning. The roots are edible when cooked or made into tea. It can have a slight sedative effect, which reduces stress. It has a high vitamin C and iron content that supports immune, joint, and bone health and helps balance the body's inflammatory response.

St. John's wort–An herb that relieves anxiety and prevents colds and fevers. As a supplement or tea, it helps lessen depression and treats insomnia, menopause symptoms, PMS, shingles pain, sciatica, and inflammation of the stomach and intestinal walls from parasites.

Strawberry leaves–The leaves of the strawberry plant have medicinal properties that help reduce upset stomach and bloating. Rich in vitamin C, they're great for hair growth and healthy skin and can relieve painful arthritis. The antifungal and antibacterial properties promote healing of the skin. Try drying some organically grown leaves to use as a tea to aid the digestive system.

Tarragon–The oil can stimulate a sluggish digestive system and stop indigestion, hiccups, and menstrual pain.

Thyme–This popular herb and spice has the power to stimulate the thymus gland and boost immunity, and thyme oil destroys parasites in the intestines. It can be consumed dry or fresh.

Tinospora cordifolia–The extract from this plant has been used since the early 1900s in Ayurvedic medicine for its immune–modulating actions. It contains a complex of polysaccharides and polyphenols that regulate key immune mediators and stimulate macrophage activity to strengthen the immune system. It also can provide relief to allergy sufferers from sneezing, nasal discharge, and nasal obstruction.

Turmeric–A potent anti–inflammatory that is, according to some studies, as effective as ibuprofen for treating osteoarthritis in the knees. Turmeric is a superstar that improves brain health, digestion, liver health, immune system strength, metabolism, and insulin sensitivity. It also reduces oxidative stress, which can lead to major diseases, and supports healthy levels of cholesterol. It is a wonder healer that can be used in cooking or taken in supplement form.

Valerian–Valerian is noted for promoting sleep and relaxation and makes a wonderful and soothing evening tea. In herb form, it lowers blood pressure and improves digestion. Valerian is one of the few plants prescribed by doctors for sleep and anxiety issues and for generalized anxiety disorders, thanks to research studies showing its effectiveness as equal to that of drugs like Valium. It does take a few weeks to begin working as a sleep and anxiety aid, as it builds up in the system, and does have mild side effects like headache, upset stomach, palpitations, and dizziness. Because of its sedative effects, it should never be taken with alcohol or other sedating medications.

Vanilla–It makes a nice remedy for a fever and acts as an aphrodisiac.

Wheatgrass–Balances the body's pH levels and reduces acidity in the blood to help maintain a good alkaline–acid ratio. This helps relieve digestive issues such as gas, constipation, ulcers, ulcerative colitis, and diarrhea.

White willow bark–White willow bark is a natural pain reliever and fever reducer once used by Native Americans. Aspirin is made with similar ingredients.

Yarrow–A body of scientific research indicates that this common perennial herb, found growing wild in fields, pastures, and roadsides, is an antiseptic, anti-inflammatory, anti-spasmodic, astringent medicinal for fighting off colds and flus, healing stomach ulcers, reducing fevers, treating urinary tract infections, reducing high blood pressure, and stopping abdominal cramping; externally, yarrow oil treats wounds and stops excessive blood flow when used in a salve or poultice form. Yarrow has a slight sedative effect, so drink the tea form at night before bedtime.

Yellow dock–A weed that promotes the flow of bile to keep the liver clear and aids in digesting fats. It is bitter to the taste but can normalize bowel function in the intestinal tract when consumed.

Yerba mate–A South American herb that boosts energy like coffee and gives you more stamina without the caffeine jitters. It also aids weight loss by preventing excess fat accumulation in the body. The polyphenols in this herb are anti-inflammatory and fight allergy symptoms, reduce bad cholesterol, and may reduce the progression of arteriosclerosis. You can drink it in hot or cold teas, coffee-style drinks, or in any of the energy drinks the herb is found in, but keep consumption of energy drinks with caffeine low, as they have been linked to heart attacks and strokes in younger people.

Ylang ylang–This flower is considered an aphrodisiac and can be used as an essential oil for sensual massage.

Yucca–Parts of the plant can be rubbed on the skin to treat wounds and other skin issues. Yucca is a medicinal, and the fruits, seeds, and flowers are all edible and good for their high antioxidant properties and vitamin C to boost the immune system and stimulate the production of white blood cells, which fight diseases and infections.

INDEX

Note: (ill.) indicates photos and illustrations